Advance Praise for *Systems Thinking for Global Health*

'A remarkable collection of diverse Global Health issues where systems thinking approaches are harnessed in the design and evaluation of interventions. This book is illuminative and timely for an age where the world is contending with complex health issues arising from exogenous shocks such as wars and pandemics.'

Agnes Rwashana Semwanga,
Associate Professor of Information Systems and Deputy Principal,
College of Computing and Information Sciences, Makerere University, Uganda

'Both an erudite text and an incredibly hands-on guide, Systems Thinking for Global Health *is useful out-of-the-box thinking for health practitioners and policy-makers alike.'*

Ronald Labonté,
Professor and Distinguished Research Chair,
University of Ottawa, Canada

'Very timely and ambitious! Addressing a wide range of key challenges in Global Health, this book will be of great value for policymakers, researchers, and healthcare practitioners across the world.'

Kiyoshi Kurokawa, MD,
Professor Emeritus of the University of Tokyo, Tokai University,
and National Graduate Institute for Policy Studies, Japan

SYSTEMS THINKING FOR GLOBAL HEALTH

How can systems-thinking contribute to solving key challenges in Global Health?

Edited by

FIONA LARKAN

Assistant Professor and Course Director, Centre for Global Health, Trinity College Dublin, Ireland

FRÉDÉRIQUE VALLIÈRES

Associate Professor of Global Health Director, Trinity Centre for Global Health, UK

HASHEEM MANNAN

Associate Professor, University College Dublin Visiting Professor, FLAME University, Ireland

NAONORI KODATE

Associate Professor, University College Dublin, Ireland

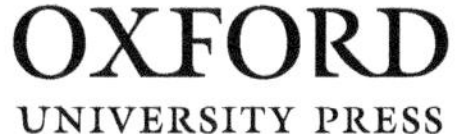

UNIVERSITY PRESS

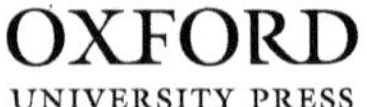

Great Clarendon Street, Oxford, OX2 6DP,
United Kingdom

Oxford University Press is a department of the University of Oxford.
It furthers the University's objective of excellence in research, scholarship,
and education by publishing worldwide. Oxford is a registered trade mark of
Oxford University Press in the UK and in certain other countries

First Edition published in 2023

Impression: 1

Published in the United States of America by Oxford University Press
198 Madison Avenue, New York, NY 10016, United States of America

British Library Cataloguing in Publication Data
Data available

Library of Congress Control Number: 2022931242

ISBN 978–0–19–879949–8

DOI: 10.1093/oso/9780198799498.001.0001

Printed and bound by
CPI Group (UK) Ltd, Croydon, CR0 4YY

Dedication

This book is lovingly dedicated to our close friend and colleague, Dr. Fiona Larkan.

Fiona completed her BA, MA, and PhD (2007) at Maynooth University in the Department of Anthropology and served as the Director of the MSc Global Health in Trinity College Dublin from 2010 until her untimely death in 2017. Fiona embodied systems thinking; she instinctively understood that any strong system succeeds or fails based on the people within it. In her family life this meant nurturing a fun and loving family home by cultivating the love and friendship of her husband, Brad, and that of their two boys, Cían and David. As an academic and widely respected medical anthropologist, Fiona devoted her career to sharing the voices and experiences of people living with HIV and AIDS in South Africa and Ireland to advocate for more inclusive healthcare for some of society's most marginalized populations. As a teacher and the Director of the MSc Global Health, she counselled hundreds of students, inspiring them to think critically and to question systems that promote existing inequities, and thus offered the world the gift of a future generation of capable and responsible global health researchers. Fiona amassed an extraordinary circle of friends—as diverse as it was large—at the center of which was one of the most affable and welcoming individuals we were ever fortunate enough to know. Ar dheis Dé go raibh a hanam.

Contents

Dedication v
Contributors xi

1. An Introduction to Systems Thinking 1
Domhnall McGlacken-Byrne, Fiona Larkan, Hasheem Mannan, Frédérique Vallières, and Naonori Kodate

2. A Systematic Review of the Use of Systems-Thinking Frameworks in Health Systems Strengthening 18
Savyasachee Jha, Deepak Thomas, Steve Thomas, and Charles Normand

3. Applying Systems Thinking to Health Workforce Development: Lessons from Sudan 39
Ayat Abu-Agla and Elsheikh Badr

4. Supportive Supervision for Community Health Workers: A Systems-Thinking Approach 54
Camille Coyle, Áine Travers, Mary Creaner, Damen Haile-Mariam, and Frédérique Vallières

5. Applying Systems Thinking to Understand the Process of Decentralization: A Malawi Case Example 67
Kingsley Rex Chikaphupha, Thomasena O'Byrne, Linda Nyondo-Mipando, Isabel Kazanga Chiumia, Mairéad Finn, and Frédérique Vallières

6. A Systems-Thinking Approach to the Training and Supervision of Community Healthcare Workers in Kenya 77
Niall Winters, Anne Geniets, and Alice Lakati

7. Unpacking Complexity: Systems Thinking for Communities 86
Brynne Gilmore, Henry Mollel, Nazarius Mbona Tumwesigye, and Eilish McAuliffe

8. Applying Systems Thinking to Health Information Systems: Lessons from South Africa and Tanzania 96
Annariina Koivu, Margunn Aanestad, and Nima Shidende

9. Assistive Technology: The Importance of a Systems-Thinking Approach 107
Jessica Power, Emma M. Smith, Ikenna D. Ebuenyi, and Malcolm MacLachlan

10. Responding to Health Needs in War and Armed Conflict: What Can Systems Thinking Contribute to Best Practice? 120
Marion Birch, Maria Kett, and Mike Rowson

11. Governance in Conflict-affected Fragile States: Systems Thinking for Collaborative Decision-making in Reproductive Health 133
Khalifa Elmusharaf, Elaine Byrne, and Diarmuid O'Donovan

12. Implementing Systems Thinking for Global Mental Health during Humanitarian Emergencies 145
Frédérique Vallières, Mohamed Elshazly, Jihane Bou Sleiman, Rony Abou Daher, Caoimhe Nic a Bháird, Ruth Ceannt, Philip Hyland, and Peter Ventevogel

13. Innovative Education Pathways for Refugees to Strengthen Health Systems 158
Minerva Rivas Velarde

14. Using Systems Thinking as a Heuristic in the Design of Interventions for Social Inclusion: "Including the excluded is a complex challenge" (World Bank, 2013) 173
Tessy Huss, Euan Mackway-Jones, and Malcolm MacLachlan

15. Using a Systems Approach to Understand Quality Improvement in a Nursing Home in Japan: Robotics-aided Care and Organizational Culture 188
Naonori Kodate, Kazuko Obayashi, Hasheem Mannan, and Shigeru Masuyama

16. Capability Approach to Aid Systems-Thinking in Addressing Right to Health of Persons with Disabilities 202
Thilo Kroll and Hasheem Mannan

17. How Can Systems-Thinking Address the Barriers to Implementing the Right to Health and Rehabilitation in South Africa 218
Meghan Hussey, Malcolm MacLachlan, and Gubela Mji

18. Systems Thinking for Global Health Initiatives (GHIs) in Sub-Saharan Africa 234
Amanuel Kidane and Lillian Mwanri

19. Systems Thinking for Pastoral Health: Challenges and Prospects in Ethiopia 246
Mirgissa Kaba

20. Systems Thinking in the Implementation of the Framework Convention on Tobacco Control: Lessons from ASEAN 253
Tikki Pang and Gianna Gayle Herrera Amul

21. The Planetary Health Imperative to Eradicate Nuclear Weapons 265
Tilman Ruff

22. Learning from Case Studies in Global Health 285
Joseph Rhatigan

23. Statelessness, the Right to Health, Policy, and Case Law: The Potential Role of Feminist Development Education and the Campaign for Universal Birth Registration 293
Patricia Erasmus

24. Systems Thinking to Combat Malaria: A Literature Review of Building Blocks 306
Savyasachee Jha and Anjula Gurtoo

25. The Utility of Systems Thinking in the Context of Infectious Disease Surveillance in India 322
Rosemary James, Anish Jammu, Annabel Taks, Tapashi Adhikary, Hasmik Nazaryan, Sreya Abraham, Upasna Gaba, Zeenath Roohi, Alexandra Humpert, and Isabel Foster

26. Human Rights and Social Inclusion in Health Policies: HIV/AIDS, Tuberculosis, and Malaria Policies across Namibia, Malawi, South Africa, and Sudan 342
Mutamad Amin, Malcolm MacLachlan, Hasheem Mannan, Durria M. Elhussein, Leslie Swartz, Alister Munthali, Gert Van Rooy, and Joanne McVeigh

27. Stillbirth: The Hidden Global Mortality Burden 360
Margaret M. Murphy, Rakhi Dandona, Hannah Blencowe, Paula Quigley, Susannah Hopkins Leisher, Claire Storey, Dimitrios Siassakos, Alexander Heazell, and Vicki Flenady, on behalf of the International Stillbirth Alliance

Index 375

Contributors

Margunn Aanestad Department of Information Systems, University of Agder, Agder, Norway

Sreya Abraham Manipal Academy of Higher Education, Manipal, India

Ayat Abu-Agla Trinity Centre for Global Health, University of Dublin, Trinity College, Dublin, Ireland

Tapashi Adhikary Manipal Academy of Higher Education, Manipal, India

Mutamad Amin Research and Grants Unit, Ahfad University for Women, Omdurman, Sudan

Gianna Gayle Herrera Amul Research for Impact, Singapore; Institute of Global Health, University of Geneva, Switzerland

Elsheikh Badr Sudan Medical Specialization Board, Khartoum, Sudan

Caoimhe Nic a Bháird Save the Children International, London, UK

Marion Birch Institute for Global Health, University College London, London, UK

Hannah Blencowe London School of Hygiene and Tropical Medicine, London, UK

Jihane Bou Sleiman International Medical Corps Lebanon, Beirut, Lebanon

Elaine Byrne Institute of Leadership, Royal College of Surgeons in Ireland, Dublin, Ireland

Ruth Ceannt Health Service Executive, Dublin, Ireland

Kingsley Rex Chikaphupha Research for Equity and Community Health (REACH) Trust, Lilongwe, Malawi

Camille Coyle Health Research Board, Dublin, Ireland

Mary Creaner School of Psychology, University of Dublin, Trinity College Dublin, Dublin, Ireland

Rony Abou Daher TABYEEN Centre, Beirut, Lebanon

Rakhi Dandona University of Washington, and Professor at the Public Health Foundation of India, New Delhi, India

Ikenna D. Ebuenyi Assisted Living and Learning Institute, Department of Psychology, Maynooth University, Maynooth, Ireland

Durria M. Elhussein Ahfad University for Women Biomedical Research Laboratory, Omdurman, Sudan

Khalifa Elmusharaf School of Medicine, University of Limerick, Limerick, Ireland, and Reproductive and Child Health Research Unit, University of Medical Sciences and Technology, Khartoum, Sudan

Mohamed Elshazly United Nations High Commission for Refugees, Cox's Bazar sub-Office, Dhaka, Bangladesh

Patricia Erasmus Courts Service, Dublin, Ireland

Mairéad Finn Trinity Centre for Global Health, University of Dublin, Trinity College, Dublin, Ireland

Vicki Flenady Mater Research, University of Queensland, Brisbane, Australia

Isabel Foster McMaster University, Hamilton, Canada

Upasna Gaba Manipal Academy of Higher Education, Manipal, India

Anne Geniets University of Oxford, Oxford, UK

Brynne Gilmore School of Nursing, Midwifery and Health Systems, Health Sciences Centre, University College Dublin, Dublin, Ireland

Anjula Gurtoo Department of Management Studies, Indian Institute of Science, Bangalore, India and Centre for Society and Policy, Indian Institute of Science, Bangalore, India

Alexander Heazell Tommy's Stillbirth Research Centre, University of Manchester, Manchester, UK

Susannah Hopkins Leisher International Stillbirth Alliance, New Jersey, USA

Alexandra Humpert Maastricht University, Maastricht, The Netherlands

Tessy Huss Trinity Centre for Global Health, University of Dublin, Trinity College, Dublin, Ireland

Meghan Hussey Special Olympics Inc., Washington, DC, USA

Philip Hyland Maynooth University, Maynooth, Ireland

Rosemary James Maastricht University, Maastricht, The Netherlands

Anish Jammu McMaster University, Hamilton, Canada

Savyasachee Jha Department of Management Studies, Indian Institute of Science, Bangalore, India

Mirgissa Kaba Department of Preventative Medicine, School of Public Health, Addis Ababa University, Addis Ababa, Ethiopia

Isabel Kazanga Chiumia Department of Health Systems and Policy, College of Medicine, University of Malawi, Zomba, Malawi

Maria Kett Institute of Epidemiology and Healthcare, University College London, London, UK

Amanuel Kidane School of Public Health and Community Medicine, University of New South Wales, Sydney, Australia

Naonori Kodate School of Social Policy, Social Work and Social Justice, University College Dublin, Dublin, Ireland; Hokkaido University Public Policy School Research Centre, Sapporo, Hokkaido, Japan

Annariina Koivu Tampere Center for Child, Adolescent, and Maternal Health Research: Global Health Group, Tampere University, Tampere, Finland

Thilo Kroll School of Nursing, Midwifery and Health Systems, Health Sciences Centre, University College Dublin, Dublin, Ireland

Alice Lakati School of Health Sciences, Amref International University, Nairobi, Kenya

Fiona Larkan Trinity Centre for Global Health, University of Dublin, Trinity College, Dublin, Ireland

Euan Mackway-Jones Independent Consultant, Paris, France

Malcolm MacLachlan Department of Psychology and Assisting Living and Learning Institute, Maynooth University; and National Clinical Programme for People with Disability, Ireland

Hasheem Mannan School of Nursing, Midwifery and Health Systems, Health Sciences Centre, University College Dublin, Dublin, Ireland; School of Liberal Education, Department of Social Sciences, FLAME University, Pune, India

Damen Haile-Mariam Department of Community Health, Addis Ababa University, Zambia St, Addis Ababa, Ethiopia

Shigeru Masuyama Tokyo Medical University, Shinjuku, Tokyo

Eilish McAuliffe School of Nursing, Midwifery and Health Systems, Health Sciences Centre, University College Dublin, Dublin, Ireland

Domhnall McGlacken-Byrne Royal College of Physicians in Ireland, Dublin, Ireland

Joanne McVeigh Department of Psychology and Assisting Living and Learning (ALL) Institute, Maynooth University, Maynooth, Ireland

Gubela Mji Centre for Rehabilitation Studies, Stellenbosch University, Stellenbosch, South Africa

Henry Mollel Centre of Excellence in Health Monitoring, Department of Health System Management, Mzumbe University, Morogoro, Tanzania

Alister Munthali Centre for Social Research, University of Malawi, Zomba, Malawi

Margaret M. Murphy School of Nursing and Midwifery, University College Cork, Cork, Ireland

Lillian Mwanri College of Medicine and Public Health, Flinders University, Adelaide, Australia

Hasmik Nazaryan McMaster University, Hamilton, Canada

Charles Normand Centre for Health Policy and Management, Trinity College Dublin, Dublin, Ireland

Linda Nyondo-Mipando School of Public Health and Family Medicine, College of Medicine, Blantyre, Malawi

Thomasena O'Byrne Trinity Centre for Global Health, University of Dublin, Trinity College, Dublin, Ireland

Diarmuid O'Donovan School of Medicine, Dentistry and Biomedical Sciences, Queens University, Belfast, UK

Kazuko Obayashi Nihon Fukushi University, Mihama, Aichi, Japan/Tokyo Seishin-kai, Nishitokyo, Tokyo

Tikki Pang Yong Loo Lin School of Medicine, National University of Singapore, Singapore

Jessica Power Trinity Centre for Global Health, University of Dublin, Trinity College, Dublin, Ireland

Paula Quigley International Stillbirth Alliance; Co-founder, Women in Global Health, Dublin, Ireland

Joseph Rhatigan Harvard Medical School, Harvard School of Public Health, BWH-Division of Global Health Equity, Boston, MA, USA

Minerva Rivas Velarde School of Medicine, University of Geneva, Geneva, Switzerland

Zeenath Roohi Manipal Academy of Higher Education, Manipal, India

Mike Rowson Faculty of Population Health Sciences, University College London, London, UK

Tilman Ruff Officer of Order of Australia Nossal Institute for Global Health, School of Population and Global Health, University of Melbourne, Melbourne, Australia; Co-President, International Physicians for the Prevention of Nuclear War (Nobel Peace Prize 1985), Boston, USA; Founding Chair, Australian Committee Member, International Campaign to Abolish Nuclear Weapons, Geneva, Switzerland (Nobel Peace Prize 2017)

Nima Shidende College of Informatics and Virtual Education, Dodoma University, Dodoma, Tanzania

Dimitrios Siassakos University College London and University College Hospital, London, UK

Emma M. Smith Assisting Living and Learning Institute, Department of Psychology, Maynooth University, Ireland

Claire Storey International Stillbirth Alliance, Bristol, UK

Leslie Swartz Department of Psychology, Stellenbosch University, Stellenbosch, South Africa

Annabel Taks Maastricht University, Maastricht, The Netherlands

Deepak Thomas Trinity Centre for Global Health, University of Dublin, Trinity College, Dublin, Ireland

Steve Thomas Trinity Centre for Global Health, University of Dublin, Trinity College, Dublin, Ireland

Áine Travers Trinity Centre for Global Health, University of Dublin, Trinity College, Dublin, Ireland

Nazarius Mbona Tumwesigye Department of Epidemiology and Biostatistics, Makerere University, Kampala, Uganda

Frédérique Vallières Trinity Centre for Global Health, University of Dublin, Trinity College, Dublin, Ireland

Gert Van Rooy Multidisciplinary Research Centre, University of Namibia, Windhoek, Namibia

Peter Ventevogel United Nations High Commissioner for Refugees, Geneva, Switzerland

Niall Winters Department of Education, University of Oxford, Oxford, UK

1
An Introduction to Systems Thinking

Domhnall McGlacken-Byrne, Fiona Larkan, Hasheem Mannan, Frédérique Vallières, and Naonori Kodate

Introduction

A holistic perspective, systems thinking is fundamentally different from traditional forms of analysis that seek to explain an entity purely in terms of its constituent parts. Whereas "analysis," derived from the Greek *análusis*, literally means "to unravel" or "to break into parts" (Aronson, 1996), systems thinking focuses on *both* specific parts and on the relationships and broader contextual patterns of organization within any social, biological, physical, or other complex system (Cabrera, Colosi, & Lobdell, 2008). As Senge explains, "systems thinking is a framework for seeing interrelationships rather than things, for seeing patterns rather than static snapshots ... a set of general principles spanning fields as diverse as physical and social sciences, engineering and management." Thus, systems thinking is the idea that the nature and behavior of a complex system is best explained in terms of the connections between its parts, relative to a common purpose. Hitchins (n.d.) illustrated this by comparing a drystone wall—easily dismantled and easily reconstructed—to a dismantled human, the pile of organs, bones, and sinews having permanently lost the collective capacity to be human.

With intellectual origins in biology, anthropology, physics, psychology, mathematics, management, and computer science, systems thinking expanded rapidly as a field of enquiry in the twentieth century. For this book, we sought contributions from experts and colleagues, located all over the world, spanning several disciplines, to lend their experience toward answering the question: "How can systems-thinking contribute to solving existing challenges in global health?" In this introductory chapter, we clarify the defining characteristics of systems thinking and systems more generally, offer some background on the development of systems thinking as a discipline over time, and briefly outline the core concepts and tools which can be applied within the field of global health. As such, we consider a system within the context of health to be a group of interdependent factors that, when understood together, determines the health and well-being outcomes of individuals and societies.

What Is a System?

Distinct from a mere collection of objects, a system, whether social, physical, biological, or conceptual, is defined by a number of key traits:

- *Systems have purpose.* Crucially, this purpose applies to the whole and not to any of the parts. For example, while a health system exists to promote healthy

Domhnall McGlacken-Byrne, Fiona Larkan, Hasheem Mannan, Frédérique Vallières, and Naonori Kodate, *An Introduction to Systems Thinking* In: *Systems Thinking for Global Health.* Edited by: Fiona Larkan, Frédérique Vallières, Hasheem Mannan, and Naonori Kodate, Oxford University Press. © Oxford University Press 2023. DOI: 10.1093/oso/9780198799498.003.0001

societies, this purpose cannot be detected in just the hospital or in a research laboratory or in medical technician training course.

- *All parts of a system must be present for it to fulfill this purpose.* As (Peters, 2014) notes, this characteristic of a system is reflected in the Greek work from which it is derived, *sunistanai*, meaning "to cause to stand together." Furthermore, if there are two parts of a system which are not related, these are in fact distinct systems, or subsystems.
- *Systems are tightly linked.* The arrangement of the parts of a system affects its performance overall. In a system such as a hospital, the hospital's performance would likely be adversely affected if, for instance, the surgeons decided to switch places with the pharmacists. In contrast, the nature of a collection of medical books is not affected by the order in which they are stacked.
- *Systems are constantly changing, but tend toward stability, via interactions, feedback, and adjustments between their constituent parts.* The human body is a complex system which maintains a fixed temperature. If we increase our level of exertion, our sweat glands will be activated, seeking to cool our bodies via perspiration back to the norm; when the need for cooling has subsided, the sweat glands will be inhibited again, via feedback. So, while our body temperature rises and falls on a regular basis, *over time* the system remains stable.
- *Systems are self-organizing.* System dynamics arise spontaneously from internal structure (de Savigny & Taghreed, 2009). In this way, no individual or agent determines the nature of a system, which is instead defined by the dynamic interaction of its parts and with other systems.
- *Systems exhibit non-linear causality.* Relationships within a system cannot be deconstructed to simple input–output lines but instead often exhibit what is termed circular causality. As such, the consequences of introducing of an intervention into a system are unpredictable.
- *Systems are resistant to change.* The non-linearity of systems, coupled with the complexity of their interactions, render them difficult to manipulate without astute understanding. Interventions may have no effect or the opposite effect to what was intended, and systems are sometimes referred to as "policy resistant."
- *Every system has a boundary to the surrounding environment, which is more or less permeable.* The human body here, again, continuously responds to our surrounding environment, permeable through our skin, and associated mucous membranes.
- *Individual system elements might be considered as whole subsystems, while the system itself may be an element of a larger system.* While hospital divisions, or departments, may operate as sub-systems (e.g., maternity wards, emergency departments), they are all part of a larger hospital system, which in turn, are part of a larger health care delivery system.

A Brief History of Systems Thinking

While the precise beginning of systems thinking is unknown, its intellectual roots extend back to the holism propounded in various forms by philosophers from Lao

Tsu, to Aristotle and his teachers. This holistic world view, however, runs counter to the reductionist paradigm which subsequently prevailed in all areas of science up until the early twentieth century. While the prevailing reductionist paradigm may have generated enormous success for all areas of science in recent centuries, Mingers (Mingers, 2015) cites three fields of study in which this approach failed to translate into the "ultimate" theories sought. In biology, although great success had been made in deconstructing organisms down to the biochemical and molecular levels, science could not yet explain the complex behavior and differentiation of cells and organism. In response, "organicism" (Ritter, 1919) developed as an alternative, which held that it was primarily the interaction of the parts of an organism which enabled the complexity of living things. In psychology, meanwhile, the Gestalt school argued that perceptions and thoughts were wholes in themselves and could not be broken up into parts. In atomic physics, finally—the "bastion of reductionism"—scientists found that wholeness at the subatomic level is derived as much from discrete particles as from networks of fundamental forces, with Heisenberg (1963) ultimately declaring that "the world is not divided into different groups of objects, but rather into different groups of relationships. The world thus appears as a complicated tissue of events."

It is worth noting that Heisenberg's famous uncertainty principle, showing that the results of enquiry into the external world were always, at least in part, due to the act of observation itself, maps directly onto the central plank of soft systems methodology: that an observer must be recognized as part of a system and different stakeholders in a complex social system—for example, a hospital—are very likely, depending on their roles, to have contrasting perspectives on the same system. As McConnell points out, "the *weltanschauung* that systems are 'in the eye of the beholder', or only relevant from the point of view of an observer [means] the very idea that systems can be engineered is problematic … This contrasts with the realist view that the knower can attain knowledge of a really existing world and can then use this knowledge to modify the world" (McConnell, 2002: 95).

Developed by Jay Forrester and others (Forrester, 1961), the field of system dynamics was instrumental in the development of the field of system dynamics. Based on advancements in the theory of information systems and the use of computer-based and mathematical models to simulate complex systems during and after World War II, proponents of systems dynamics sought a better way to test ideas about social and other complex systems. Others have since made a vast array of contributions to the growing field of systemic enquiry. While detailing their individual contributions is beyond the scope of this book, we would be remiss to exclude them. These include Coyle (1977, 1996), Richardson and Pugh (1981), Roberts et al. (1997), Wolstenholme and Coyle (1983), Senge (1990), Richardson (1991), Mohapatra et al. (1994), Morecroft and Sterman (2000), and Richmond and Petersen (1997). Especially notable among these is Peter Senge, who is acknowledged as having introduced and popularized the concepts of system dynamics to a wide management audience with *The Fifth Discipline* in 1990.

Systems Thinking for Global Health

In 2009, the World Health Organization (WHO) produced a flagship report (de Savigny & Taghreed, 2009), *Systems Thinking for Health Systems Strengthening*. Within

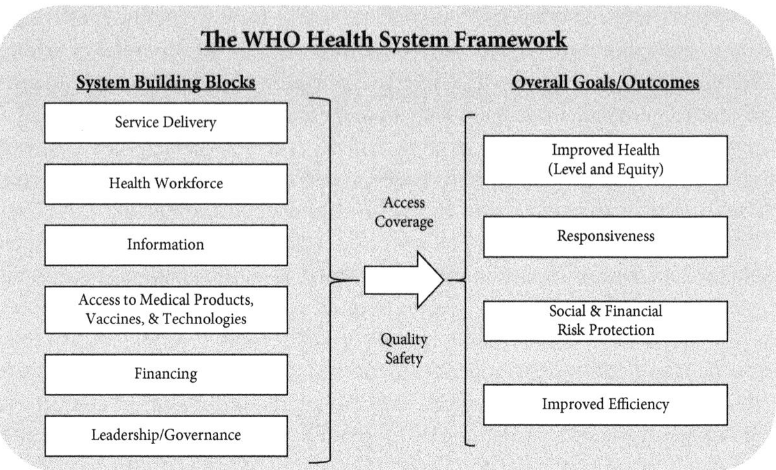

Figure 1.1 The building blocks of the health system: aims and attributes

Reproduced with permission from de Savigny, D., & Taghreed, A. (Eds.) (2009). *Systems thinking for health systems strengthening*. Geneva: World Health Organization. Retrieved from https://apps.who.int/iris/handle/10665/44204

this report, the WHO presents its influential *Framework for Action*, which describes six discrete health system 'building blocks' of any functioning health system (see Figure 1.1). Seen in a systems-thinking context, these building blocks map, approximately, to the predominant subsystems of a complex health system. Vaz et al. (2020) further developed and operationalized systems thinking, applying it to monitoring the quality of health interventions.

Classifying Systems

Broadly speaking, systems can be classified into "hard" and "soft." In truth however, these are two ends of a scale and rarely can a system be designated unequivocally as either a hard system or a soft system. Typically, a hard system is associated with well-defined systems in which technical or mechanical factors are predominant. Hard systems are thus associated with fields such as systems engineering, operations research and computing. Furthermore, a Hard System Approach (HAS) assumes that there exists an ideal solution to the problem at hand, whereby problems can be precisely defined. For example, a "bug" in a computer system. In contrast, soft systems are subject to the unpredictable influences of social structures, people, and human intentionality, of which human structures such as a health system or an economy are examples. The Soft Systems Approach (or Soft Systems Methodology; SSM) therefore accepts that most organizational problems cannot be defined exactly, often because different stakeholders in a system will interpret a problem differently. As such, SSM adopts a creative, flexible approach to problem-solving, the desired outcomes of which are learning, better understanding of the system at hand, and progress overall.

Defined in more abstract terms, Checkland and Holwell (1998) usefully characterize soft systems as moving away from "ontological commitment"—that is, assuming systems are truly part of the real world—toward an epistemological, phenomenological position in which a systemic approach is a "useful intellectual device" which merely enables us as observers to describe and to talk about the world in a higher-quality fashion. Correspondingly, as Mingers outlines (2015), quantitative systems research applies most easily to hard systems, generating measurable data from an underlying deterministic model, which "from an empiricist or positivist viewpoint, is really the only valid form of scientific research." In contrast, qualitative methods generating information of a non-measurable nature—such as interviews, ethnography, and hermeneutics—are generally "underwritten by interpretivist philosophical assumptions," congruent to the approach of SSM.

As Mingers and White (2009) note however, the distinction between hard and soft systems has come under scrutiny (Lane & Oliva, 1998; Pidd, 2010), with some arguing that the distinction itself is artificial (van de Water, Schinkel, & Rozier, 2007). Instead, it has been suggested that the real distinction lies in the approach used when evaluating and describing a system, which can be solely analytical and modelling-based, or incorporate the principles of SSM, or integrate both approaches (Lehaney & Paul, 1996). In the 1980s, a debate as to which approach should be used, and when, culminated in recognizing the value of employing both hard and soft methods together, termed multimethodology (Mingers, 2000) or coherent pluralism (Jackson, 1999).

In addition to distinguishing between "hard" and "soft," systems can also be classified by their level of complexity. A simple system has relatively few elements, does not affect and is not affected by the external environment, and where interactions between elements, which are well-defined, are few and do not evolve over time. A complex system, on the other hand, would include most human and biological systems. The nature of a complex system, with its many variables, thus involves many factors at play and multifaceted interactions, which change over time and gives rise, as Anderson and Johnson (1997) describe, to specific types of problems. These include *conflicting goals*, whereby subsystems have goals which compete with or diverge from those of the overall system. This, in turn, can give rise to the *centralization-decentralization dilemma*, in which a large system—such as a health system—can swing back and forth between local and centralized decision-making. Additional problems include *distortion of feedback* between subsystems, either by inaccurate transmission or inaccurate interpretation, and *lack of predictability*. As previously mentioned, the latter is highly characteristic of a complex system and arises from its internal governing mechanisms. For example, the endurance of a market economy compared to a tightly controlled economy is countered by the former's greater unpredictability.

Core Concepts and Tools in Systems Thinking

(i) Systems thinking is a language, with several useful traits

The analogy of systems thinking as a language has been articulated in numerous settings (elucidated in detail by Richmond (2001)). As a language, systems-thinking possesses several useful traits that describe and attempt to resolve complex systemic issues. Most notably, systems thinking:

- *Is circular rather than linear*, focusing on what are termed "closed-interdependencies," or a circular causal relationship between elements.
- *Has precise terminology*, reducing the scope for ambiguity and miscommunication when different stakeholders are describing an issue.
- *Is highly visual*, enabling complex issues to be conveyed in both a precise and a reasonably accessible fashion.
- *Enforces explicitness during a modelling process*, often revealing subtle yet significant differences in values and viewpoints between stakeholders. In this way, the process itself of generating a representation of a complex problem satisfactory to all stakeholders fosters consensus and mutual understanding.

(ii) Systems thinking is a way of thinking, characterized by a number of specific key thinking skills

Systems thinking offers us several useful tools. To employ these tools successfully requires that we change our way of thinking, in what the WHO (de Savigny & Taghreed, 2009) describes as "a paradigm shift." A number of key thinking skills clarify what this shift means:

- *Dynamic thinking, instead of static.* Systems thinking frames a problem in terms of patterns of behavior over time; conventionally, we think in terms of particular events.
- *System-as-cause thinking, instead of system-as-effect.* Systems thinking places responsibility for the behavior of a system predominantly on actors within it, who manage the policies and "plumbing" of the system. Contrastingly, system-as-effect thinking views the behaviors of a system—especially problematic ones—as being driven by external forces. Richmond imagines a slinky, held with two hands, which then oscillates up and down when the supporting hand is removed: what is the cause of the oscillation? Two instinctive answers are gravity, and removal of our hand. System-as-cause thinking, however, argues that the inherent nature of the slinky predisposes it to oscillatory behavior, making the cause the slinky.
- *Forest thinking, instead of tree-by-tree.* Systems thinking emphasizes understanding the context of relationships, whereas traditional analysis seeks to know something by focusing on its details.
- *Operational thinking, instead of factors thinking.* Operational thinking focuses on causality and how a behavior is generated, instead of simply listing factors that correlate with some result.
- *Loop thinking, instead of straight-line thinking* views causality as an ongoing process, with effect feeding back to influence the causes, rather than viewing causality as running in a single, linear direction.
- *10,000-meter thinking* is analogous to the view one gets when looking out the window of an airplane: a horizontal expanse, but little vertical detail (as to the

gradient and finer features of the land); 10,000-meter thinking prefers a "big picture" overview of a system to fine discriminations of detail.

(iii) There are multiple, hierarchical levels into which we can systemically organize our thinking about the world

A key paradigm within systems thinking is the hierarchical way we can view the world on different levels, corresponding to different modes of action and orientations of time (Senge, 1990; Kim, 1994; Leveson, 2004), termed "the iceberg" (Figure 1.2).

We are regularly exposed to information from a plethora of sources: news, weather, stock market activity. Most of this information is on an events level. Events are thus the occurrences encountered within a system on a day-to-day basis: a fire in a city, a machine breaks down, an arrival in the Emergency Room. As such, we tend to expend most energy focused firmly in the present tense, on events and how to deal with them: we are operating reactively.

Patterns, however, refer to trends and changes in events over time. Patterns are thus our accumulated memories of events. Pattern-based thinking enables us to interpret present events in the context of the past and to modify behavior in anticipation of the forthcoming future: we can act adaptively.

On a deeper level again, we might think in a systemic, structural fashion. Systemic structures refer to the parts of a system which generate the patterns and events described—for example, while treating a lung cancer case (i.e., an event) is certainly appropriate, it is unlikely to do anything to avert future lung cancer. If one thinks systemically, however, one might notice a particular part of a county with seemingly large numbers of lung cancer cases (i.e., patterns), and subsequently uncover that this region contains high exposure to work and environmental hazards, high rates of smoking, and too few primary care physicians. By deepening the level of understanding to the systemic level, one's capacity to exert influence successfully on a system is increased. By, for example, establishing more stringent health and safety regulations together with launching a smoking-cessation program, we are thinking into the future again; we are operating creatively.

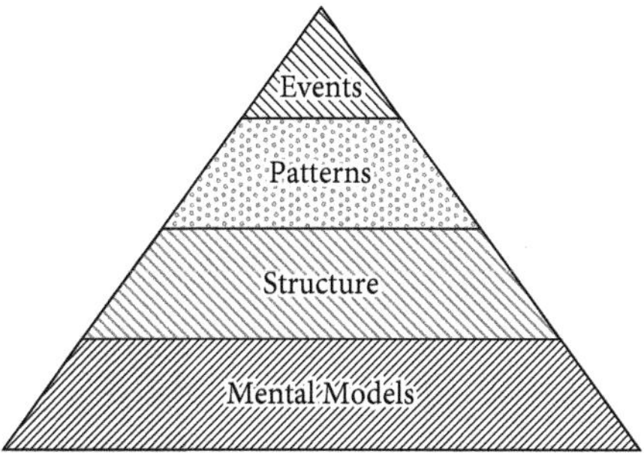

Figure 1.2 The 'iceberg'

Adapted with permission from Senge, P. (1990). *The fifth discipline: The art & practice of the learning organization*. New York, NY: Currency Doubleday.

Finally, one's stated and unstated visions and mental models contribute to the systemic structures of which one is a part. For example, a collective decision to enact more stringent health and safety regulations is born of a shared value of the importance of human lives and the right to live and work in safe and healthy environments. An understanding of the complex interactions and patterns of relationships (e.g., teamwork, communications) in health systems can assist health policy-makers and practitioners in determining key areas of intervention, the impact of these interventions on the system, and the potential intended and unintended consequences of change (Anderson et al., 2019). By clarifying shared vision and values, stakeholders in a system can act generatively.

(iv) A complex system typically contains leverage points

Complex adaptive systems typically contain what are known as leverage points, or "tipping" points, at which a supposedly small intervention can give rise to a disproportionately significant set of consequences in the system. As noted by the WHO report, *Systems Thinking for Health Systems Strengthening* (de Savigny & Taghreed, 2009), this is particularly relevant to actions on complex systems associated with unpredictable behavior, such as an economy, ecosystem or health system—in which "a seemingly minor event (e.g., freezing salaries) may tip the system into large-scale change or crisis (e.g., provoking a strike)."

While it is difficult to identify leverage points in advance, where possible a leverage point can be utilized positively to yield synergies which improve the workings of the system. As noted by Meadows (1999), in complex, multi-unit systems, high leverage points are particularly associated with two subsystems—governance and information—which, in the context of health systems, are known to receive the least attention from interventionists (WHO, 2008). Specifically, poor information flow has been described as the most common cause of system malfunction (Meadows, 2008) and so, for better or worse, might be considered an ideal example of a high-influence leverage point on the rest of the system.

(v) There are structural limits to how fast a system can respond to intervention

When systemically considering any decision, it is valuable to attempt to anticipate both short-term and delayed, long-term consequences. A key tenet of systems thinking is that behavior accruing short-term desired consequences can often yields subtle, delayed consequences which abrogate or fully negate initial benefits if insufficiently anticipated. Kim (1999) describes four basic types of delay: physical, transactional, informational, and perceptual. A *physical* delay refers to time spent for physical items to change from one place or role in a system to another. A *transactional* delay refers to any decision-making process, from a brief phone call to protracted contract negotiations. *Informational* delays refer to the time spent successfully communicating information about changes in a system, including both delays in transmission and in comprehension of the information. Finally, and easily forgotten, *perceptual* delays can extend beyond physical, transactional, or informational periods and refer to the slow changing of beliefs and assumptions of stakeholders in a system in response to change. As Kim notes, importantly, "delays are neither good nor bad; it's how we handle them that determines whether they'll cause trouble." In the domain of safety science, there are a series of methods (e.g., Functional Resonance Analysis Method; FRAM) (Hollnagel, 2012) that can be utilized to examine how an adverse event occurred, looking for hazards or bottlenecks, and checking the feasibility of proposed solutions or interventions.

(vi) The use of models to clarify one's perceptions of a complex system is fundamental to systems thinking

> "Perfection is attained not when there is nothing left to add, but when there is nothing left to take away." de Saint Exupéry (1939: 59)

Systems modelling is the primary tool of systems thinkers. A model might be defined as a method by which we can compactly and accurately represent an object, phenomenon, or system. A model serves as a proxy for a system in the real world which enables us to predict the consequences of our decisions before they are implemented. As Peters (2014) notes, any time one predicts how an event will turn out—be it a biological experiment or complex social process—we use our knowledge about the elements of the system and the connections between them to construct a mental model that tells us, within the bounds of what we know, what to expect. In systems thinking, we are encouraged to formulate assumptions based on known data to construct an explicit model (see Figure 1.3).

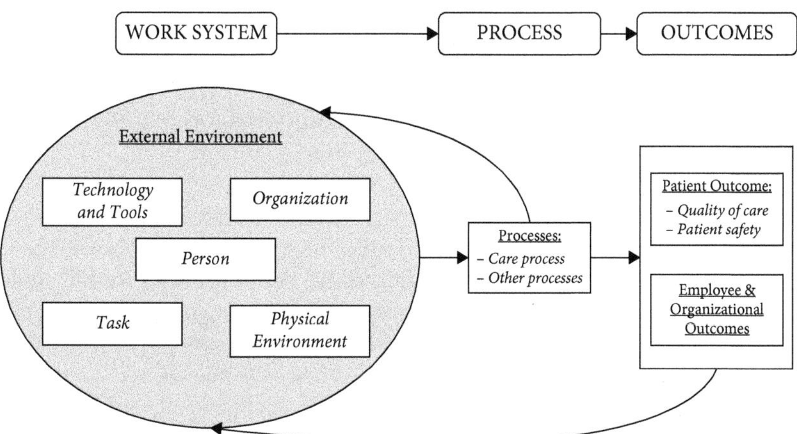

Figure 1.3 The Systems Engineering Initiative for Patient Safety (SEIPS) model

Adapted with permission from Carayon, P., et al.. (2006). Work system design for patient safety: The SEIPS model. *BMJ Quality Safety*, *15*(suppl 1), i50–ii8. doi:10.1136/qshc.2005.015842

Forrester argues when a thorough model is built from observed and agreed-upon evidence, and assumptions are clarified fully, a model can adequately reflect the behavior of even a complex system (Forrester, 1994). For example, the predictions of Forrester's "world model" (Forrester, 1971)—modelling the global economy over fifty years and reducing its complexity to a limited set of informed assumptions and five major variables—have largely been shown to be accurate (Turner, 2008). Importantly, Freeman, Yearworth, Jones, and Cherruault (2013) note that complex sociotechnical systems—or "system of systems," or soft system—are challenging to model accuracy, and emphasize the importance of "soft variables," which are those for which numerical metrics are unavailable (such as morale, investor optimism, and collective belief systems).

Moreover, in what Sterman (2000) terms "double loop learning," the very process of iteratively improving the accuracy of mental models as we test them in the real world and use new information to clarify our understanding is evidence of the tenet that decision-makers are within the system and decision-making affects the system. Accordingly, Checkland and Scholes (1999) stress the inherent subjectivity of any model and the importance of clarifying each stakeholder's unique perspective on the system, emphasizing the delineation between hard and soft systems, their respective bases in the ontological and epistemological outlook, and the importance of the role of the observer particularly in the latter.

For example, the Systems Engineering Initiative for Patient Safety (SEIPS) framework represented in Figure 1.3 was developed to examine a work system within an organization in healthcare, to improve quality of care and enhance the resilience of the system. Using systems thinking and resilience engineering, a new concept of safety (Safety-II) has been proposed. Reflecting the conventional view that health is the absence of disease or illness, the conventional view of safety was the absence of accidents and incidents. Safety-II, on the other hand, is additionally defined as the ability of individuals, teams, and organizations to succeed under varying conditions (Braithwaite, Wears, & Hollnagel, 2015).

(vii) By deploying the full range of concepts and tools proposed by systems thinking, we acquire the ability to work on a system, rather than in it

Kim (1999) emphasizes the holistic approach of the systems thinker with the question: who has the greatest impact on the safety and comfort of your average flight with an airline? Instinctive answers might include: the pilots, who handle take-offs, landings, and your general safety; or flight attendants, who maintain contact with you throughout, and without whom you would have no information. However, Kim argues that the designers of the aircraft exert the greatest influence, who designed the parameters within which the pilots, flight attendants, and passengers operate: the aircraft designers work on the system, rather than merely operating within it. By fully deploying the concepts, tools, and holistic way of thinking propounded by systems thinking, one can learn to exert influence as designers of the system at hand, rather than merely operating within it.

(viii) Theories and methodologies which come under the broad scope of systems thinking

While a full explanation of the various theories and methodologies that are prominent under the scope of systems thinking is beyond the scope of this book, what follows is a selection of notable theories, models and tools proposed in recent decades relevant to systems thinking taken from Peters (2014) (see Table 1.1).

Table 1.1 Systems thinking theories, methods, and tools

Name	Purpose and description	Key reference
Theories		
Catastrophe theory	A theory in mathematics and geometry to study how small changes in parameters of a non-linear system can lead to sudden and large changes in behavior of a system.	Poston & Stewart (1978)
Cybernetics	Historically used as a synonym for systems theory, it is a field of study of the communication and control of regulatory feedback in both living and non-living systems (e.g., organizations, machines).	Ashby (1956)
Chaos theory	A field of study in mathematics with applications in a wide number of disciplines to explain a dynamic system and that is highly sensitive to the initial conditions, so that small changes in initial conditions produce wildly different results. The changes occur through fixed rules about changing relationships, and without randomness.	Strogatz (1994)
General systems theory	Less of a theory than a way of finding a general theory to explain systems in all fields of science. It was not intended to be a single theory of systems, but more of a systematic inquiry into different domains of philosophy, science, and technology.	von Bertalanffy (1950), von Bertalanffy (1968)
Learning organizations theory	A description of organizations that facilitate learning by its members and continuously transforms itself. Systems thinking approaches are the conceptual basis for understanding the organization in its environment, and provides a basis for other key characteristics, namely a process of learning (personal mastery), the challenging and building of mental models, and the development of a shared vision and team learning.	Senge (1990)
Path dependency theories	Occurs in economics, social sciences, and physics, and refers to the explanations for why processes can have similar starting points yet lead to different outcomes, even if they follow the same rules, and outcomes are sensitive not only to initial conditions, but also to bifurcations and choices made along the way.	Arthur (1994)

(continued)

Table 1.1 Continued

Name	Purpose and description	Key reference
Punctuated equilibrium (in social theory)	Theory inspired from evolutionary biology (Eldredge & Gould, 1972) to explain long periods of stasis interrupted by rapid and radical change, particularly as applied to the evolution of policy change or conflict.	Baumgartner & Jones (1993)
Methods		
Agent-based modelling (ABM)	ABMs are used to create a virtual representation of a complex system, modelling individual agents who interact with each other and the environment. Although the interactions are based on simple, pre-defined rules, in a complex system these simulations allow for the identification of emergence and self-organization.	Epstein (2006)
Network Analysis (or Social Network Analysis)	Network analysis uses graphical methods to demonstrate relations between objects. Grounded in computer science, it has applications in social, biological, and physical sciences. Social network analysis involves application of network theory to social entities (e.g., people, groups, organizations), demonstrating nodes (individual actors within a network), and ties (the type of relationships) between the actors, and uses a range of tools for displaying the networks and analyzing the nature of the relationships.	Newman (2013); Valente (2010)
Scenario planning	This is a strategic planning method that uses a series of tools to identify and analyze possible future events and alternative possible outcomes. These can involve quantitative projections and/or qualitative judgments about alternatives. The value lies more in learning from the planning process than the actual plans or scenarios.	Schoemaker (1993)
Systems dynamics modelling	Not a single method, but an approach that uses a set of tools to understand the behavior of complex systems over time. The methods focus on the concepts of stocks and flows and feedback loops. They are designed to solve the problem of simultaneity (mutual causation) by being able to change variables over small periods of time while allowing for feedback and various interactions and delays. The common tools include causal loop diagrams and stock and flow diagrams.	Forrester (1968)

Table 1.1 Continued

Name	Purpose and description	Key reference
Tools		
Causal loop diagrams (CLDs)	CLDs are a system dynamics tool that produces qualitative illustrations of mental models, focused on highlighting causality and feedback loops. Feedback loops can be either reinforcing or balancing, and CLDs can help to explain the role of such loops within a given system. CLDs are often developed in a participatory approach. The drawings can be further developed by categorizing the types of variables and quantifying the relationships between variables to form a stock and flow diagram.	Williams & Hummelbrunner (2010)
Innovation (or change management) history	Innovation or change management history aims to generate knowledge about a system by compiling a systematic history of key events, intended and unintended outcomes, and measures taken to address emergent issues. It involves in-depth interviews with as many key stakeholders as possible to build an understanding of the performance of the system from a number of different points of view.	Douthwaite & Ashby (2005)
Participatory Impact Pathways Analysis (PIPA)	PIPA is a workshop-based approach that combines impact pathway logic models and network mapping through a process involving stakeholder engagement. PIPA workshops aim to help participants to make their assumptions and underlying mental models about how projects run explicit and to reach consensus on how to achieve impact	Alvarez et al. (2010)
Process mapping	A set of tools, such as flow charts, to provide a pictorial representation of a sequence of actions and responses. Their use can be quite flexible, such as to make clear current processes, as a basis for identifying bottlenecks or inefficient steps, or to produce an ideal map of how they would like them to be.	Damelio (2011)
Stock and flow diagrams	Stock and flow diagrams are quantitative system dynamics tools used for illustrating a system that can be used for model-based policy analysis in a simulated, dynamic environment. Stock and flow diagrams explicitly incorporate feedback to understand complex system behavior and capture non-linear dynamics.	Sterman (2000)
Systems archetypes	Systems archetypes are a number of generic structures that describe common behaviors between the parts of a system. They provide templates to demonstrate different types of balancing and reinforcing feedback loops, which can be used by teams to come to a diagnosis about how a system is working, and particularly about how performance changes over time.	Kim (1993)

Reproduced with permission from Peters, D. H. (2014). The application of systems thinking in health: Why use systems thinking? *Health Research Policy and Systems*, 12, 51.

Useful Tools for Systems Thinking

To think on a systemic level, feedback, reinforcing, and balancing mechanisms within a system must be considered. A linear perspective which fails to take feedback into account us doomed to repeatedly respond with similar efforts and thus fail to effect systemic change within the organization. Systems thinking therefore values a non-linear perspective on causality; regarding a system as an interconnected set of relationships, where one element affects another, which then affects other elements. Feedback is thus an important type of interconnection; with two types of feedback being *reinforcing* processes and *balancing* processes.

A reinforcing process, or positive feedback loop, refers to change within a system which predisposes the system toward further change in the same direction. The balancing process, or loop, on the other hand, is a tendency of a system to maintain stability at some defined level of performance. A classic example of a balancing process is biological homeostasis, as outlined in the earlier example of body temperature regulation. Useful tools to elucidate these concepts (see Kim, 1994) include *loop diagrams* as well as the *behavior-over-time graph*, the latter of which accessibly depicts reinforcing, balancing and oscillatory processes within a system with respect to time. Finally, unlike causal loops, *stock and flow diagrams* depict pathways of change. This renders them useful in conveying the higher-order real-life complexity of a system, thereby facilitating computer-based modelling of a system.

Conclusion

We maintain that the best way to illustrate the utility and application of systems thinking within global health is by outlining some of its successful applications to practical, real-world problems across a diversity of disciplines and policy areas. To this end, the following chapters reflect the importance of applying a systems-thinking approach to the field of Global Health as a complex interaction of political, environmental, economic, and socio-cultural factors that cannot be viewed within an immutable framework. Specifically, the following contributions offer a series of case studies, prescriptive or retrospective reflections, conceptual pieces, interventions, and methodological approaches to systems thinking. However, and given that systems-thinking requires that attention be paid to the dynamic architecture and interconnectedness of the health system building blocks, organizing a book of this nature brings its own challenges. Specifically, any organization of this book inherently imposes a linear structure on what is a fluid and interdependent process. Therefore, we encourage readers to approach this book by jumping across the various chapters as well as reading them in a linear fashion.

References

Alvarez, S., Douthwaite, B., Thiele, G., Mackay, R., Córdoba, D., & Tehelen, K. (2010). Participatory impact pathways analysis: A practical method for project planning and evaluation. *Development in Practice, 20*(8), 946–958. https://doi.org/10.1080/09614524.2010.513723

Anderson, V., & Johnson, L. (1997). *Systems thinking basics. From concepts to causal loops.* Waltham, MA: Pegasus Comm., Inc.

Anderson, J. E., Ross, A. J., Lim, R., Kodate, N., Thompson, K., Jensen, H., & Cooney, K. (2019). Nursing teamwork in the care of older people: A mixed methods study. *Applied Ergonomics, 80*, 119–129.

Aronson, D. (1996). *Overview of systems thinking. Systems thinking.* Retrieved from http://www.stefanibardin.net/wp-content/uploads/2017/01/Overview-of-Systems-Thinking.pdf

Arthur, W. B. (1994). *Increasing returns and path dependency in the economy.* Ann Arbor, MI: University of Michigan Press.

Ashby, W. R. (1956). *An introduction to cybernetics.* London: Chapman & Hall Ltd. Retrieved from http://pespmc1.vub.ac.be/books/IntroCyb.pdf.

Baumgartner, F., & Jones, B. D. (1993). *Agendas and instability in American politics.* Chicago, IL: University of Chicago Press.

Braithwaite, J., Wears, R. L., & Hollnagel, E. (2015). Resilient health care: Turning patient safety on its head. *International Journal of Quality in Health Care, 27*(5), 418–420.

Cabrera, D., Colosi, L., & Lobdell, C. (2008). Systems thinking. *Evaluation and Program Planning, 31*(3), 299–310. https://doi.org/10.1016/j.evalprogplan.2007.12.001

Carayon, P., Schoofs Hundt, A., Karsh, B-T., Gurses, A. P., Alvarado, C. J., Smith, M., & Flatley, B. P. (2006). Work system design for patient safety: The SEIPS model. *Quality & Safety in Health Care, 15*(Suppl I), i50–i58. doi:10.1136/qshc.2005.015842

Checkland, P., & Holwell, S. (1998). *Information, systems and information systems making sense of the field.* Chichester: Wiley.

Checkland, P., & Scholes, J. (1999). *Soft Systems Methodology in Action.* Wiley.

Coyle, R. G. (1977). *Management system dynamics.* London: Wiley.

Coyle, R. G. (1996). *System dynamics modelling: A practical approach.* London: Chapman & Hall.

Damelio, R. (2011). *The basics of process mapping* (2nd ed.). Boca Raton, FL: CRC Press.

de Saint-Exupéry, A. (1939). *Terre des hommes.* Gallimard. Paris, France.

de Savigny, D., & Taghreed, A. (Eds.) (2009). *Systems thinking for health systems strengthening.* Geneva: World Health Organization. Retrieved from https://apps.who.int/iris/handle/10665/44204

Douthwaite, B. (2002). *Enabling Innovation: A Practical Guide to Understanding and Fostering Technological Change.* Zed Books Ltd. London, UK.

Eldredge, N., & Gould, S. J. (1972). Punctuated equilibria: An alternative to phyletic gradualism. In T. J. M. Schopf (Ed.), *Models in paleobiology* (pp. 82–115) San Francisco, CA: Freeman Cooper.

Epstein, J. M. (2006). *Generative social science studies in agent-based computational modeling.* Princeton, NJ: Princeton University Press.

Forrester, J. W. (1961). *Industrial dynamics.* Cambridge, MA: MIT Press.

Forrester, J. W. (1968). *Principles of systems* (2nd ed.). Portland, OR: Productivity Press.

Forrester, J. W. (1971). *World dynamics.* Williston, VT: Pegasus Communications.

Forrester, J. W. (1994). System dynamics, systems thinking, and soft OR. *System Dynamics Review, 10*(2–3), 245–256. https://doi.org/10.1002/sdr.4260100211

Freeman, R., Yearworth, M., Jones, L., & Cherruault, J. Y. (2013). *Systems thinking and system dynamics to support policy making in DEFRA (final report).* London: UK Department for Environment, Food & Rural Affairs.

Heisenberg, W. (1963). *Physics and philosophy*. London: Allen and Unwin.

Hitchins, D. (n.d.) System thinking. Retrieved from https://systems.hitchins.net/systems/systems-thinking/systems-thinking.html

Hollnagel, E. (2012). *FRAM—the functional resonance analysis method: Modelling complex socio-technical systems*. Farnham: Ashgate.

Jackson, M. (1999). Towards coherent pluralism in management science. *Journal of the Operational Research Society, 50,* 12–22.

Kim, D. H. (1994). *Systems thinking tools: A user's reference guide.* Cambridge, MA: Pegasus Communications.

Kim, D. H. (1999). *Introduction to systems thinking.* Cambridge, MA: Pegasus Communications.

Lane, D. C., & Oliva, R. (1998). The greater whole: Towards a synthesis of system dynamics and soft systems methodology. *European Journal of Operational Research, 107*(1), 214–235.

Lehaney, B., & Paul, R. J. (1996). The use of soft systems methodology in the development of a simulation of outpatient services at Watford General Hospital. *Journal of the Operational Research Society, 47*(7), 864–870.

Leveson, N. (2004). A new accident model for engineering safer systems. *Safety Society, 42,* 237–270.

McConnell, G. R. (2002). Emergence: A partial history of systems thinking. *Proceedings of the 12th Annual INCOSE International Symposium, 12*(1), 90–98. International Council on Systems Engineering (INCOSE). Orlando, FL.

Meadows, D. (1999). *Leverage points: Places to intervene in a system.* Hartland, WI: The Sustainability Institute.

Meadows, D. (2008). *Thinking in systems: A primer.* White River Junction VT: Chelsea Green Publishing.

Mingers, J. (2000). Variety is the spice of life: Combining soft and hard OR/MS methods. *International Transactions in Operational Research, 7*(6), 673–691.

Mingers, J. (2015). *Systems thinking, critical realism and philosophy: A confluence of ideas (ontological explorations).* Abingdon-on-Thames: Routledge.

Mingers, J., & White, L. (2009). A review of recent contributions of systems thinking to operational research and management science. Working Paper 197, Canterbury, UK: Kent Business School.

Mohapatra, P. K. J., Mandal, P., & Bora, M. C. (1994). *Introduction to System Dynamics Modeling.* Universities Press.

Morecroft, J. D. W., & Sterman, J. D. (2000). *Modeling for Learning Organizations.* Taylor & Francis.

Newman, M. (2013). *Networks: An introduction.* Princeton, NJ: Princeton University Press.

Peters, D. H. (2014). The application of systems thinking in health: Why use systems thinking? *Health Research Policy and Systems, 12,* 51.

Pidd, M. (2010). Making sure you tackle the right problem: linking hard and soft methods in simulation practice. In *Conceptual Modelling for Discrete-Event Simulation.* Taylor and Francis. Boca Raton, FL.

Poston, T., & Stewart, I. N. (1978). *Catastrophe theory and its applications.* London: Pitman.

Richardson, G. P. (1991). *Feedback thought in social science and systems theory.* Philadelphia, PA: University of Pennsylvania Press.

Richardson, G. P., & Pugh, A. L. (1981). *Introduction to system dynamics modeling with DYNAMO*. Cambridge, MA: MIT Press.

Richmond, B. (2001). *An introduction to systems thinking: STELLA software*. Hanover, NH: High Performance System, Inc.

Richmond, B., & Peterson, S. (1997). *An introduction to systems thinking*. Hanover, NH: High Performance System, Inc.

Ritter, W. E. (1919). *The unity of the organism, or the organismal conception of life*. Boston, MA: Gorham Press.

Saint-Exupéry, A. de. (1939). *Terre Des Hommes*. Gallimard.

Schoemaker, P. J. H. (1993). Multiple scenario developing: Its conceptual and behavioral basis. *Strategic Management Journal, 14*, 193–213.

Senge, P. (1990). *The fifth discipline: The art & practice of the learning organization*. New York, NY: Currency Doubleday.

Sterman, J. D. (2000). *Business system dynamics: Systems thinking and modeling for a complex world*. Boston, MA: McGraw-Hill Companies, Inc.

Strogatz, S. H. (1994). *Nonlinear dynamics and chaos*. New York, NY: Persius Books Publishing, LLC.

Turner, G. (2008). A comparison of the limits to growth with 30 years of reality. *Global Environmental Change, 18*, 397–411.

Valente, T. M. (2010). *Social networks and health: Models, methods, and applications*. Oxford: Oxford University Press.

van de Water, H., Schinkel, M., & Rozier, R. (2007). Fields of application of SSM: a categorization of publications. *Journal of the Operational Research Society, 58*(3), 271–287.

Vaz, L. M. E., Franco, L., Guenther, T., Simmons, K., Herrera, S., & Wall, S. N. (2020). Operationalising health systems thinking: A pathway to high effective coverage. *Health Research Policy and Systems, 18*, 132.

von Bertalanffy, L. (1950). The Theory of Open Systems in Physics and Biology. *Science*, 111(2872), 23–29.

von Bertalanffy, L. (1968). *General system theory: Foundations, development, applications*. New York, NY: George Braziller.

Williams, B., & Hummelbrunner, R. (2010). *Systems concepts in action: A practitioner's toolkit*. Stanford, CA: Stanford University Press.

Wolstenholme, E. F., & Coyle, R. G. (1983). The development of system dynamics as a methodology for system description and qualitative analysis. *Journal of the Operational Research Society, 7*, 569–581.

World Health Organization. (2008). *Neglected health systems research: Governance and accountability. Alliance for Health Policy and Systems Research, Research Issues No. 3*. Retrieved from http://www.who.int/alliance-hpsr

2
A Systematic Review of the Use of Systems-Thinking Frameworks in Health Systems Strengthening

Savyasachee Jha, Deepak Thomas, Steve Thomas, and Charles Normand

Introduction

Health systems ought to strive to improve public health and increase equity within healthcare in ways that are responsive, financially fair, and make most efficient use of available resources. The World Health Organization (WHO) has stated that strong health systems are fundamental to improving health outcomes and accelerating the goals of reducing maternal and child mortality, combating HIV, malaria, and combating other communicable and non-communicable diseases (de Savigny & Adam, 2009). In order to achieve this goal, health systems must be designed to respond quickly to dynamic changes in patterns of ill-health within the parameters of public health. However, most jurisdictions have existing health systems that are constrained by manifold factors such as history, politics, and resources. The question of strengthening these health systems thus becomes one of extreme value.

Health systems strengthening is defined as the process of identifying and implementing changes in policy and practice in a country's health system so that the country can respond better to its health and health system challenges (World Health Organization, 2010). Various approaches have been proposed and used for this goal. The WHO developed a framework for action to meet the critical and immediate need to improve and strengthen health systems (World Health Organization, 2007). However, as the then Director General of the WHO pointed out, health systems being context-specific means there is no single template solution for improvement. As this chapter shows, many frameworks and approaches have been developed to work around issues present in the different building blocks of health systems and some seek to work with elements from other systems such as the biological ecosystem, environment, and the socio-economic ecosystem as well.

In particular, this chapter examines the process of designing a systems-thinking framework to strengthen health systems and gather various approaches used to achieve this goal. Specific care was taken to identify frameworks which had been applied practically and were portable between jurisdictions. While many selected studies worked within the six building blocks of the WHO systems-thinking framework, namely service delivery, workforce, information services, access to medical technologies, financing, and leadership and governance (see Chapter 1 for details),

Savyasachee Jha, Deepak Thomas, Steve Thomas, and Charles Normand, *A Systematic Review of the Use of Systems-Thinking Frameworks in Health Systems Strengthening* In: *Systems Thinking for Global Health.* Edited By: Fiona Larkan, Frédérique Vallières, Hasheem Mannan, and Naonori Kodate, Oxford University Press.
DOI: 10.1093/oso/9780198799498.003.0002

some studies looked beyond these building blocks and sought to include other factors in their ambit (see Table 2.1 for details).

Methodology

The primary motivation of this study was to identify and evaluate the use of systems-thinking frameworks and models. Both published and grey literature were searched, and a bespoke wide-ranging search strategy was employed with a modification after a trial (scoping search). This was done using PubMed initially and extrapolated to fit the other databases. The PubMed search strategy was as follows:

1. Systems thinking[tiab] OR systems analysis[tiab] OR systems theor*[tiab] OR "Systems Theory"[Mesh] OR "Systems Analysis"[Mesh]
2. "Models, Theoretical"[Mesh] OR framework*[tiab] OR model*[tiab] OR paradigm*[tiab] OR example*[tiab] OR approach[tiab] OR lens[tiab]
3. "Global Health"[Mesh] OR "Developing Countries"[Mesh] OR Global health[tiab] OR international health[tiab] OR public health[tiab]
4. health delivery[tiab] OR healthcare delivery[tiab] OR health care delivery[tiab] OR health polic*[tiab] OR health system*[tiab] OR health service*[tiab] OR "Delivery of Health Care"[Mesh] OR "Health Services"[Mesh]
5. #1 AND #2 AND #3 AND #4

All reviewed studies were either interventional, for evaluation, or exploratory in nature and included theoretical concepts. There were no restrictions placed on any of these categories to maximize inclusion of extant literature in the search. The studies reviewed were all in English and there were no further filters for study design. They were subjected to a title and abstract screening followed by full-text screening. The CASP (Critical Appraisal Skills Program) criteria were utilized to judge studies (Singh, 2013). A study must have had the following for inclusion:

1. Statement of research aims
2. Appropriate qualitative methodology
3. Justification of the research process
4. A statement of findings
5. A systems-thinking framework that has been or can be used (as per research question) and optionally a description of the same
6. Mention and/or description of appropriate system thinking tools or implication in the study that systems tools were employed but not necessarily described as such

Studies were given a quality rating according to the points above. A study given a quality rating of "strong" would satisfy all six points. A "moderately strong" study would satisfy the first five points, but not the last. A "moderate" study would fail to satisfy the sixth point as well as any one other point.

A total of 2081 articles were identified as being potentially relevant using the search strategy. On combined title and abstract screening, 1904 articles were found not to be

Table 2.1 Results of the systematic review

Authors	Type of Article/ Focus	Country/ Region	Main Theme(s)	Objective(s)	Methodology	Result(s) & Conclusion(s)	Quality Rating
All six building blocks (WHO framework)							
Abdullah & Shaikh (2014)	• Review • Intervention evaluation	Pakistan	All WHO building blocks	• Discuss evidence-based solutions for controlling the spread of HIV in Pakistan to provide a holistic way forward	• Narrative review • Pakistan's National AIDS Control Program, Global Fund to Combat AIDS, TB and Malaria, and the WHO used as information sources • Six WHO building blocks used for review	• Multiple solutions for each building block specified with emphasis on legislative solutions	Moderate
Adam (2014)	• Editorial • Examination of WHO systems framework	None	All WHO building blocks	• Offer a selection of tools and strategies used for systems-thinking purposes • Introduce article series on systems thinking	• Narrative review • Papers accepted for series used as sources for review	• Multiple papers targeting WHO building blocks are introduced • An introduction to the usage of abstract systems-thinking tools for strengthening health systems was given	Moderate
Best et al. (2016)	• Original Research • Examination of WHO systems framework	British Columbia (Canada)	All WHO building blocks	• Examine mechanisms that enable and constrain the implementation of clinical guidelines across various clinical settings	• General model of complex adaptive systems, realist evaluation, and systems dynamics mapping frameworks were used	• Themes for managing large-scale clinical change included: Creating context to prepare clinicians for change, strengthening shared	Strong

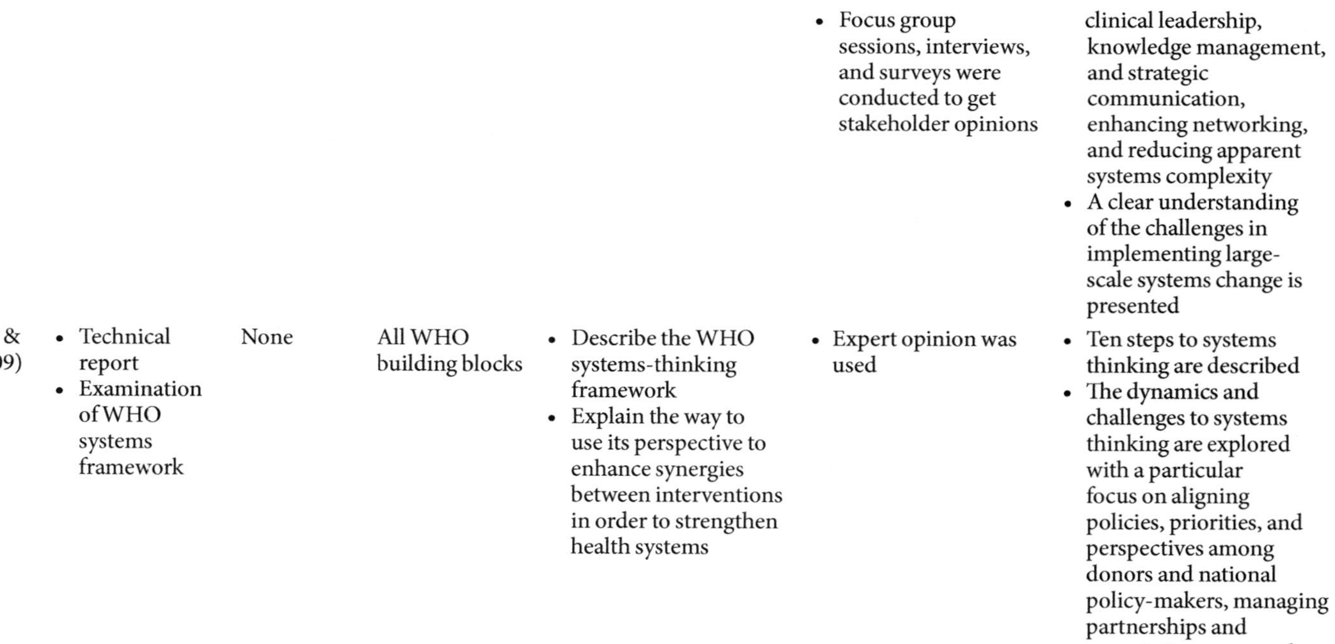

					• Focus group sessions, interviews, and surveys were conducted to get stakeholder opinions	clinical leadership, knowledge management, and strategic communication, enhancing networking, and reducing apparent systems complexity • A clear understanding of the challenges in implementing large-scale systems change is presented	
de Savigny & Adam (2009)	• Technical report • Examination of WHO systems framework	None	All WHO building blocks	• Describe the WHO systems-thinking framework • Explain the way to use its perspective to enhance synergies between interventions in order to strengthen health systems	• Expert opinion was used	• Ten steps to systems thinking are described • The dynamics and challenges to systems thinking are explored with a particular focus on aligning policies, priorities, and perspectives among donors and national policy-makers, managing partnerships and expectations among the various stakeholders, and building systems capacity	Strong

(*continued*)

Table 2.1 Continued

Authors	Type of Article/ Focus	Country/ Region	Main Theme(s)	Objective(s)	Methodology	Result(s) & Conclusion(s)	Quality Rating
One or multiple building blocks (WHO framework)							
Agyepong (2014)	• Original Research • Intervention evaluation	West Africa	Financing	• The Ebola outbreak in West Africa was analyzed from a systems perspective to draw out meaningful lessons	• Causal loop diagram created • Relationship between Ebola virus and elements of the system identified	• Low national incomes ought not to become obstacles to financing • Investment in surveillance and sanitation systems required • Multi-agency and multi-sector weaknesses need to be addressed	Strong
Allender et al. (2019)	• Review • Intervention evaluation	Victoria, Australia	Service delivery, information systems, leadership and governance	• Report on the development, implementation and evaluation of Whole of Systems Trial of Prevention Strategies for Childhood Obesity, which is a two-year systems-based childhood obesity prevention program	• Cluster-randomized trial in ten communities • Foster-Fishman's framework's four principle steps for transformative change applied to evaluate intervention from a systems-thinking perspective	• Intervention analyzed from the perspective of systems norms, financial resources, human resources, social resources, regulations, and operations • Framework is able to engage communities which are targeted by this intervention	Strong

Cave & Willis (2016)	• Case study presentation and original research • Examination of specific health subsystems	England, UK	Workforce	• Describe how systems thinking and systems dynamics are integrated into an in-house framework used for developing workforce management policies in the healthcare and social welfare systems	• High-level description of the frameworks and resultant models are provided • Two case studies are presented • Causal loop diagrams and stock and flow diagrams are used	• Systems thinking and systems dynamics approaches are described • The in-house framework is described • Workforce-model development is described • The resultant framework is shown to integrate horizon scanning, scenario generation and workforce modelling • The inclusion of systems thinking is shown to enhance collaboration between stakeholder groups	Strong
Fahey et al. (2004)	• Original research • Health system design evaluation/ enhancement	United Kingdom	Information Systems	• To show how systems modelling may be used to convert the complex input of the UK's public health network into an actionable plan	• Checkland's seven-stage soft systems methodology is used • Causal loop diagrams and stock and flow diagrams are used	• Cybernetic model was used to developed to provide an overview of the network • Models for the various perspectives of the public health network were produced • Models for network functions were created • Input/Output process model was developed to form the basis of an actionable plan	Strong

(*continued*)

Table 2.1 Continued

Authors	Type of Article/ Focus	Country/ Region	Main Theme(s)	Objective(s)	Methodology	Result(s) & Conclusion(s)	Quality Rating
Jahanmehr et al. (2015)	• Original research • Health system design evaluation/ enhancement	Iran	Leadership and governance	• Design a conceptual framework according to the policies and priorities of the Ministry of Health to evaluate public health and primary care performance and evaluate their relationship	• Literature review was performed • Expert opinions were solicited • Identification of fifty-one indicators from a possible 602 was done	• A conceptual framework was created to define the area of responsibility of health deputies and define a chain of results consisting of input, output, process, and outcome indicators • Five dimensions were defined to evaluate the performance of a health deputy: efficiency, effectiveness, equity, access, and improvement of health status	Moderately strong
Johnston, Matteson, & Finegood (2014)	• Review • Exploration of specific health outcomes	Canada, United States	Service delivery, medical technologies, leadership and governance	• Review the use of systems-based frameworks to assess solutions to complex problems, in particular obesity	• Literature review was used to identify documents of interest • The intervention-level framework (ILF) was used	• The utility of ILF for analyzing systems was demonstrated • It was seen that the interventions analyzed focused on elements dealing directly with affected individuals and not on more high-level systems components • The importance of weight-related stigma and bias was not emphasized by the studies selected	Strong

Knai et al. (2018b)	• Original research • Exploration of specific health outcomes	None	Leadership and governance	• Explore the value of systems thinking to understand non-communicable diseases (NCDs) as an emergent property of a dynamic system	• Meadows's systems-thinking framework is utilized to analyze commercial determinants of NCDs and unhealthy commodity industries	• Unhealthy commodity industries design and shape the policy system for NCDs, intervening at different levels to gain agency over the policy development process, and legitimize their presence in these areas	Strong
Lee, Chang, & Kim (2019)	• Original research • Intervention evaluation	South Korea	Information systems, leadership and governance	• Analyze the relationships between specialists and the direction and management of diesel fuel (which causes an increase in particulate matter concentration leading to worse healthcare outcomes)	• Interviews with specialists • Q-methodology • Causal loop diagrams	• Main reasons for ineffective diesel policy are dysfunction in ministries, lack of stakeholder engagement, and uncertainty regarding citizen engagement • Recommendations to improve this are: creating a mediating group among stakeholders, rethinking the roles and functions of ministries, and increasing cooperation with neighbouring countries	Strong
Lembani et al. (2018)	• Original research • Health system design evaluation/ enhancement	South Africa	Service delivery, workforce, leadership and governance	• Understand the reason behind poor health service indicators in South Africa	• Semi-structured interviews • Participatory group model-building exercise • Inter-relationship diagraphs • Causal loop diagrams	• Quality of leadership was a major factor overall systems performance, and was linked directly with staff motivation and capacity building • Staff motivation was linked directly with quality of care	Strong

(*continued*)

Table 2.1 Continued

Authors	Type of Article/ Focus	Country/ Region	Main Theme(s)	Objective(s)	Methodology	Result(s) & Conclusion(s)	Quality Rating
						• Quality of care influenced patient attendance, which itself fed staff motivation • Improved leadership and staff support lead to positive effects on staff competence and attitudes • Patient waiting times and satisfaction, and staff workload are extremely important variables which work independently of staff attitudes and competence	
Littlejohns et al. (2018)	• Original research • Health system design evaluation/ enhancement	Australia	Service delivery, workforce, information systems, financing, leadership and governance	• Examine the key factors that influenced health promotion policy and practice in a multisectoral health system in Australia	• Schema which incorporated health policy goals, actions, and strategies with WHO building blocks • Analysis of government documents • Detailed interviews with stakeholders	• The majority of feedback mechanisms identified were vicious cycles which inhibited health policy and practice • Some virtuous cycles were also identified • Leadership and governance featured extremely prominently in most cycles	Strong

					• Establishment of causal pathways and feedback loops • Causal loop diagram	• The importance of reducing vicious cycles, encouraging virtuous cycles, and the central role of leadership and governance was brought out using causal loop diagrams	
Mikkelsen-Lopez, Wyss, & de Savigny (2011)	• Review • Subsystem reform	None	Leadership and governance	• Review contemporary health sector frameworks which focus on defining and developing indicators to assess governance in the health sector	• Literature review	• Theoretical approach to creating a new framework for assessing governance in health systems was created	Moderately strong
Mutale et al. (2017)	• Original research • Intervention evaluation	Zambia	Workforce, access to medical technologies	• Report the system-wide effects of a complex health system intervention called Better Health Outcome through Mentorship and Assessment (BHOMA) that aimed to improve service quality	• BHOMA is a cluster randomized trial being implemented in three different districts • Interviews and focus group discussion with relevant stakeholders • Qualitative analysis of the interviews • Causal loop diagrams	• Framework for empirical systems strengthening was developed • It was found that BHOMA intervention increased the quality of service at health facilities as well as in community follow-up of patients • The introduction of new filing systems led to reducing barriers in health systems access • Community health workers were found to be key drivers of the intervention	Strong

(*continued*)

Table 2.1 Continued

Authors	Type of Article/ Focus	Country/ Region	Main Theme(s)	Objective(s)	Methodology	Result(s) & Conclusion(s)	Quality Rating
						• Many unintended consequences were identified • BHOMA interventions often increased burden in participating health centers	
Newell et al. (2017)	• Original research • Intervention evaluation	United Kingdom	Service delivery	• Understand the reasons patients were preferring to self-medicate instead of using emergency rooms at hospitals for asthmatic issues	• Soft systems methodology	• Multiple reasons were found for patients fearing coming to emergency rooms • A stakeholder-based solution was created involving patients as well as members of the healthcare system	Strong
Renmans, Holvoet, & Criel (2017)	• Original research • Subsystem reform	Uganda	Workforce, financing	• Combine theoretical approaches with systems thinking to link outcomes with various factors within health systems	• Semi-structured interviews with health workers and key informants • Causal loop diagrams	• Systems thinking framework was created to assess the workforce • Performance-based financing has the potential to attract more patients to facilities due to better work environment and financial accessibility • It is thought that performance will increase until the facility is saturated	Strong

						• The role of the supervisor was seen to be a very major one: a more formative supervision was preferred over a checklist based one	
Semwanga et al. (2016)	• Original research • Exploration of specific health outcomes	Uganda	Service delivery, workforce, financing	• Apply alternate solutions to the problem of neonatal mortality in Africa	• Dynamic systems methodology • Quantitative simulation model • Validation of the model through brainstorming with stakeholders • Strategies tested using "what if" analysis • Sensitivity analysis for determining strategies which would have a great impact on neonatal mortality	• A neonatal health simulation model was developed with four sectors: population, demand for services, health of the mothers. and choices of clinical care • The effects of various interventions were tested: health education campaigns, free delivery kits, motorcycle coupons, kangaroo mother care, improving neonatal resuscitation and labor management skills, and interventions to improve the mother's health • Free delivery kits and motorcycle coupons were found to be the most effective strategies	Strong

(continued)

Table 2.1 Continued

Authors	Type of Article/ Focus	Country/ Region	Main Theme(s)	Objective(s)	Methodology	Result(s) & Conclusion(s)	Quality Rating
Williams et al. (2005)	• Original research • Exploration of specific health outcomes	United States	Information systems	• Review initial twenty-four modelling efforts in immunization and cancer registries and present a case to apply business modelling approaches to analyze and improve public health processes	• Business modelling using activity diagrams, domain diagrams, and business rules	• Implementation of business modelling led to improved analysis and best practices	Strong
Other frameworks and models							
Atun et al. (2010)	• Commentary • Theoretical framework creation	None	Elements of system as described in methodology	• Describe an analytical approach for defining health systems integration • Describe a conceptual framework to analyze and map for the nature of integration and the factors influencing it	• Six building blocks used in analytical framework: governance, financing, planning, service delivery, monitoring and evaluation, and demand generation • Conceptual framework uses five building blocks: nature of the problem, intervention, adoption system, system characteristics, and context	• Analytical approach may be used for understanding purpose, integration of intervention into critical health system functions, and classification of the extent and nature of integration into the health system • Conceptual framework may be used for literature reviews, program reviews, case studies, or program planning at national/ sub-national levels in two dimensions: diagnostic and formative	Moderately strong

Bunch (2016)	• Case study presentation and original research • Examination of specific health subsystems	Canada, India, Nepal	Relationship between health systems and the environment/ society	• Explain ecohealth systems framework • Provide three illustrative case studies	• Multiple Causal loop diagrams used • Case studies from Nepal, India, and Canada used to illustrate approach	• Links between ecosystems and health systems explained • Links between poverty, environmental degradation, and zoonotic disease in the Bishnumati Valley (Nepal) clarified • Links between lack of access to government services, illiteracy, unemployment, substance abuse, and cholera outbreaks in Chennai (India) explained • Importance of watershed management for both ecosystem strengthening and healthcare was explained	Strong
Clarke, Swinburn, & Sacks (2018)	• Original research • Intervention evaluation	Victoria (Australia)	Leadership and governance and the effect of external actors on health policy formulation	• Investigation of the Achievement Program, a key pillar of the obesity prevention program in Victoria, Australia	• Semi-structured interviews were used to gather data • Relevant documentation was gathered from people interviewed • Advocacy coalition framework and multiple streams theory were used for analysis • Causal loop diagrams were used for visualization	• Factors found to influence obesity prevention policy include issues in problem prioritization, political risks associated with action, and framing used by policy advocates to reduce risks and highlight opportunities	Strong

(*continued*)

Table 2.1 Continued

Authors	Type of Article/ Focus	Country/ Region	Main Theme(s)	Objective(s)	Methodology	Result(s) & Conclusion(s)	Quality Rating
Knai et al. (2018a)	• Original research • Intervention evaluation	England (United Kingdom)	Commercial determinants of service delivery	• To understand the functioning of the Health Responsibility Deal (RD) and analyze relationships between the various elements of this system	• Literature review was performed to understand the various mechanisms and effect of the RD • Causal loop diagrams were developed • Qualitative systems dynamic modelling was used to illustrate the RD as a system	• A systems thinking model of the RD was constructed • The reasons why the RD was unable to meet its objectives was examined • The production and uptake of pledges by RD partners were largely driven by the interests of partners, allowing wider business systems to resist change	Strong
Mutingi & Mbohwa (2014)	• Original research • Theoretical framework creation	None	Holistic satisfaction focusing on patient, staff, employer, and other stakeholders	• Create a systems-thinking approach toward understanding sustainability in healthcare systems	• Identification of variables pertaining to satisfaction and sustainability in health systems through literature search • Systems dynamics • Causal loop diagram	• A systems-thinking model was created which used sustainability indices to satisfy environmental, social, and economic aspects of health systems • The model seeks to lead policy-makers to an approach for satisfying all stakeholders	Strong
Williams et al. (2015)	• Commentary • Intervention evaluation	United States	Goals, feedback loops, input, throughout, and environment as defined by the ABCD model	• Examine the Affordable Care Act (ACA) using systems thinking	• ABCD system model	• The ACA was broken down into its constituent parts and each part was examined separately	Strong

relevant and 177 articles were identified for full text screening. Of these the authors were unable to access six articles. Thus 171 articles underwent full text screening. A total of 145 articles were excluded, and twenty-six articles were selected as appropriate and underwent data extraction.

Results

Out of twenty-six articles presented here, seven were not focused on any country or region, five were based in a region within a country, while the others focused on one or more countries. All twenty-six papers either mentioned the use of system thinking derived frameworks or advocated a framework or model developed to look at health system strengthening in the context of the WHO health building blocks.

These studies may be classified thus:

- Four reviews
- One editorial
- Two commentaries
- One technical report
- Sixteen original research studies
- One case study presentation
- Two studies combining original research with case study presentation

The articles were further categorized into three groups (Table 2.1). The first group A (4 articles) cover all the six building blocks (service delivery, workforce, information services, access to medical technologies, financing, and leadership and governance) from the WHO framework. The second group B (16 articles) deals with one or a few of the six building blocks, and the third group C (6 articles) discussed different frameworks or models from the WHO's.

Nine of these studies critically examined specific interventions. Abdullah and Shaikh (2014) use the WHO framework to review and understand the challenges and shortcomings of the systems used to combat human immunodeficiency virus (HIV) in Pakistan. Five studies utilized parts of the WHO model to create their own evaluation framework. Agyepong (2014) analyzes the Ebola outbreak of West Africa and the systemic failures which caused it to become very deadly; Allender et al. (2019) report on the "Systems Trial of Prevention Strategies for Childhood Obesity" program in Victoria, Australia; Lee, Chang, and Kim (2019) examine the role of specialists in the failure of clean air policies in South Korea; Mutale et al. (2017) explore the system-wide effects of Zambia's Better Health Outcome through Mentorship and Assessment program; and Newell, Corrigan, Punshon, and Leary (2017) seek to understand the failure of patients in utilizing emergency rooms at hospitals during severe asthmatic episodes in the United Kingdom.

The final three out of those nine studies (the ones in Group C) did not use the WHO systems-thinking framework at all. Clarke, Swinburn, and Sacks (2018) investigate the Achievement Programme, a key pillar of the obesity prevention program in Victoria, Australia using a specifically created framework in order to improve understanding of the role of external policy actors in the formation of health policy in this area. Knai et al. (2018a) explore the reasons why England's Health Responsibility Deal was judged to have been a failure using qualitative systems dynamic modelling. Williams et al. (2015) examine the United States Affordable Care Act through an application of the ABCD system model.

Two other studies examine certain health subsystems through the ambit of systems thinking. Cave and Willis (2016) utilize a case study to explain healthcare and social service workforce management in England, resulting in a management framework which can be generalized to other jurisdictions. Bunch (2016) uses the eco-health systems framework to understand the relationship between health systems and the environment and society and present three case studies of the same.

Four studies seek to explore specific outcomes as a function of health systems interventions. Johnston, Matteson, and Finegood (2014) seek to do this with levels of obesity in Canada and America, Knai et al. (2018b) seek to model obesity as an emergent property of a complex system in a theoretical manner, Semwanga, Nakubulwa, and Adam (2016) examine the root of the issue of high neonatal mortality in South America, and Williams, Lyalin, and Wingo (2005) present a case to apply business modelling approaches to improve public health processes in the case of building immunization and cancer registries in the United States.

Four studies create frameworks for evaluating, changing, or enhancing the design of health systems. Fahey, Carson, Cramp, and Muir Gray (2004) seek to use systems modelling to create actionable plans from the UK's public health network, Jahanmehr et al. (2015) create a framework to evaluate the relationship between public health and primary care in Iran through the evaluation of health deputies, Lembani et al. (2018) design an evaluation framework which seeks to understand the reason behind poor health service indicators in South Africa, and Littlejohns, Baum, Lawless, and Freeman (2018) examine the key factors that influenced health promotion policy and practice in Australia.

Out of the remaining studies, three explain the WHO systems-thinking framework in depth (de Savigny & Adam, 2009; Adam, 2014; Best et al., 2016). Two studies seek to create new approaches toward assessing certain aspects in the healthcare system as defined by the WHO. Mikkelsen-Lopez, Wyss, and de Savigny (2011) focus on leadership and governance, and Renmans, Holvoet, and Criel (2017) try to link workforce outcomes with various factors in a health system. Finally, two studies remain independent of the categorization discussed previously. Mutingi and Mbohwa (2014) design a framework to maximize stakeholder satisfaction which has some overlap with parts of the WHO framework (service delivery and workforce), and Atun, de Jongh, Secci, Ohiri, and Adeyi (2010) create two frameworks: an analytical framework for defining health systems integration, and a conceptual framework to analyze its nature and factors surrounding it, both independent of the WHO framework.

Discussion

The number of studies using systems thinking in the spirit encapsulated by the WHO, regardless of whether they use its health systems strengthening framework or not, has increased over the past few years as a growing number of jurisdictions begin to integrate systems thinking into their planning and evaluation frameworks. This remarkable adoption of systems thinking speaks to its great power of analysis. The twenty-six studies reviewed in this chapter cover a large number of countries whose socio-economic indicators differ widely. Their health systems are also at different levels of maturity. This speaks to the versatility of the tools used for designing these frameworks.

Most authors emphasize the role of systems thinking in designing strong integrations between different elements of a health system, though not all of them define systems thinking in the same manner. The term has been used fairly broadly across literature, often getting mixed with concepts like systems dynamics. This is both a strength and a weakness. On the one hand, it allows this paradigm to be used for multiple problems using similar tools (the most common being causal loop analysis), but on the other, it becomes extremely hard to define and conceptualize a single framework, or at times, a single paradigm which all of these studies follow.

This creates a lot of variation in this area, giving one a glimpse of the power of systems thinking in exploring relationships between the elements of various types of health interventions. Different frameworks, tools, and variables have been utilized in a systematic manner to create frameworks which explore certain facets of extremely varied programs. However, the specificity of these frameworks is not universally a good thing. Greater specificity has the potential to lead to a better understanding and more detailed evaluation of a health system. Unfortunately, this very specificity may lead to a loss of universality of the tool as well as the findings.

It also leads to a narrowing of focus. Only one of nine studies focusing on specific interventions (Abdullah & Shaikh, 2014) considered all aspects of a health system during evaluation. However, the authors did not evaluate the relationships between the different building blocks and created no conceptual model. The other eight studies did evaluate the relationships between building blocks but reduced the number of blocks they targeted. Their focus may accurately be described as trying to understand the strengthening of certain aspects of a health system.

Various other studies seek to delve into the working of individual subsystems without the clouding lens of an intervention. These studies model their targeted subsystems as complete systems with varying results. At times they increase complexity by adding elements which the WHO framework does not consider (Mutingi & Mbohwa, 2014; Bunch, 2016), but others remain within the boundaries of the WHO (Mikkelsen-Lopez, Wyss, & de Savigny, 2011; Cave and Willis, 2016; Renmans, Holvoet, & Criel, 2017). These studies all work with the same implicit assumption, namely the strengthening of certain parts of a health system will lead to the strengthening of the whole. While this assumption is not unjustified by the very nature of systems thinking, few authors seek to justify it or try to add other aspects of the health system into the frameworks they design.

This is most visible in studies which try to understand certain health intervention outcomes using systems thinking. Their usage of published metrics and documents often presupposes the angle of their study. Semwanga et al. (2016) go the furthest in trying to overcome this problem by employing a quantitative simulation model (Rwashana, Nakubulwa, Nakakeeto-Kijjambu, & Adam, 2014). Unfortunately, their choice of variables remains informed by past literature which was not influenced by systems thinking.

This issue is minimized in studies which seek to look at specific parts of a health system in order to evaluate them or recommend changes. While their outlook is similar to other studies, the nature of their inquiries means that their focused approach is a net positive. One study in particular (Littlejohns et al., 2018) looked at five out of six WHO building blocks, giving it a wide range of variables to consider while remaining extremely focused.

This immediately leads us to identify a gap within existing literature: very few studies try to analyze an entire health system, even for the sake of a single intervention. The complex nature of health systems means that increasing the number of variables and detail in a study results in its focus narrowing, causing a loss of understanding of a wider set of relationships and interconnections. A larger team of researchers, the definition of a systems-thinking framework taking into account the opinions of a larger number of stakeholders, a wider variety of variables, and a greater set of recognized interconnections may lead to greater insight into the deeper workings of complex health systems.

On the other hand, theoretical studies, namely the ones which seek to create new theoretical frameworks or review existing ones, are largely immune from this criticism because they are free from the work of actually collecting data for their variables themselves and can hence target many building blocks and variables. Unfortunately, justification for these frameworks cannot come until these frameworks are applied, which brings one back to the requirement of data collection and analysis.

Conclusion

Systems thinking has become an extremely important framework for examining different aspects of a health system. However, its definition differs from author to author. Similarly, different authors define health systems differently. We have collected twenty-six studies to highlight this diversity while simultaneously showing the similarity of process between them. The different frameworks in use have all been created with a small number of specialized tools (viz. causal loop analysis).

Nevertheless, current frameworks appear to have a relatively narrow scope in order to explain low-level interconnections. The WHO's building blocks are often redefined as systems themselves, leading to a loss of higher systems-level information. Other frameworks have similar problems: broader frameworks tend to be defined only theoretically, whereas those which are actually used for analysis and evaluation tend to be defined much more narrowly. It is imperative that new systems-thinking frameworks be designed which are more universal in their outlook so as to cover a wider range of health subsystems while remaining sufficiently practical to be applied to make impact on the ground.

References

Abdullah, M. A., & Shaikh, B. T. (2014). Confusion and denial: Need for systems thinking to understand the HIV epidemic in Pakistan. *Journal of Ayub Medical College, Abbottabad, 26*(3), 396–400.

Adam, T. (2014). Advancing the application of systems thinking in health. *Health Research Policy and Systems, 12*. doi:10.1186/1478-4505-12-50

Agyepong, I. A. (2014). A systems view and lessons from the ongoing Ebola Virus Disease (EVD) outbreak in West Africa. *Ghana Medical Journal, 48*(3), 168–172.

Allender, S., Brown, A. D., Bolton, K. A., Fraser, P., Lowe, J., & Hovmand, P. (2019). Translating systems thinking into practice for community action on childhood obesity. *Obesity Reviews, 20*(S2), 179–184.

Atun, R., de Jongh, T., Secci, F., Ohiri, K., & Adeyi, O. (2010). Integration of targeted health interventions into health systems: A conceptual framework for analysis. *Health Policy and Planning, 25*(2), 104–111.

Best, A., Berland, A., Herbert, C., Bitz, J., van Dijk, M.W., Krause, C., Cochrane, D., Noel, K., Marsden, J., McKeown, S., & Millar, J. (2016). Using systems thinking to support clinical system transformation. *Journal of Health Organization and Management, 30*(3), 302–323.

Bunch, M. J. (2016). Ecosystem approaches to health and well-being: Navigating complexity, promoting health in social–ecological systems. *Systems Research and Behavioral Science, 33*(5), 614–632.

Cave, S., & Willis, G. (2016). Applying system dynamics and systems thinking methods to the development of robust workforce policies for the health and social care system in England. *International Journal of Applied Systemic Studies, 6*(3), 239–257.

Clarke, B., Swinburn, B., & Sacks, G. (2018). Understanding health promotion policy processes: a study of the government adoption of the Achievement Program in Victoria, Australia. *International Journal of Environmental Research and Public Health, 15*(11), 2393.

de Savigny, D., & Taghreed, A. (Eds.) (2009). Systems thinking for health systems strengthening. Geneva: World Health Organization. Retrieved from https://apps.who.int/iris/handle/10665/44204

Fahey, D. K., Carson, E. R., Cramp, D. G., & Muir Gray, J. A. (2004). Applying systems modelling to public health. *Systems Research and Behavioral Science, 21*(6), 635–649.

Jahanmehr, N., Rashidian, A., Khosravi, A., Farzadfar, F., Shariati, M., Majdzadeh, R., … Mesdaghinia, A. (2015). A conceptual framework for evaluation of public health and primary care system performance in Iran. *Global Journal of Health Science, 7*(4), 341.

Johnston, L. M., Matteson, C. L., & Finegood, D. T. (2014). Systems science and obesity policy: A novel framework for analyzing and rethinking population-level planning. *American Journal of Public Health, 104*(7), 1270–1278. doi:10.2105/AJPH.2014.301884

Knai, C., Petticrew, M., Douglas, N., Durand, M. A., Eastmure, E., Nolte, E., & Mays, N. (2018a). The public health responsibility deal: Using a systems-level analysis to understand the lack of impact on alcohol, food, physical activity, and workplace health sub-systems. *International Journal of Environmental Research and Public Health, 15*(12), 2895.

Knai, C., Petticrew, M., Mays, N., Capewell, S., Cassidy, R., Cummins, S., … Katikireddi, S.V. (2018b). Systems thinking as a framework for analyzing commercial determinants of health. The Milbank Quarterly, *96*(3), 472–498.

Lee, H., Chang, I., & Kim, B. H. (2019). Specialist perception on particulate matter policy in Korea: causal relationship analysis with Q-methodology and system thinking. *The Annals of Regional Science, 63*(2), 341–373.

Lembani, M., de Pinho, H., Delobelle, P., Zarowsky, C., Mathole, T., & Ager, A. (2018). Understanding key drivers of performance in the provision of maternal health services in eastern cape, South Africa: a systems analysis using group model building. *BMC Health Services Research, 18*(1), 1–12.

Littlejohns, L. B., Baum, F., Lawless, A., & Freeman, T. (2018). The value of a causal loop diagram in exploring the complex interplay of factors that influence health promotion in a multisectoral health system in Australia. *Health Research Policy and Systems, 16*(1), 126.

Mikkelsen-Lopez, I., Wyss, K., & de Savigny, D. (2011). An approach to addressing governance from a health system framework perspective. *BMC International Health and Human Rights, 11*, 13. doi:10.1186/1472-698X-11-13

Mutale, W., Ayles, H., Bond, V., Chintu, N., Chilengi, R., Mwanamwenge, M. T., ... Balabanova, D., (2017). Application of systems thinking: 12-month postintervention evaluation of a complex health system intervention in Zambia: the case of the BHOMA. *Journal of Evaluation in Clinical Practice, 23*(2), 439–452.

Mutingi, M., & Mbohwa, C. (2014) Understanding sustainability in healthcare systems: A systems thinking perspective. In Pervaiz K. Ahmed, Roger Jiao, Pei-Lee Teh, Min Xie (Eds.), *2014 IEEE International Conference on Industrial Engineering and Engineering Management* (pp. 597–601). Selangor, Malaysia: IEEE.

Newell, K., Corrigan, C., Punshon, G., & Leary, A. (2017). Severe asthma: emergency care patient driven solutions. *International Journal of Health Care Quality Assurance, 30*(7), 628–637.

Renmans, D., Holvoet, N., & Criel, B. (2017). Combining theory-driven evaluation and causal loop diagramming for opening the "black box" of an intervention in the health sector: a case of performance-based financing in Western Uganda. *International Journal of Environmental Research and Public Health, 14*(9), 1007.

Rwashana, A. S., Nakubulwa, S., Nakakeeto-Kijjambu, M., & Adam, T. (2014). Advancing the application of systems thinking in health: understanding the dynamics of neonatal mortality in Uganda. *Health Research Policy and Systems, 12*(1), 36.

Semwanga, A.R., Nakubulwa, S., & Adam, T. (2016). Applying a system dynamics modelling approach to explore policy options for improving neonatal health in Uganda. *Health Research Policy and Systems, 14*(1), 35.

Singh, J. (2013). Critical appraisal skills programme. *Journal of Pharmacology and Pharmacotherapeutics, 4*(1), 76.

Williams, J. C. (2015). A systems thinking approach to analysis of the patient protection and affordable care act. *Journal of Public Health Management and Practice, 21*(1), 6–11.

Williams, W., Lyalin, D., & Wingo, P. A. (2005). Systems thinking: What business modeling can do for public health. *Journal of Public Health Management and Practice, 11*(6), 550–553.

World Health Organization (2007). *Everybody's business—strengthening health systems to improve health outcomes: WHO's framework for action.* Geneva: World Health Organization.

World Health Organization (2010). Health system strengthening—current trends and challenges. Executive Board (EB128/37). Retrieved from http://apps.who.int/gb/ebwha/pdf_files/EB128/B128_37-en.pdf

3

Applying Systems Thinking to Health Workforce Development

Lessons from Sudan

Ayat Abu-Agla and Elsheikh Badr

Introduction

The health workforce is the cornerstone for health systems and pivotal for healthcare and population health. Health workers spearhead health production, linking knowledge, skills, and technology (e.g., medical devices and medicines) to the person in need. Research has demonstrated a positive correlation between the health workforce's density and population health outcomes (Anand & Barnighausen, 2004). Evidence also suggests that investment in the health workforce through scaling up health employment lends itself to inclusive economic growth and is vital for realizing universal health coverage (UHC) and contributing to attaining the Sustainable Development Goals (Buchan, Dhillon, & Campbell, 2017). However, the centrality of the health workforce has only recently been highlighted, with the realization that people-centered health systems cannot be achieved without adequate and competent health workers (de Savigny 2009; George et al., 2018). The advent of the COVID-19 pandemic has further highlighted the centrality of the health workforce and has exposed the lack of adequate investment in the human capacity of health systems (Bourgeault et al., 2020). Notwithstanding rising attention to health workforce issues, greater efforts are required at country level and internationally to ensure adequate investment in health workforce development for stronger and more resilient health systems.

Systems Thinking to Address Health Workforce Complexity

With its holistic, dynamic, and interconnected approach, systems thinking is best suited to study and analyze complex fields such as health systems. In contrast to a reductionist approach, a systems-thinking paradigm views problems in context and appreciates the linkages of events, patterns, and structures (see Chapter 1). Unlike mechanical systems in which component parts interact linearly to produce a predictable output; the health system is characterized by non-linear, dynamic, and unpredictable nature (Lipsitz, 2012). This is because the health system has social and political dimensions in addition to the technical aspects. The multiple and iterative interactions

Ayat Abu-Agla and Elsheikh Badr, *Applying Systems Thinking to Health Workforce Development* In: *Systems Thinking for Global Health*. Edited by: Fiona Larkan, Frédérique Vallières, Hasheem Mannan, and Naonori Kodate, Oxford University Press. DOI: 10.1093/oso/9780198799498.003.0003

among the various health system components (levels of care, funding, governance, technical and human resources) that are shaped by sociocultural and political processes thus necessitate a systems-thinking approach, or a soft system methodology (see Chapter 1) to disentangle complexity and ensure the desired outcomes.

Systems thinking is also highly relevant to the health workforce domain as a key component of the health system. As the health workforce is underpinned by human nature and human relationships, it is arguably more complex than other health system building blocks such as information and medicines. The health workforce further involves multiple stakeholders with different roles, including educational institutions, regulatory bodies, employment agencies, funding entities, and professional associations, which contribute even more complexity. Additionally, the policies and decisions related to the health workforce within these institutions may lack alignment and consistency, further necessitating systems thinking.

Frameworks developed for analyzing the health workforce over the last two decades emphasize the continuity and interconnected nature of the health workforce functions. The framework proposed by the World Health Organization (WHO) in 2006, for example, introduces the concept of a *working lifespan approach* to analyze the health workforce across three stages: entry, active workforce, and exit, and entails a systems perspective (World Health Organization, 2006). The framework therefore seeks to counteract the practice of *ad hoc* single-event interventions to address health workforce challenges, which tend to create more problems than solutions (Buchan et al., 2017). For instance, a country might raise the standard of educating its health workers to internationally comparable levels without addressing retention aspects, only to find its graduates migrating to other countries, leaving behind gaps in service coverage and quality. Such an example highlights the need to plan strategically for the sector to safeguard against the unintended effects of otherwise desired health workforce strengthening interventions, consistent with a systems-thinking approach. The political economy of health systems further adds complexity to addressing health workforce issues as wider contextual dimensions are needed to support technical solutions (Fieno, Dambisya, George, & Benson, 2016). When labor market dynamics are considered in isolation, severe and counter-productive consequences might result. For example, if a country scales up production of the health workforce to address a shortage—as a good and commonly adopted strategy—but fails to provide for adequate jobs to absorb the graduates; frustration, emigration, or industrial actions against the state as a result of unemployment usually ensue. Taken together, the above examples evidence the need for more systems-thinking approaches to addressing critical gaps and requirements for a more robust health workforce.

Sudan's Health System

Sudan, situated in East Africa, is a member of the WHO's Eastern Mediterranean Region, with 40.7 million population growing at a rate of 2.8% per annum (Federal Ministry of Health, 2017). The country depends on agricultural and livestock economy with some contribution from oil resources. Politically, since 1990, Sudan has adopted a devolved three-tier system of governance with federal level and 18 state governments in addition to over 180 localities. The country is currently undergoing a major political transformation, following the downfall of the regime that ruled Sudan for the past thirty years. The political outlook is still unclear with a transitional period that is supposed to lead to general elections in 2023 (Harshe, 2020).

The primary health challenges in Sudan include communicable diseases, coupled with rising trends of non-communicable diseases, in addition to health emergencies. With an infant mortality rate of fifty-seven per 1,000 live births, a maternal mortality ratio of 216 per 100,000 live births and malaria as one of the leading causes of death; the country's progress toward Millennium Development Goals was judged to be below optimum (Federal Ministry of Health, 2017).

The country's health system is decentralized, where states have substantial authority in various aspects including health workforce decisions. Nationally, the Federal Ministry of Health (FMoH) and State Ministries of Health spearhead the overall system. Whereas the former is responsible for policy and strategic planning, the latter is mandated with operational planning and implementation. National authorities regulate pharmaceuticals, supplies, and equipment although challenges exist in availability, supply chain, and unregulated prescription of drugs, in addition to a lack of an effective health technology assessment, (i.e., systems for appraisal for equipment purchase). The national health information system depends on facility-level reporting, supplemented by national surveys. There are, however, limitations in data coverage, quality, and analysis. The system also faces the challenges of fragmentation, with many health programs developing and using separate systems for data collection and reporting. A recently adopted strategy aims to move the country toward a more integrated system, with an electronic interface (Federal Ministry of Health, 2017). In addition to the FMoH, there are other stakeholders, including Police and Army health services, and a national health insurance fund. More recently, the country has seen an expansion of private sector institutions, both in terms of service provision and professional training of healthcare workers. Governance for health in Sudan is challenged by fragmentation and lack of effective coordination among major players in the health arena (Public Health Institute, 2016a).

On the health financing front, Sudan spends almost 6.5% of its gross domestic product (GDP) on health, while total government health expenditure is 9% (Public Health Institute, 2016b). Despite the improvement in public allocation for health over the last period, Sudan still falls short of the target of 15% from the Abuja Declaration to which Sudan is a signatory. A social health insurance scheme is developing in the country, with an estimated 54% coverage (Federal Ministry of Health, 2017). However, 70% of total health expenditure comes from out-of-pocket expenditure, representing a daunting challenge for attaining universal health coverage's financial protection dimension (Public Health Institute, 2016b).

Sudan's Health Workforce

The health workforce sector in Sudan comprises over 150,000 health workers of various categories (Federal Ministry of Health, 2012), with recent years witnessing increased production across all cadres. Most of the health workforce serves in the public sector, although dual practice, whereby health workers also maintain an involvement in private sector work, is prominent. The Federal Ministry of Health spearhead the policy and leadership arena for the health workforce. Other essential human resources for health stakeholders include the higher education sector, regulatory councils, syndicates, and professional associations. Problems of coordination and synergy among these stakeholders, however, are not uncommon in the country.

Professional health worker education is deeply rooted in Sudan, with nursing, midwifery, and allied health personnel schools dating back to the early 1900s (Bayoumi, 1979). The first medical school in Tropical Africa was established in Khartoum, the capital of Sudan, in 1924. Within the North Africa region, the medical school in Khartoum ranked second only to Kasr Al Aini Medical School in Egypt in having a comprehensive syllabus (Haseeb, 1967). The subsequent evolution of professional health worker education generated a two-tier educational system, whereby medical education came under the responsibility of the Ministry of Higher Education and requiring university accreditation, and nursing, midwifery, and paramedic education remained within vocational schools under the Federal Ministry of Health. Under this educational divergence, doctors, dentists, and pharmacists became regulated by the Sudan Medical Council (SMC). At the same time, nurses, midwives, and others fell under auspices of the National Council for Medical and Health Professions (NCMHP).

As early as 1976, Sudan led the implementation of important initiatives to develop their primary healthcare workforce, notably medical assistants and community health workers, which helped to extend the coverage of health services in a country with vast land and dispersed populations (Bayoumi, 1979). The experience of the midwifery program, which introduced modern training for midwives in support of better maternal and childcare in Sudan, contributed toward Sudan's much lower morbidity and mortality compared to other countries in the region (Bella, 2011). The robust foundations for professional health education and the strong civil service structure, both legacies form Sudan's colonial period, bolstered the availability, quality, and performance of the Sudan health workforce. However, over the years, and especially following the economic crisis of the 1980s, Sudan started to experience difficulties with its health workforce sector. Specifically, in 1990s the country faced a health workforce shortage and a geographical misdistribution of its health workforce, whereby 70% of health workers served only 30% of Sudan's population (Federal Ministry of Health, 2012). Skill mix imbalances also emerged with severe shortages in nurses and allied health professionals (National Human Resources for Health Observatory, 2006; Federal Ministry of Health, 2017). Sudan also faced imbalances of its health labor market, represented by inadequate budget allocation for health sector jobs and low wages for civil servants, including health workers, resulting in increased emigration trends (Abuagla, Yousif, & Badr, 2013). By the year 2000, Sudan had lost nearly 60% of its medical doctors to emigration, mainly to destinations in the Gulf area and Europe (Badr, 2005). In addition to the health workforce challenges mentioned earlier, scarcity of resources, contradicting health policies, and poor working environments adversely influenced health worker retention, performance, and productivity (Abuagla, 2013). Taken together, absenteeism, an increase in dual practice, especially in rural and remote areas, weak leadership, lack of synergies, and conflicting policies among health workforce stakeholders, and insufficient funding, represent underlying factors that have contributed to the neglect of the health workforce sector in Sudan, resulting in numerical shortages, skill mix imbalances, inequitable geographic distribution, and massive emigration (Badr, Mohamed, Afzal, & Bile, 2013).

The Need for Reform and Transformation

The year 2001 witnessed a leadership change in the FMoH that brought ideas and momentum for health sector reform. The Ministry initiated a comprehensive move toward identifying and addressing the significant challenges facing the country's health system. The FMoH and stakeholders opted for a national reform agenda based on health system analysis reports, including policy development, strategic planning, organizational change, and capacity-strengthening efforts. As one of the building blocks of the health system, the health workforce was therefore included as an object for reform, as part of the broader health sector movement. This provided an enabling context to initiate and implement a transformational initiative in the health workforce domain.

The Health Workforce Transformation Initiative

A cardinal sign of the health workforce transformation agenda in Sudan is the paradigm shift in how the country's health workforce's analysis and development is approached. This shift was brought forward by a few health workforce champions, with support from the technical and political leadership in the health sector. A policy dialogue initiated in 2001 generated momentum among stakeholders and helped to develop a national framework to address the challenges of the country's health workforce, based on a single strategic vision. This dialogue resulted in a broad consensus of main philosophies and principles and represented a shift away from more traditional toward a more transformative agenda (see Box 3.1).

The transformation initiative in the health workforce sector in Sudan thus introduced a new philosophy and policy direction emphasizing a holistic, strategic, and systems approach to enable change. The interconnected nature of the health workforce's function has since been more broadly appreciated, paving the way for a better understanding of this complex sector, and allowing for collective and streamlined efforts by relevant stakeholders.

Box 3.1 Ten identifying features of the health workforce paradigm shift in Sudan

1. Transforming the thinking around the health workforce from a personnel administration view to a broader health workforce development perspective.
2. Strategically positioning health workforce agenda, structures, and dialogue.
3. Moving from numerical operational planning for the health workforce to the broader arena of strategic planning and policies emphasizing both quantitative and qualitative dimensions.
4. Taking health workforce development beyond medical doctors and devoting attention to addressing the broader health workforce, including different categories of health workers.
5. Appreciating the role of evidence in informing health workforce policies, plans, and decision-making.
6. Taking health workforce issues beyond the health ministry boundaries by reaching out to the broader stakeholders, and enabling partnerships to promote the health workforce, emphasizing full engagement of state and non-state actors.
7. Appreciating the role of capacity building for strategic health workforce development across the system, institutional, and individual levels.
8. Developing the health workforce domain as a field of knowledge and science, moving away from the traditional normative view for the domain as a routine function.
9. Recognizing the techno-political nature of health workforce issues as requiring political engagement and commitment hand in hand with the technical dimension.
10. Appreciating the regional and global dimensions of the health workforce crisis and the need for concerted action beyond the national remits.

Setting the Stage for Health Workforce Interventions

The health workforce transformation initiative introduced in Sudan yielded many achievements for the health system and population health. Based on the policy shifts emphasizing a strategic perspective, a systems-thinking approach has further supported a concerted and comprehensive strategy to address the country's health workforce issues over the past two decades. In order to level the playing field for effective and systematic interventions for health workforce development, the transformation movement also paved the way for improvements to health workforce governance.

Shortly following the inception of the 2001 reform, the unit responsible for health workforce development in the FMoH was upgraded to a General Directorate, enabling strategic positioning and additional resources and staff to be mobilized. Health workforce structures within the country's eighteen states were also upgraded and systematically linked to the national health workforce apparatus. An expert group was formed around the General Directorate for Health Workforce Development to work on policy development and strategic planning. The following aspects were also realized:

- An evidence-generation movement, resulting in the first-ever national health workforce census in the country, with results published in 2005.
- The development of health workforce priority policies including a training policy, deployment and retention policies, and career pathways.
- The establishment in 2006 of a national health workforce observatory to act as a hub for health workforce information and evidence, and to facilitate stakeholder coordination.
- The introduction of a national health workforce stakeholder forum, involving over twenty entities related to health workforce issues. The forum brought in partners across the public and private sectors and organized periodic meetings and events leading to more coordinated actions.
- Increased political leverage and visibility for the health workforce agenda through the formation of the health workforce committee in 2007, as one of three permanent committees under the highly positioned National Council for Health Care Coordination. This committee has been pivotal in driving critical decisions in favor of health workforce development.
- The development of the first-ever comprehensive health workforce strategic plan in the country, covering the period 2012–2016. This strategy was based on thorough situation analyses and involved developing robust strategic objectives and interventions covering the interconnected health workforce dimensions. The strategy development process was highly participatory, with stakeholders demonstrating active engagement and support.
- The introduction of a capacity building program resulted in establishing a national public health institute in 2007 and more effective partnerships with Western universities for training individuals in health systems and health workforce development. Starting from 2001, Sudan trained over 200 public health professionals in key health system and health workforce areas through mainly international scholarships. As a result, the country succeeded in developing a critical mass of leaders, champions, and technical staff in the field of health workforce development subsequently termed "the health workforce brigade."

Achievements on Health Workforce Development

The health workforce governance interventions outlined above represent both achievements and facilitators for interventions to address specific domains related to health workforce development. The *Working Lifespan* framework has been used to guide and inform efforts to analyze and strengthen the Sudanese health workforce (World Health Organization, 2006). The entry stage entails planning education and recruitment of health workers, while in the active stage issues of regulation and performance pertain. The exit stage captures the move of health workers out of the health sector through retirement, migration, or death. The WHO life span framework thus represents a systems-thinking approach as it delineates vital entry points for intervention and represents a logical continuum for considering the interlinkages across the three stages of health workforce development.

The following section describes interventions implemented in Sudan which aimed to strengthen the health workforce across the three stages (entry, workforce, and exit) of the health workforce working lifespan framework.

Entry Stage

The entry phase includes essential functions, such as education and training, recruitment, and regulation. Sudan realized substantial progress across all these domains, including:

- The scaling up of professional health worker education and production: The number of university-level educational institutions increased rapidly to reach over 319 schools and institutes in 2019, compared to seventy-three in 2001, including the substantial growth of medical schools from twenty-five in 2001 to sixty-nine in 2019. This was enabled through both public and private investment in the education of health workers. This scale-up resulted in an increasing number of graduates across all healthcare cadres, but largely an increase in medical doctors.
- The establishment of the Academy of Health Sciences (AHS) in 2005, under the auspices of the FMoH as a response to emerging skill mix imbalance, and with the mandate to address the categorical shortage in health workforce production. The AHS represented a key achievement by enrolling over 40,000 students across nursing, midwifery, and allied health professions. Thus far, with over 25,000 graduates, the AHS succeeded in bringing balance to the skill mix of the Sudanese health workforce and scaling up health service coverage across the country.
- Effective decentralization of professional health education enabled more capacity for training across the country, increasing retention by encouraging students to remain in the settings where they were trained. There is currently at least one public medical school in each of the country's eighteen states, with other types of schools showing a more balanced geographic distribution.
- Despite economic constraints and restrictions on employment, recruitment and job creation for health workers has remained a priority at national and subnational levels. Records suggest that over 90% of graduates from the AHS were employed at their training place across different states.
- The revitalization of a comprehensive regulatory system for health workers, covering all health professions and enhancing quality and professionalism. In 2010, new legislation was endorsed, resulting in the promotion and autonomy of the NCMHP. The newly renovated council led to the regulation of nurses, midwives, and allied health professions. Following the foot-steps of the long-standing SMC responsible for regulating medical doctors, dentists, and pharmacists. Along the lines of enhancing health workforce quality, the SMC launched an accreditation program for medical, dental, and pharmacy schools in 2006, leading to

the development of national standards and system for institutional accreditation. This program has resulted in tangible improvements in terms of adopting quality structures and practices, and the SMC has ultimately received recognition by the World Federation of Medical Education as a competent national authority for accreditation (World Federation of Medical Education, 2018).

Active Workforce Stage

The workforce's active stage includes aspects such as geographic balance, retention, performance, and productivity. Continuing professional development (CPD) and specialty training are also included under this stage. As part of the transformation initiative, Sudan has successfully introduced:

- A more balanced geographic distribution through the decentralized education system, effective deployment, and targeted policies. The typical picture of 70% of health workers serving 30% of the population witnessed a positive change with access to healthcare (and health workers) reaching up to 95% of the population in 2017 (Federal Ministry of Health, 2017).
- The introduction of effective retention strategies and initiatives leading to sustainable and more consistent staffing at decentralized health facilities. A targeted national scheme introduced in 2013 succeeded in increasing the number of medical specialists in states other than Khartoum's capital area from 450 to over 1,200 specialist doctors. State-level initiatives supported by federal subsidies further helped retain primary healthcare workers across states and remote areas. The collective approach in health workforce governance has also helped streamline the mandatory national service scheme managed by the military sector to improve rural and remote health facilities' staffing.
- The introduction of a CPD system and practice to ensure health workers acquire new and evolving knowledge, strategies, skills, and technologies within health. In 2007, the FMoH established a national center for CPD which subsequently extended its remit to states in the form of branches. Other providers of CPD also emerged, including centers and institutes in both the public and private sectors. Consequently, coverage of CPD improved from 24% in 2005 to 67% in 2012 (Badr et al., 2013), becoming even more commonplace in subsequent years.
- A reform of postgraduate specialty training was also implemented to better respond to health system needs and the challenge of emigration. In 2014, the Sudan Medical Specialization Board (SMSB) introduced a significant transformation program resulting in the expansion of medical specialties; the introduction of professional specialty programs for nurses, midwives, and allied health professions; decentralized training; and quality enhancement through the accreditation of multiple training sites (Sudan Medical Specialization Board, 2019). Specifically, specialty programs increased from thirty-three in 2013 to fifty-nine in 2019, and the number continues to evolve. Likewise, the number of candidates sitting their SMSB entry exam increased from 2,150 in 2005 to 11,000 in 2019, representing a massive scaling up in postgraduate training to

match the expanding undergraduate professional health education and to address health needs.

Exit Stage

This final stage reflects when health workers leave their practice settings due to emigration, retirement, change of career, or death. As a country with a high emigration rate, Sudan introduced policies to mitigate the exit of its health workforce. Specifically, the health workforce transformation initiative led to the introduction of:

- A robust program aimed at health worker mobility management to maximize gains and mitigate emigration's adverse effects. Sudan is among the pioneering countries to integrate the Global Code of Practice for International Recruitment of Health Personnel, adopted by the World Health Assembly (WHA) in 2010 (Abuagla & Badr, 2016). Subsequently, Sudan developed a national policy on health workforce mobility involving a three-pronged strategy: targeted retention, bilateral agreements with destination countries, and mobilizing the diaspora to support healthcare and training in Sudan. Implementation records suggest progress along these three strategies, with national support for retaining the specialist workforce and a successful diaspora mobilization program (Abdalla, Omar, & Badr, 2016, Badr, Abdalla, & Abuagla, 2016). Additionally, Sudan entered into effective bilateral agreements with central destination countries such as Saudi Arabia and the Republic of Ireland. These agreements enjoyed effective implementation and brought in benefits to the country and health workers. The agreements involved regulating mobility through formal arrangements and providing placements for training and professional development.
- Extension of retirement age from sixty years to sixty-five years, in addition to allowing a flexible employment modality for universities. These arrangements, brought in by a 2011 Presidential Decree, have been instrumental in retaining senior and experienced health workers and academics to support healthcare and training of younger generations. They also helped to boost the number and capacity of the health workforce in the country.

Adopting the health workforce lifespan model enabled a holistic approach and a more coherent strategy to address health workforce development in Sudan. This systems-thinking methodology helped identify connections and interlinkages among different entry points for strengthening the health workforce. In such a manner, it was possible to avoid counterproductive actions and to rectify side effects of some otherwise desired interventions. One example is the introduction of the AHS to restore the skill mix imbalance resulting from the proliferation of medical schools, at the expense of nursing and allied health professional training institutions. By keeping the overall picture in sight, systems thinking improves coherence and identifies irregularities, thus providing a guide to corrective strategies.

Challenges and How They are Addressed

Despite the successes of the health workforce transformation in Sudan, several challenges and bottlenecks remain, including:

- The economic situation in Sudan continues to adversely affect the stability and performance of the health workforce. Wages in the public sector remain poor, leading to high turnover at all levels and fueling emigration. In the face of these challenges, health authorities opted to allow and regulate dual practice to retain the critical mass of health workers. Arrangements based on public–private partnerships in the health sector and joint appointment policies for academic staff show promising results in stabilizing the health workforce amid significant emigration trends.
- Challenges of sustaining stakeholder commitment and buy-in, causing difficulties in fully harmonizing and synchronizing actions in the health workforce arena. In a culture characterized by working in silos, adopting strategies such as periodic meetings, participative planning, and multiple entry points to stakeholders are showing promise in maintaining collective stakeholder action for health workforce development.
- A devolved system of decentralization, where states have substantial authority in health workforce decisions, has at times hampered retention and adversely affected health workers' equitable distribution. Less privileged states find themselves in a weak position, competing with wealthier states over the employment of qualified staff. To tackle this challenge, the national government opted to dictate some national schemes to deploy and incentivize health workers in remote states and promote dialogue for more collective and coordinated health workforce interventions across the country.
- Reaching out to private sector institutions has always been a challenge in a country where government oversight and capacity are not optimized. Extending dialogue to private sector entities and representative groups, besides promoting public–private partnerships, are examples of strategies adopted to address an expanding private sector's role in the country.
- Harmonization of regulation across health professions remains a challenge, hampering teamwork and inter-professional practice. A national framework for collaborative practice is currently being promoted through transparent dialogue involving all health professions to address this critical dimension.
- Performance and productivity of the health workforce is still an area of minimum evidence and intervention in Sudan. Wide variations in the work environment standardization and the lack of adequate evidence hamper the use of performance management strategies. To approach the problem, the FMoH has embarked on a policy to address performance and productivity, focusing on reducing absenteeism and moonlighting.
- Loss of investment and capacity through massive emigration of health workers has jeopardized coverage and quality of healthcare services in the country. The

recently developed and adopted mobility management policy carries the promise of addressing this dimension through rationing emigration and allowing diaspora mobilization to support the health system and healthcare coverage and quality.

Lessons Learnt

Throughout the past two decades of the health workforce transformation initiative in Sudan, some vital insight and learning emerged. Lessons learnt to inform action on health workforce development in the country and beyond include:

- The realization that health workforce issues are complex, multidimensional, and interconnected, thereby warranting a systems approach.
- The health workforce domain is a multi-stakeholder endeavor, and the systematic engagement of several stakeholders is a prerequisite for success in any intervention.
- The role of evidence is pivotal in informing planning and decision-making for health workforce development. Figures and statistics proved to be a powerful advocacy tool for mobilizing support and action.
- Political leverage is required and fundamental to address health workforce issues and challenges; technical expertise alone cannot suffice.
- Health workforce leadership and the role of champions is fundamental to progress the transformation agenda for health workforce development.
- Innovation and atypical solutions are critical dimensions for addressing health workforce issues, especially in challenging and resource-constrained environments.

Conclusions and Prospects

The employment of a systems-thinking model for addressing the complex health workforce issues in Sudan has proven successful and promising. The national momentum transforming the health workforce has resulted in a strategic perspective, a comprehensive approach, and a collective thrust that enabled a structured course of interventions along the health workforce continuum. Challenges, however, still abound in Sudan. The country would need to reflect critically on its experience to improve identification and addressing of bottlenecks and enable further progress along with the health workforce development agenda. Regional and global movements and initiatives for the health workforce represent opportunities for Sudan to share its experience and learn from other contexts working toward improvements in health workforce development and ultimately health system strengthening and population health improvement.

References

Abdalla, F. M., Omar, M. A., & Badr, E. E. (2016). Contribution of Sudanese medical diaspora to the healthcare delivery system in Sudan: Exploring options and barriers. *Human Resources for Health, 14,* 28. Retrieved from https://doi.org/10.1186/s12960-016-0123-x

Abuagla, A. (2013). *Magnitude, trends and implications of health professional out migration in Sudan 2012.* (Medical Doctorate in Community Medicine, Sudan Medical Specialization Board).

Abuagla, A., Yousif, N., & Badr, E. (2013). *Understanding the labour market of human resources for health in Sudan.* Department for Health Systems Policies and Workforce World Health Organization. Geneva, Switzerland.

Abuagla, A., & Badr, E. (2016). Challenges to implementation of the WHO Global Code of Practice on International Recruitment of Health Personnel: The case of Sudan. *Human Resources for Health, 14*(26), 5–10. Retrieved from https://doi.org/10.1186/s12960-016-0117-8

Anand, S. A. & Barnighausen, T. (2004). Human resources and health outcomes: Cross-country econometric study. *The Lancet, 364,* 1603–1609.

Badr, E. (2005). Brain drain of health professionals in Sudan: Magnitude, challenges and prospects for solution. (MA thesis, University of Leeds).

Badr, E., Abdalla, F., & Abuagla, A. (2016). Supporting medical specialty training in Sudan: A framework for systematic engagement of diaspora. *International Journal of Sudan Research, 6,* 103–112.

Badr, E., Mohamed, N., Afzal, M., & Bile, K. (2013). Strengthening human resources for health through information, coordination and accountability mechanisms: the case of the Sudan. *Bulletin of the World Health Organization, 91,* 868–873.

Banati, P., & Moatti, J. P. (2008). The positive contributions of global health initiatives. *Bulletin of the World Health Organization, Nov; 86*(11), 820–821.

Bayoumi, A. (1979). *The history of Sudan health services.* Nairobi: KLB.

Bella, H. (2011). *The Sudan barefoot doctors: A successful story that impressed the world.* Khartoum: Khartoum University Press

Bourgeault, I. L., Maier, C. B., Dieleman, M., Ball, J., MacKenzie, A., Nancarrow, S., Nigenda, G., & Sidat, M. (2020). The COVID-19 pandemic presents an opportunity to develop more sustainable health workforces. *Human Resources for Health, 18,* 83. Retrieved from https://doi.org/10.1186/s12960-020-00529-0

Buchan, D. I., Dhillon, I. S., & Campbell, J. (2017). *Health employment and economic growth: An evidence base.* Geneva: World Health Organization.

Buse, K., & Walt, G. (2002). Globalisation and multilateral public-private health partnerships: issues for health policy. In K, Lee, K, Buse, & S, Fustukian (Eds.) *Health policy in a globalizing world* (pp. 41–62). Cambridge: Cambridge University Press.

Campbell, M., Fitzpatrick, R, Haines, A, Sandercock, P., & Tyer, P. (2000). Framework for design and evaluation of complex interventions to improve health. *British Medical Journal, 321*(7262), 694–696.

de Savigny, D., & Taghreed, A. (Eds.) (2009). Systems thinking for health systems strengthening. Geneva: World Health Organization. Retrieved from https://apps.who.int/iris/handle/10665/44204

Federal Ministry of Health. (2012). *National Health Sector Strategic Plan 2012–2016.* Khartoum, Sudan: Federal Ministry of Health.

Federal Ministry of Health. (2017). *National Health Policy for Sudan 2017–2030*. Khartoum, Sudan: Federal Ministry of Health.

Federal Ministry of Health. (2017). *National Health Policy 2017–2030*. Khartoum, Sudan: Federal Ministry of Health.

Fieno, J. V., Dambisya, Y. M., George, G., & Benson, K. (2016). A political economy analysis of human resources for health (HRH) in Africa. *Human Resources for Health, 14*, 44. Retrieved from: https://human-resources-health.biomedcentral.com/track/pdf/10.1186/s12960-016-0137-4.pdf

George, A. S., Campbell, J., Ghaffar, A., & HPSR HRH reader collaborators. (2018). Advancing the science behind human resources for health: Highlights from the health policy and systems research reader on human resources for health. *Human Resources for Health, 16*, 35.

Hanefeld, J. (2008). How have global health initiatives impacted on health equity? *Journal of Education and Health Promotion, 15*(1), 19–23.

Harshe, R. (2020). *Interpreting the unprecedented political transition in Sudan*. Raisina Debates, Observer Research Foundation. Retrieved from https://www.orfonline.org/expert-speak/interpreting-unprecedented-political-transition-sudan/

Haseeb, M. A. (1967). Medical education in the Sudan. *Journal of Medical Education, 42*, 666–672.

Holden, L. M. (2005). Complex adaptive systems: concept analysis. *Journal of Advanced Nursing, 52*(6), 651–657.

Labonte, R., & Schreker, T. (2006). The G8 and global health: What now? What next? *Canadian Journal of Public Health, Jan-Feb;97*(1), 35–38.

Lipsitz, L. A. (2012). Understanding health care as a complex system: The foundation for unintended consequences. *Journal of the American Medical Association, 308*(3), 243–244. Retrieved from https://www.ncbi.nlm.nih.gov/pmc/articles/PMC3511782/pdf/nihms422926.pdf

Murray C. J. L., Frenk, J., & Evans, T. (2007). The global campaign for the health MDGs: Challenges, opportunities, and imperative of shared learning. *The Lancet, 370*(9592), 1018–1020. doi: https://doi.org/10.1016/S0140-6736(07)61458-5

National Human Resources for Health Observatory. (2006). *National Human Resources for Health Survey 2006*. Khartoum, Sudan: Federal Ministry of Health.

Pawson. R. G. T., Harvey, G, & Wallshe, K. (2005). Realist review—a new method of systematic review designed for complex policy interventions. *Journal of Health Services Research & Policy, Jul;10*, (Suppl 1), 21–34.

Public Health Institute. (2016a). *Strengthening primary health care in Sudan through a family health approach: Policy options*. Khartoum, Sudan: Public Health Institute.

Public Health Institute. (2016b). *Health finance policy options for Sudan*. Khartoum, Sudan: Public Health Institute.

Samb, B., & World Health Organization Maximizing Positive Synergies Collaborative Group. (2009). An assessment of interactions between global health initiatives and country health systems. *The Lancet, 373*(9681), 2137–2169.

Schieber, G. P., Fleisher, L. K., & Leive, A. A. (2007). Financing global health: Mission unaccomplished. *Health Affairs (Millwood), Jul-Aug;26*(4), 921–934.

Sterman, J. D. (2006). Learning from evidence in a complex world. *American Journal of Public Health, 96*(3), 505–514.

Sudan Medical Specialization Board. (2019). *Annual report of the Sudan Medical Specialization Board*. unpublished Sudan Medical Specialization Board. Khartoum-Sudan.

World Federation for Medical Education. (2018). *Sudan Medical Council (SMC) awarded Recognition Status*. World Federation for Medical Education. Retrieved from https://wfme.org/news/sudan-medical-council-smc-awarded-recognition-status/

World Health Organization. (2006). Working Together for Health. World Health Report. Geneva: World Health Organization.

World Health Organization. (2017). *A health policy and systems research reader on human resources for health*, Geneva: World Health Organization.

Yu, D., Souteyrand, Y., Banda, M. A, Kaufman, J., & Perriëns, J. H. (2008). Investment in HIV/AIDS programs: Does it help strengthen health systems in developing countries? *Global Health, 4*, 8. https://doi.org/10.1186/1744-8603-4-8

4

Supportive Supervision for Community Health Workers

A Systems-Thinking Approach

Camille Coyle, Áine Travers, Mary Creaner, Damen Haile-Mariam, and Frédérique Vallières

Introduction

Community health workers (CHWs) form the core of the health workforce in many countries. They are typically the first point of contact between their communities and the wider health system. CHWs often work on a volunteer basis, although in some contexts they receive salaries, and the length and content of their training varies widely between countries. Most CHWs work either individually or in teams of two, and their supervisors can be nurses, public health officers, environmental health officers, district health officers, or non-governmental organization (NGO) staff. While CHWs were traditionally tasked with providing basic healthcare in the form of preventive health services, they are increasingly trained to deliver curative care as well. They are seen as a cost-effective means of delivering evidence-based care, through culturally acceptable and community-centered approaches (Vaughan, Kok, Witter, & Dieleman, 2015).

CHWs were perceived as crucial to the Millennium Development Goals (Singh & Sachs, 2013) and they remain a key strategy in achieving universal health coverage and the Sustainable Development Goals, specifically Goal 3—ensure healthy lives and promote well-being for all at all ages (United Nations, 2015). Effective CHW programs are also consistent with a rights-based approach to health (United Nations Committee on Economic, Social and Cultural Rights, 2000) by helping to increase the availability, accessibility, and acceptability of health services. Understanding the critical components of effective CHW programs is therefore crucial if their expansion is to have a lasting impact on health outcomes.

Supervision of Community Health Workers

Supervision is an essential component of CHW programs (Chen et al., 2006; Rowe, Onikpo, Lama, & Deming, 2010; World Health Organization, 2006). Many CHWs work in rural and remote areas, and their supervisor is often their only link to the wider health system. Yet, supervision has been identified as particularly challenging

Camille Coyle, Áine Travers, Mary Creaner, Damen Haile-Mariam, and Frédérique Vallières, *Supportive Supervision for Community Health Workers* In: *Systems Thinking for Global Health.* Edited by: Fiona Larkan, Frédérique Vallières, Hasheem Mannan, and Naonori Kodate, Oxford University Press. © Oxford University Press 2023. DOI: 10.1093/oso/9780198799498.003.0004

to implement, often due to limited resources and low institutional commitment (Crigler, Gergen, & Perry, 2013). Historically, CHW supervision systems within primary healthcare programs have focused on an "overseer" model, where fault-finding, inspection, and control are employed as means to drive individuals to perform their duties. This approach to supervision focuses on checklists and outputs and is not typically open to dialog and consultation between supervisor and supervisee (Clements, Streefland, & Malau, 2007). In management theory, this is sometimes referred to as Theory X management style (McGregor, 1989), an approach characterized by the use of rewards and punishment as professional motivators, based on the assumption that workers are inherently unmotivated and resistant to work.

Recent years have seen a shift toward more supportive forms of CHW supervision, emphasizing regular and consistent interactions characterized by constructive feedback and joint problem-solving (Strachan et al., 2012). Supportive supervision focuses on identifying the needs of individual CHWs by building mutually trusting and collegial relationships. This represents a shift in the dynamics of power between supervisor and supervisee toward more equal engagement, in which CHWs are treated as colleagues rather than subordinates. This approach is more consistent with the Theory Y style of management (McGregor, 1989), in which instead of believing that individuals wish to avoid work, it is assumed that they are intrinsically motivated by work, are ambitious, and have a desire to perform well. In the Theory Y approach, it is the manager's duty to nurture these qualities in individuals and to try to promote the conditions they require to work at their optimal level.

While the concept of supportive supervision for health workers has existed for over thirty years (Devgan, 1990), it began to be discussed more widely in primary healthcare programs in the early 2000s. In 2002, it was defined as "an approach to supervision that emphasizes joint problem-solving, mentoring and two-way communication between the supervisor and those being supervised" (Marquez & Kean, 2002: 3). In 2013, Crigler et al. (2013) noted that supportive supervision for community health workers is "a process of guiding, monitoring, and coaching workers to promote compliance with standards of practice and ensure the delivery of quality care" (p. 2).

Research has shown that supportive supervision is positively associated with motivation (Ndima et al., 2015), work engagement, job satisfaction (Vallières et al., 2018), and improved performance among CHWs and other health workers (Frimpong, Helleringer, Awoonor-Williams, Yeji, & Phillips, 2011; Mubyazi et al., 2012; Fatti et al., 2013). Joint problem-solving is a particularly important component of supportive supervision and has been found to increase health workers' motivation and confidence (Uys, Minnaar, Reid, & Naidoo, 2004; Suh, Moreira, & Ly, 2007; Bradley et al., 2013). In light of these findings, many primary healthcare programs are increasingly shifting toward supportive supervision for CHWs (Hill et al., 2014). Additionally, supportive supervision is specifically cited as the preferred approach to supervision within task-shifting frameworks by the World Health Organization (WHO), which has further bolstered its uptake (World Health Organization, President's Emergency Plan for AIDS Relief, & Joint United Nations Programme on HIV and AIDS, 2007).

Supportive Supervision as Systems Thinking

In this chapter we will demonstrate that supportive supervision represents a systems-thinking approach. Both supportive supervision and systems thinking are ways of addressing problems that take a broad range of factors into account, including contextual factors. A multitude of factors influence an individual CHW's knowledge, skills, engagement, motivation, and, ultimately, performance (Kok et al., 2014). Supportive supervision takes these multiple factors into account by focusing on collaboration within the supervisory relationships, whereby a supervisor works closely with a CHW to identify their individual needs, existing challenges, and how to address these in the best way possible. Within traditional supervision, supervisors identify faults in CHWs' services with the expectation that as a result, CHWs will provide improved health services. The move away from traditional supervision and toward supportive supervision represents a shift toward a systems-thinking paradigm, in that supportive supervision aims to address the complex interplay of factors that influence CHWs' performance.

Moreover, we argue that as a complex problem, applying a systems-thinking approach to supportive supervision can enhance its ability act as a key leverage point within health systems to promote positive change by helping to improve quality of care and service delivery. We apply the WHO's health system building blocks—health workforce; health information; service delivery; medical products, vaccines, and technologies; health system financing; and leadership and governance—as a framework with which to examine the key elements that interact with supportive supervision. We aim to demonstrate that (i) supportive supervision in primary healthcare programs exemplifies key aspects of systems thinking and (ii) the implementation of supportive supervision, in turn, benefits from a systems-thinking approach.

Human Resources for Health and Supportive Supervision

Estimates suggest that the projected demand for health workers will rise to 45 million by 2030. If current trends continue, this represents a deficit of 14.5 million health workers by 2030 globally, with a 3.7 million deficit in sub-Saharan Africa (World Health Organization & Global Health Workforce Alliance, 2014; World Health Organization, 2016). Indeed, the vast majority of the deficit will predominantly be felt in low- and middle-income countries where the need and burden of disease is arguably greatest. Retaining existing CHWs in their current posts is therefore paramount to ensure that they continue to serve their communities in the face of the global deficit of health workers. Supportive supervision, as a key determinant of CHW performance and retention, is therefore an important strategy to ensure the delivery of essential services. Specifically, by providing a structure for recognition, feedback, and problem-solving (Jaskiewicz & Tulenko, 2012), supportive supervision represents a system-level response to the need to identify what motivates individual CHWs in the context of their community.

Unfortunately, many CHW programs face high rates of staff turnover. Driven by the complex interaction of multiple and varying individual, organizational, and socio-economic factors, attrition poses a consistent threat to primary healthcare service delivery. These factors include the absence of remuneration or poor remuneration, high opportunity costs for CHWs, insufficient resources (including essential medicines, equipment, and transport), loss of motivation, inadequate community recognition, and lack of refresher training and career development opportunities (Rahman et al., 2010; Abbey et al., 2014). Although supportive supervision cannot address structural barriers such as chronic underfunding and lack of essential resources, implementing supportive supervision constitutes a sustainable use of existing resources which can act as a leverage point to help to address retention.

Research has demonstrated that supportive supervision is associated with improvements in motivation, work engagement, job satisfaction, performance, and creating a sense of community and organizational commitment (Kok et al., 2014). In this way, supportive supervisors promote the use of a systems-thinking approach, by identifying patterns of behavior rather than incidents, and viewing causality as an ongoing process (Richmond, 2010). The emphasis in supportive supervision on strengthening relationships also correlates with the concept in systems thinking that in order to understand a complex problem you must understand the relationships that underlie it (Richmond, 2010). Indeed, research suggests that while regular interactions between supervisors and CHWs are important, it is the approach to supervision experienced or perceived by the CHW that determines important indicators of retention (Vallières et al., 2018). Similarly, health workers in Ghana who felt supported by their manager were significantly more productive in comparison to those who had not been supervised, as well as to those who had been supervised but did not feel supported (Frimpong et al., 2011). Likewise, a review of twenty-two CHW impact papers suggests that improving supervision quality has a greater impact than increasing the frequency of supervision alone (Hill et al., 2014). As such, supportive supervision, which emphasizes identifying the individual needs of CHWs through respectful engagement, in addition to regular contact, may help mitigate the high turnover rates of CHWs. This would make important contributions to maintaining the current global workforce of CHWs, which is crucial in the face of the growing global deficit in human resources for health.

Health Information and Supportive Supervision

Supervisors often personify the health system for CHWs, acting as their primary and sometimes exclusive link with information channeled through the formal health system. Crucially, it can facilitate the transfer of accurate and timely health information. Trust and openness in the supervisory relationship could also lead CHWs to feel more comfortable passing on accurate health information. Moreover, because supportive supervision focuses on fostering relationships that can strengthen CHWs' skills and performance, supportive supervision represents an important strategy to strengthen communication between communities, CHWs, and the wider health system (Jaskiewicz & Tulenko, 2012). Indeed CHWs, who are themselves community members, have been shown to be effective conduits of behavior change and health messaging, as evidenced by reductions in delays in treatment-seeking behaviors and increased uptake of services offered within health facilities (i.e., maternal and child health services, immunization, and voluntary counselling and testing for human immunodeficiency virus (HIV)) (Gilmore & McAuliffe, 2013). In addition, CHWs have been shown to play a key role in rapidly relaying urgent and important health messaging, rectifying dangerous health myths, and helping to curb the spread of disease in emergency settings, including the 2014–2015 Ebola outbreak in West Africa (Miller et al., 2018) and more recently, in the COVID-19 pandemic (Bhaumik, Moola, Tyagi, Nambiar, & Kakoti, 2020). Finally, CHWs can act as an important source of health information gathering, including through regular household surveys and adequately maintained community health and activity records. CHWs are a particularly valuable source of reliable health information among those households who are least likely to access health centers, where health information is most commonly gathered. By engaging in respectful, open dialogue and regular communication with their supervisors, CHWs may internalize such approaches to communication and take the same approach as they engage with their communities.

Supportive supervision, which emphasizes the importance of joint problem identification, can also make use of such health information to promote joint problem-solving. Joint problem-solving approaches are considered particularly important in contexts where there are two parallel, sometimes competing, health systems: traditional health systems and formal health systems. Traditional health systems comprise influential cadres such as traditional birth attendants and traditional healers, whom CHWs know and encounter regularly in their community. Formal health systems comprise cadres such as nurses, physicians, and pharmacists. Supportive supervision represents an important opportunity to build trust across the two systems, whereby CHWs act as a bridge between both health systems.

CHWs have also benefited from advancements in mobile health (mHealth) technologies, such as CommCare. Such programs leverage mobile phones to facilitate regular monitoring of community health data, communication between CHWs and their supervisors, and follow-up with households in need of regular care (i.e., in cases of pregnancy or acute child malnutrition). Such technological solutions also have potential to enable the scaling up of training and supportive supervision for CHWs. For example, evidence from a randomized controlled trial in Pakistan that investigated the impact of the "Technology-Assisted Cascaded Training and Supervision system" (TACTS) (Rahman et al., 2019) on the competence of CHWs in delivering the "Thinking Healthy" psychological program found that TACTS produced results that were equally as effective as when CHWs were trained and supervised face-to-face by a specialist. The TACTS model uses a training application that can be downloaded to a phone and includes interactive activities and videos of role plays and examples. Supportive supervision is then provided remotely by a non-specialist trainer, who in turn has been trained by a master trainer. This type of approach demonstrates how systems thinking can be applied to improve supervision practice, with limited personnel, training, and technology-assisted knowledge-transfer between professionals ensures an efficient use of resources and time.

Technology can also be used to complement face-to-face supervision. For example, a randomized controlled trial conducted in Mali (Whidden et al., 2018) showed that using a personalized feedback dashboard within sessions enhanced the performance of CHWs. The personalized dashboard assisted supervisors in providing supervisees with specific and meaningful feedback and allowed the accurate tracking of supervisees' progress over time.

Service Delivery and Supportive Supervision

Effective implementation of supportive supervision has potential to improve the quality of a range of services within a health system (Marquez & Kean, 2002). For example, a cluster randomized trial in Kyrgyzstan found that implementation of supportive supervision within a hospital setting significantly improved the quality of pediatric care and enhanced practitioners' adherence to WHO guidelines (Lazzerini et al., 2017). Similarly, a randomized field trial from Georgia demonstrated an improvement in immunization program indicators associated with the implementation of a supportive supervision approach (Djibuti et al., 2009). The shift in supportive supervision from a controlling dynamic toward a respectful and trusting supervisory relationship is thus critical to ensuring effective service delivery. Indeed, a systematic review by Bailey et al. (2016) demonstrated that a trusting supervisory relationship is fundamental to the effectiveness of supportive supervision in improving quality of care in CHW programs. This is particularly important for CHWs, who often work in isolated and remote areas.

A major challenge in global health has been the replication and expansion of interventions found to be effective in specific settings. While supportive supervision has been found to increase CHWs' motivation and performance effectively in some settings, as it is implemented more widely the complex realities of target contexts must be understood. Therefore, a systems-thinking approach is highly suitable to scaling up supportive supervision in a way that ensures it is implemented in a contextually appropriate manner.

Medical Products, Vaccines, Technologies, and Supportive Supervision

Supervisors play a key role in ensuring that CHWs have consistent stocks of medical products and technologies. For example, supply chains for community case management programs, which employ a quality improvement approach to strengthening supply chain practices and supporting standardized resupply procedures, are heavily reliant on CHWs and supportive supervision systems. In particular, in these programs supportive supervision allows CHWs to identify gaps in product resupply procedures, identify root causes of supply chain bottlenecks, and ensure that stock cards reflect accurate required quantities. Supervisors also train and support CHWs in administering medical products and technologies and provide oversight regarding their safe use. As such, supportive supervision is integral to ensuring that communities have access to safe and effective medications, vaccines, and medical technologies.

Health System Financing and Supportive Supervision

Supportive supervision programs provide a crucial link between CHWs and the wider health system. As previously mentioned under the health information building block, this creates potential for consistent upward flow of information regarding the on-the-ground needs of the population. This, in turn, and in the presence of strong leadership, can help ensure that health financing is more responsive to contextual realities and can allow resources to be redirected to those most in need.

Additionally, donors are increasingly acknowledging the importance of supportive supervision as a key component of CHW training, now viewing supervision as a crucial element of sustaining the effects of training into the longer term (Perera et al., 2021). Supervision is necessary to enable skill building following knowledge acquisition during training, and it is therefore vital that it is reflected accordingly in budgets. By building capacity in this way, supervision acts as a crucial leverage point that can increase long-term capacity and thus enhance health service sustainability within communities and the wider health system.

However, lack of resources is a major barrier to the implementation of supportive supervision of CHWs (e.g., Ndima et al., 2015). Consistent with a systems-thinking perspective, it is important not to place the sole burden of responsibility for implementing supportive supervision practice on supervisors alone. Supervisors require training in supportive supervision practice, and there are certain resources—such as having designated time and space for supervision—that are prerequisites to its implementation. The responsibility for creating these conditions depends on levels of the health system that are higher than individual supervisors. Similarly, although supportive supervision addresses some barriers to staff motivation and well-being, there are other barriers relating to rôle satisfaction that are even more directly related to financing, such as appropriate remuneration and timeliness of salary payments (Renggli et al., 2019). These factors should be addressed alongside supportive supervision implementation as part of a holistic approach to staff well-being and retention in community health programming.

Leadership and Governance and Supportive Supervision

The governance of CHW programs has been a challenge in many countries, as evidenced by low levels of institutional commitment in terms of both structural support and resources (Crigler et al., 2013), despite commitments to supportive supervision in policy documents. In order for supportive supervision to be effectively translated from policy into practice, leadership and governance are essential.

Leadership in particular plays a pivotal role in the application of systems thinking (Best & Holmes, 2010). In order for CHWs to contribute meaningfully to universal health coverage through the delivery of primary healthcare at scale, CHW programs require strong national and/or district-level leadership. This is particularly important because leadership plays a pivotal role in establishing the structures of CHW programs, including the architecture of programs, relationships between key actors, and ownership of decision-making (Lewin & Lehmann, 2014). Ensuring that supportive supervision is embedded within CHW program architecture and, where applicable, situated within national frameworks and policies, is thus key to ensuring that supervisors are adequately trained in supportive approaches and are given both the time and the resources (both financial and physical) required to carry out supportive supervision. This, however, requires that leaders build collective visions and mobilize commitment across multiple stakeholders (Schneider & Nxumalo, 2017), including CHWs, community leaders, health workers, district health management teams, and national-level government officials. Moreover, research on supportive supervision for CHWs has shown that supervisors' ability to effectively carry out their role is enhanced by being supported themselves (Daniels, Nor, Jackson, Ekström, & Doherty, 2010), evidencing the importance of collaborative leadership at every level of a health system.

Transformational leadership in particular has been identified as having high potential to lead to change in complex health systems (Swanson et al., 2012). Transformational leadership, which emphasizes collaborative engagement toward a shared vision of efficiency and equity in health systems (Swanson et al., 2012), parallels the focus in supportive supervision on two-way communication and joint problem-solving. Consistent with a shift away from more traditional approaches to supervision toward more supportive approaches, Best and Holmes have also noted that systems thinking requires collaborative leadership, which they define as "a shift in leadership style from "command and control" leading and managing to facilitating and empowering, from delegation to participation" (Best & Holmes, 2010: 152). Supportive supervision empowers supervisors to demonstrate both transformational and collaborative leadership.

The Role of Supportive Supervision for Community Health Workers in the Context of COVID-19

CHWs have potential to play a crucial role in managing and suppressing the community spread of coronavirus SARS-CoV-2 (Palafox et al., 2020). Knowledge of their communities, access to vulnerable groups, and experience in responding to public health initiatives and emergencies place CHWs in a unique outreach position, provided they receive adequate training, resources, and supportive supervision (Barnard, 2020; Ballard et al., 2020). As mentioned earlier, supervisors have a central role in ensuring that CHWs are optimally resourced, however supervisors in turn need health system support to work effectively. In the context of COVID-19, health systems need to facilitate additional training in pandemic response measures and provide resources for increased supportive supervision where necessary (Palafox et al., 2020). Lessons learned from other pandemics and public health crises indicate that CHWs experience psychosocial stress including isolation, social stigma, and burnout (Deng & Naslund, 2020). CHWs are vulnerable to the same challenges in the current pandemic. As frontline workers, they are also a high-risk population for contracting COVID-19 and access to adequate personal protective equipment is essential (Bhaumik et al., 2020).

Health workers the world over are facing unprecedented pressure in the context of COVID-19 and demands on the health workforce will increase as vaccines against COVID-19 are rolled out globally. Supportive supervision has enormous potential to engage and empower an increasingly overburdened and exhausted health workforce. As a result, the implementation of supportive supervision for CHWs is more urgent than ever. COVID-19 is unequivocally a complex problem, and systems thinking demonstrates that in order to address complex problems effectively, related contextual factors and their interactions must be examined. As we have demonstrated, supervision is a crucial aspect of healthcare provision, and therefore it ought to be a key priority in community health worker programs to safeguard the health and well-being of CHWs, if the COVID-19 pandemic is to be effectively addressed.

Conclusion

The WHO has noted that communication, sharing, and problem-solving between health system actors are integral to systems thinking in health system strengthening (de Savigny & Adam, 2009). The structures of supportive supervision—characterized by joint problem-solving, mentoring, and constructive feedback—represent a common framework in which CHWs and supervisors work together toward the shared goal of expanding universal access to essential health services. With consistent calls for more research on supportive supervision in CHW programs (Marquez & Kean, 2002; Rohde, 2006; Rowe et al., 2010; Hill et al., 2014; Bailey et al., 2016) and the expansion of CHW programs throughout the world, CHW programs would benefit from taking a systems-thinking approach to understanding the complex problem of implementing supportive supervision. There are a number of ways in which this could happen. Supervisors could be trained in how to address the supervision needs of CHWs by focusing on patterns of behavior over time. This could involve problem-solving through the identification of opportunities for improving the structure of the health system. For instance, if supervisors were to view CHWs' behavior as a consequence of their environment over time, they could consequentially see that an individual CHW who lacked motivation does not operate in a vacuum. Additionally, training could encourage supervisors to identify systemic factors that might be contributing to a CHW's lack of motivation so that these factors could be addressed in a cohesive way.

By analyzing supportive supervision through the lens of WHO's health system building blocks, we have demonstrated the key role that supportive supervision can play in ensuring high-quality care and service delivery in CHW programs. In doing so, we have also shown that supportive supervision systems in primary healthcare programs exemplify key aspects of systems thinking, and, in turn, that the implementation of supportive supervision for CHWs would benefit from a systems-thinking approach. Doing so has the potential to increase motivation, engagement, and performance among CHWs, thereby allowing CHWs to reach their potential and thrive in their efforts to improve the health of their communities.

References

Abbey, M., Bartholomew, L. K., Nonvignon, J., Chinbuah, M. A., Pappoe, M., Gyapong, M., ... van den Borne, B. (2014). Factors related to retention of community health workers in a trial on community-based management of fever in children under 5 years in the Dangme West District of Ghana. *International Health, 6*(2), 99–105. doi:10.1093/inthealth/ihu007

Bailey, C., Blake, C., Schriver, M., Cubaka, V. K., Thomas, T., & Hilber, A. M. (2016). A systematic review of supportive supervision as a strategy to improve primary healthcare services in Sub-Saharan Africa. *International Journal of Gynecology and Obstetrics, 132*(1), 117–125.

Ballard, M., Bancroft, E., Nesbit, J., Johnson, A., Holeman, I., Foth, J., ... Palazuelos, D. (2020). Prioritising the role of community health workers in the COVID-19 response. *BMJ Global Health, 5*(6), 1–7. doi:10.1136/bmjgh-2020-002550

Barnard, H. (2020). Another pandemic in Africa: Weak healthcare, strong leadership, and collective action in Africa's COVID-19 response. *Management and Organization Review, 16*(4), 753–759. doi:10.1017/mor.2020.47

Best, A., & Holmes, B. (2010). Systems thinking, knowledge and action: Towards better models and methods. *Evidence & Policy: A Journal of Research, Debate and Practice, 6*(2), 145–159.

Bhaumik, S., Moola, S., Tyagi, J., Nambiar, D., & Kakoti, M. (2020). Community health workers for pandemic response: A rapid evidence synthesis. *BMJ Global Health, 5*(6), e002769. Retrieved from https://doi.org/10.1136/bmjgh-2020-002769

Bradley, S., Kamwendo, F., Masanja, H., de Pinho, H., Waxman, R., Boostrom, C., & McAuliffe, E. (2013). District health managers' perceptions of supervision in Malawi and Tanzania. *Human Resources for Health, 11*(43).

Chen, L., Evans, D., Evans, T., Sadana, R., Stilwell, B., Travis, P. L., & World Health Organization. (2006). *Working together for health—The world health report 2006*. Geneva: World Health Organization. Accessed from: https://apps.who.int/iris/handle/10665/43432

Clements, C. J., Streefland, P., & Malau, C. (2007). Supervision in primary health care—Can it be carried out effectively in developing countries? *Current Drug Safety, 2*(1), 19–23.

Crigler, L., Gergen, J., & Perry, H. (2013). *Supervision of community health workers*. Washington, DC: United States Agency for International Development.

Daniels, K., Nor, B., Jackson, D., Ekstrom, E. C., & Doherty, T. (2010). Supervision of community peer counsellors for infant feeding in South Africa: An exploratory qualitative study. *Human Resources for Health, 8*(6).

de Savigny, D., & Adam, T. (2009). *Systems thinking for health systems strengthening*. Geneva: World Health Organization Alliance for Health Policy and Systems Research.

Deng, D., & Naslund, J.A. (2020). Psychological impact of COVID-19 pandemic on frontline health workers in low- and middle-income countries. *Harvard Public Health Review, 28*, 1–18. Retrieved from https://www.ncbi.nlm.nih.gov/pmc/articles/PMC7785092/pdf/nihms-1639166.pdf

Devgan, A. V. (1990). Supportive supervision. *The Nursing Journal of India, 81*(11), 351–352.

Djibuti, M., Gotsadze, G., Zoidze, A., Mataradze, G., Esmail, L. C., & Kohler, J. C. (2009). The role of supportive supervision on immunization program outcome—A randomized field trial from Georgia. *BMC International Health and Human Rights, 9*(S1), S11.

The Earth Institute Columbia University. (2011). *One million community health workers*. New York, NY: Columbia University.

Fatti, G., Rundare, A., Pududu, B., Mothibi, E., Jason, A., Shaikh, N., Robinson, P., Eley, B., Jackson, D., & Grimwood, A. (2013). An innovative approach to improve the quality of prevention of mother-to-child transmission of HIV programs through nurse clinical mentoring in South Africa. *Journal of Acquired Immune Deficiency Syndromes, 63*(2), 76–78.

Frimpong, J. A., Helleringer, S., Awoonor Williams, J. K., Yeji, F., & Phillips, J. F. (2011). Does supervision improve health worker productivity? Evidence from the Upper East Region of Ghana. *Tropical Medicine & International Health, 16*(10), 1225–1233.

Gilmore, B., McAuliffe, E. (2013). Effectiveness of community health workers delivering preventive interventions for maternal and child health in low- and middle-income countries: A systematic review. *BMC Public Health 13*, 847. Retrieved from https://doi.org/10.1186/1471-2458-13-847.

Greenspan, J. A., McMahon, S. A., Chebet, J. J., Mpunga, M., Urassa, D. P., & Winch, P. J. (2013). Sources of community health worker motivation: A qualitative study in Morogoro Region, Tanzania. *Human Resources for Health, 11*(52).

Hill, Z., Dumbaugh, M., Benton, L., Källander, K., Strachan, D., ten Asbroek, A., Tibenderana, J., Kirkwood, B., & Meek, S. (2014). Supervising community health workers in low-income countries—A review of impact and implementation issues. *Global Health Action, 7*(24085).

Jaskiewicz, W., & Tulenko, K. (2012). Increasing community health worker productivity and effectiveness: A review of the influence of the work environment. *Human Resources for Health, 10*(38), 1–15.

Kilminster, S. M., & Jolly, B. C. (2000). Effective supervision in clinical practice settings: A literature review. *Medical Education, 34*(10), 827–840.

Kok, M. C., Dieleman, M., Taegtmeyer, M., Broerse, J. E., Kane, S. S., Ormel, H., ... de Koning, K. A. (2015). Which intervention design factors influence performance of community health workers in low- and middle-income countries? A systematic review. *Health Policy and planning, 30*(9), 1207–1227. https://doi.org/10.1093/heapol/czu126

Lazzerini, M., Shukurova, V., Davletbaeva, M., Monolbaev, K., Kulichenko, T., Akoev, Y., ... & Boronbayeva, E. (2017). Improving the quality of hospital care for children by supportive supervision: A cluster randomized trial, Kyrgyzstan. *Bulletin of the World Health Organization, 95*(6), 397–407. https://doi.org/10.2471/BLT.16.176982

Lewin, S., & Lehmann, U. (2014). *Governing large-scale community health worker programs* (H. Perry, L. Crigler, & S. Hodgins Eds.). Baltimore. MD: USAID.

Marquez, L., & Kean, L. (2002). *Making supervision supportive and sustainable: new approaches to old problems*. Maximizing Access and Quality, Management Sciences for Health. Available from: https://usaidassist.org/sites/assist/files/maqno4final.pdf

McGregor, D. M. (1989). The human side of enterprise. In H. J. Leavitt, L. R. Pondy, & D. M. Boje (Eds.), *Readings in managerial psychology* (pp. 314–324). Chicago, IL: University of Chicago Press.

Miller, N. P., Milsom, P., Johnson, G., Bedford, J., Kapeu, A. S., Diallo, A. O., ... Papowitz, H. (2018). Community health workers during the Ebola outbreak in Guinea, Liberia, and Sierra Leone. *Journal of Global Health, 8*(2), 020601. https://doi.org/10.7189/jogh-08-020601

Mubyazi, G. M., Bloch, P., Byskov, J., Magnussen, P., Bygbjerg, I. C., & Hansen, K. S. (2012). Supply-related drivers of staff motivation for providing intermittent preventive treatment of malaria during pregnancy in Tanzania: Evidence from two rural districts. *Malaria Journal, 11*(48).

Ndima, S. D., Sidat, M., Give, C., Ormel, H., Kok, M. C., & Taegtmeyer, M. (2015). Supervision of community health workers in Mozambique: A qualitative study of factors influencing motivation and programme implementation. *Human Resources for Health, 13*(63). https://doi.org/10.1186/s12960-015-0063-x

Palafox, B., Renedo, A., Lasco, G., Palileo-Villanueva, L., Balabanova, D., & McKee, M. (2021). Maintaining population health in low- and middle-income countries during the COVID-19 pandemic: Why we should be investing in Community Health Workers. *Tropical Medicine and International Health, 26*(1), 20–22. doi:10.1111/tmi.13498. Epub 2020 Oct 12. PMID: 32985024; PMCID: PMC7537160.

Perera, C., McBride, K., Travers, Á., Tingsted Blum, P., Wiedemann, N., Dinesen, C., Bitanihirwe, B & Vallières, F. (2021). Towards an integrated model for supervision for mental health and psychosocial support in humanitarian emergencies: A qualitative study of practitioners' perspectives. *PLOS One*, *16*(10), e0256077. https://doi.org/10.1371/journal.pone.0256077

Peters, D. H. (2014). The application of systems thinking in health: Why use systems thinking? *Health Research Policy and Systems*, *12*(51). https://doi.org/10.1186/1478-4505-12-51

Rahman, A., Akhtar, P., Hamdani, S. U., Atif, N., Nazir, H., Uddin, I., … & Zafar, S. (2019). Using technology to scale-up training and supervision of community health workers in the psychosocial management of perinatal depression: A non-inferiority, randomized controlled trial. *Global Mental Health*, *6*, e8. doi:10.1017/gmh.2019.7. PMID: 31157115; PMCID: PMC6533850.

Rahman, S. M., Ali, N. A., Jennings, L., Seraji, M. H. R., Mannan, I., Shah, R., … Winch, P. J. (2010). Factors affecting recruitment and retention of community health workers in a newborn care intervention in Bangladesh. *Human Resources for Health*, *8*, 12. https://doi.org/10.1186/1478-4491-8-12

Renggli, S., Mayumana, I., Mboya, D., Charles, C., Mshana, C., Kessy, F., … & Pfeiffer, C. (2019). Towards improved health service quality in Tanzania: Contribution of a supportive supervision approach to increased quality of primary healthcare. *BMC Health Services Research*, *19*(1), 848. https://doi.org/10.1186/s12913-019-4648-2

Richmond, B. (2010). *The "thinking" in systems thinking: Seven essential skills.* In P. Communications (Ed.). https://thesystemsthinker.com/the-thinking-in-systems-thinking-how-can-we-make-it-easier-to-master/

Rohde, J. (2006). *Supportive supervision to improve integrated primary health care.* Cambridge, MA: Management Sciences for Health.

Rowe, A. K., Onikpo, F., Lama, M., & Deming, M. S. (2010). The rise and fall of supervision in a project designed to strengthen supervision of integrated management of childhood illness in Benin. *Health Policy and Planning*, *25*(2), 125–134.

Schneider, H., & Nxumalo, N. (2017). Leadership and governance of community health worker programmes at scale: A cross case analysis of provincial implementation in South Africa. *International Journal for Equity in Health*, *16*(1), 72. https://doi.org/10.1186/s12939-017-0565-3

Singh, P., & Sachs, J. D. (2013). 1 million community health workers in sub-Saharan Africa by 2015. *The Lancet*, *382*(9889), 363–365.

Strachan, D. L., Källander, K., ten Asbroek, A. H. A., Kirkwood, B., Meek, S. R., Benton, L., Conteh, L., Tibenderana, J., & Hill, Z. (2012). Interventions to improve motivation and retention of community health workers delivering integrated community case management (iCCM): Stakeholder perceptions and priorities. *The American Journal of Tropical Medicine and Hygiene*, *87*(5), 111–119.

Suh, S., Moreira, P., & Ly, M. (2007). Improving quality of reproductive health care in Senegal through formative supervision: Results from four districts. *Human Resources for Health*, *5*(26). https://doi.org/10.1186/1478-4491-5-26

Swanson, R. C., Cattaneo, A., Bradley, E., Chunharas, S., Atun, R., Abbas, K. M., Katsaliaki, K., Mustafee, N., Mason Meier, B., & Best, A. (2012). Rethinking health systems strengthening: Key systems thinking tools and strategies for transformational change. *Health Policy and Planning*, *27*(4), 54–61.

United Nations. (2015). *Transforming our world: The 2030 agenda for sustainable development.* New York, NY: United Nations.

United Nations Committee on Economic, Social and Cultural Rights (2000). *CESCR general comment no. 14: The right to the highest attainable standard of health (Art. 12).* Retrieved from https://www.refworld.org/pdfid/4538838d0.pdf.

Uys, L. R., Minnaar, A., Reid, S., & Naidoo JR. (2004). The perceptions of nurses in a district health system in KwaZulu-Natal of their supervision, self-esteem and job satisfaction. *Curationis, 27*(2), 50–56.

Vallières, F., Hyland, P., McAuliffe, E., Mahmud, I., Tulloch, O., Walker, P., & Taegtmeyer, M. (2018). A new tool to measure approaches to supervision from the perspective of community health workers: A prospective, longitudinal, validation study in seven countries. *BMC Health Services Research, 18*(1). doi:10.1186/s12913-018-3595-7

Vaughan, K., Kok, M.C., Witter, S., & Dieleman, M. (2015). Costs and cost-effectiveness of community health workers: Evidence from a literature review. *Human Resources for Health, 13*(71). doi:10.1186/s12960-015-0070-y. PMID: 26329455; PMCID: PMC4557864.

Whidden, C., Kayentao, K., Liu, J. X., Lee, S., Keita, Y., Diakité, D., ... & Holeman, I. (2018). Improving community health worker performance by using a personalised feedback dashboard for supervision: A randomised controlled trial. *Journal of Global Health, 8*(2), 020418. https://doi.org/10.7189/jogh.08.020418

World Health Organization, President's Emergency Plan for AIDS Relief, & Joint United Nations Programme on HIV and AIDS. (2007) . *Task shifting: Rational redistribution of tasks among health workforce teams: Global recommendations and guidelines*. Geneva: World Health Organization. https://apps.who.int/iris/handle/10665/43821

World Health Organization & Global Health Workforce Alliance. (2014). *A universal truth: No health without a workforce*. Geneva: World Health Organization. Retrieved from https://www.who.int/workforcealliance/knowledge/resources/hrhreport2013/en/

World Health Organization. (2016). *Global strategy on human resources for health workforce 2030*. Geneva: World Health Organization.

5

Applying Systems Thinking to Understand the Process of Decentralization

A Malawi Case Example

Kingsley Rex Chikaphupha, Thomasena O'Byrne, Linda Nyondo-Mipando, Isabel Kazanga Chiumia, Mairéad Finn, and Frédérique Vallières

What is Decentralization?

The decentralization of health systems "involves moving decision-making away from centralized control and closer to the users of health services . . . as a means to improve their responsiveness and performance (World Health Organization, 2007). Muñoz et al. (2017) have also defined decentralization as "the transfer of some managerial, technical or fiscal responsibilities from the central level to the periphery" (2017: 2). There are different forms of decentralization: devolution, where power is devolved from the central to the local level; deconcentration, where power is dispersed to lower levels within a national ministry structure only; and delegation or the dispersal of power to semi-autonomous bodies, such as hospital boards (Kolehmainen-Aitken, 2004). Globally, literature has demonstrated both positive changes and negative effects of decentralization (Liwanag & Wyss, 2018; Abimbola, Baatiema, & Bigdeli, 2019).

In the 1990s, the Malawi Department of Local Government embarked on a process of devolution (Kutengule, Kampanje, Chiweza, & Chunga, 2014), whereby administration and political authority was transferred to district and local levels (Chiweza, 2018). The process of decentralization therefore involves attempting to harmonize all components within a system—in this case, the Malawian health system. The World Health Organization's (WHO) health system building blocks therefore serve as a useful framework to facilitate insight into what has worked well and where progress remains to be achieved. In light of this, this chapter applies a systems-thinking lens as a useful tool to improve understanding of and describe the successes and challenges of this devolution process in Malawi.

Decentralization in Malawi

Malawi is a small, landlocked country in south-eastern Africa, with an estimated population of 17.5 million (National Statistics Office, 2018). The country's health system is four-tiered, consisting of community, primary, secondary, and tertiary levels. These levels have various health workforce requirements according to size, distribution, and

Kingsley Rex Chikaphupha, Thomasena O'Byrne, Linda Nyondo-Mipando, Isabel Kazanga Chiumia, Mairéad Finn, and Frédérique Vallières, *Applying Systems Thinking to Understand the Process of Decentralization* In: *Systems Thinking for Global Health.* Edited by: Fiona Larkan, Frédérique Vallières, Hasheem Mannan, and Naonori Kodate, Oxford University Press. DOI: 10.1093/oso/9780198799498.003.0005

skill mix (Zere, Moeti, Kirigia, Mwase, & Kataika, 2007) and are connected through an established referral system (Ministry of Health, 2018a). Malawi has made significant progress in improving health outcomes over the last decade yet the country's burden of disease is still high (World Bank, 2018). Non-communicable diseases are the second leading cause of death in adults in the country (Ministry of Health, 2017a). The burden is also especially high for HIV/AIDS, malaria, respiratory tract infections, perinatal conditions, and diarrheal diseases (Ministry of Health, 2017a).

A new constitution, adopted in 1994, guided government to embark on a comprehensive review of the local government system (Chiweza, 2018), leading to the enactment of both a new Local Government Act and a Decentralization Policy (Dulani, 2004). The reforms were complemented by a National Decentralization Program to mobilize resources and guide implementation in 2000. The Ministry of Local Government's vision was for devolved local government with elected councilors in a dominant role. In practice however, there was a "gradual transition to devolution with a deconcentration phase first" (Government of Malawi, 2005:20), whereby members of parliament and traditional leaders played a leading role in the affairs of district councils (Government of Malawi, 2005).

The process of decentralization, however, displays numerous challenges including ambiguous roles and responsibilities, politicized decision-making, informality, and problems of accountability in the use of resources handled at the local level (Dulani, 2004; Chiweza, 2010; Tambulasi & Common, 2011; Jagero, Kwandayi, & Longwe, 2014). In Malawi, local authorities do not have "real power" to influence decision-making, adversely impacting the potential benefits of decentralization (Roman, Cleary, & McIntyre, 2017). Moreover, the implementation of the Local Government Act and National Decentralization Programme has been rather *ad hoc* (O'Neil et al., 2014), and there remains a disconnect between the formal institutions of local government("rules-on-paper") and the ones that are actually being used ("rules-in-use") (Ostrom, Gibson, Shivakumar, & Andersson, 2001). There is also reluctance by central government to cede power to local government, funding to district levels remains inadequate, there is an absence of coordination and agreement from central level, and human and technical capacity within local authorities remains a challenge (Dulani, 2004; Chiweza, 2010; Tambulasi & Common, 2011; Jagero, Kwandayi, & Longwe, 2014).

Using the health system building block of "health workforce" as an entry point, we further examine the process of decentralization in Malawi, first through health workforce and leadership and governance, and then how these have been devolved in relation to the other building blocks of service delivery, finance, information systems, and access to medicines.

(i) Human resources for health

Malawi's health workforce is governed by a Human Resources for Health (HRH) Strategic Plan 2018–2022 to address the critical shortage and human resource crisis which is characterized by a mismatch between available skills and service needs (Ministry of Health, 2018a). For example, Malawi has around 0.51 skilled health workers per 1,000 population, substantially below the minimum threshold of 4.45 skilled health workers per 1,000 population recommended by the World Health Organization (WHO) for a country to realize Universal Health Coverage (UHC) and the Sustainable Development Goals (SDGs) (Wemos Foundation, 2018).

The HRH Strategic Plan guides the health sector in effective planning, development, management, and utilization of HRH to ensure comprehensive delivery of quality, accessible, and efficient health services for the people of Malawi (Ministry of Health, 2018a). Despite numerous efforts to increase the health workforce in Malawi, the country currently employs 37,926 staff out of a total of 62,269 staff positions available across health facilities in the country (Ministry of Health, 2018a). In 2004, to address the crisis in staff shortages, Malawi launched an Emergency Human Resources Programme (EHRP) aimed at increasing staff numbers (O'Neil et al., 2010). Though initially successful in recruiting more health workers (O'Neil et al., 2010), problems such as shortage of staff persisted, and decentralization was ultimately seen as a way to resolve this crisis (O'Neil et al., 2014).

Several factors have contributed to the shortage of health workers such as insufficient funding, low production capacity of health training institutions, high attrition rates, and poor retention due to harsh working and living conditions, among others (Ministry of Health, 2018a; Wemos Foundation, 2018). Health worker shortages are also exacerbated by increased demands on service delivery, particularly in times of crisis such as the HIV/AIDS epidemic (President's Emergency Plan for AIDS Relief, 2017). Health systems are complex and although Malawi continues to experience critical health workforce shortages and resulting concerns around quality of care, the country has displayed efforts to address these shortages through policies and strategies developed with various partners (Ministry of Health, 2017b), including through its Health Sector Strategic Plan II (HSSP) 2017–2022, as well as the HRH strategy (2018–2022). One of the remaining challenges, however, is that Malawi's devolution process retains a uniform national civil service, whereby health workers are transferred to decentralized units (e.g., districts) under centrally defined civil service terms (Kolehmainen-Aitken, 2004). The central government thus still controls who is hired and the rotation of personnel such as District Health Officers and District Nursing Officers (Chiweza, 2018), resulting in a lack of consistency and continuity at local level.

Some scholars have cautioned that there is no evidence of a direct link between decentralization and more effective management of HR (Van Lerberghe, Adams, & Ferrinho, 2002). In Malawi, the majority of Hospital Administrators have no prior training in health management which limits their knowledge of the health sector (Chimwaza et al., 2014). This observation echoes findings by Van Lerberghe, Adams, and Ferrinho (2002) who also found that in many LMICs, local health managers do not have staff adequately trained in personnel administration, nor do they have simple robust systems for managing personnel affairs (Van Lerberghe, Adams, & Ferrinho, 2002). In the case of Malawi's local health managers, not having adequately trained staff can also be attributed to a lack of alignment of strategic policies—a situation whereby different policy documents from the Ministry of Health's (MoH) directorates seem not to speak one language or reinforce each other's aspirations. For example, in 2017, the MoH published the first national community health workers strategy (Ministry of Health,

2017b). In the strategy, MoH recommended recruitment of additional 7,000 health surveillance assistants (HSAs) with clear strategies and budgets outlined (Ministry of Health, 2017b). Unfortunately, this recruitment plan, present in the Community Health Strategy, is conspicuously missing in the HRH strategy (2018–2022).

(ii) Leadership and governance

Decentralization of HRH was primarily conceptualized through the building block of leadership and governance, where issues of HRH recruitment, deployment, and remuneration were envisaged to be devolved from central to local government. Albeit with persistent weaknesses, introduction of the devolution of HRH demonstrates the strategic vision, equity/fairness, efficiency, and participation as some of the key principles necessary to attain effective intersection between leadership and governance and the health workforce blocks (Kaplan, Dominis, Palen, & Quain, 2013). Consequently, decentralization in Malawi has, to date, provoked some positive changes in HRH. District councils empowered the District Commissioner to recruit, promote, and transfer staff in the primary health care level in consultation with the Director of Health and Social Services (DHSS), providing further ownership and with the potential to increase the capacity for decision-making (Mohammed, North, & Ashton, 2016).

One of the most notable changes under decentralization, however, comes from the MoH's drive to strengthen leadership and management skills of District Health Management Teams across the country, to achieve functional and effective leadership and governance structures and systems by 2022 (Government of Malawi, 2017b). Nevertheless, resistance to cede power prevails as a result of a lack of "political equality and transparency"; politics of patronage (Chinsinga, 2008; Chiweza, 2016), and politicization of positions including marginalization of key structures (Government of Malawi, 2005). This impacts on management practices and there are challenges around implementation of reforms due to inadequate human, physical, and financial resources (Chiweza, 2018), demonstrating the connection of leadership to the health workforce. Despite initiatives to strengthen management capacity there is a need for expertise and willingness from all directorates to support a clarity of roles in pushing decentralization forward (World Health Organization, 2010).

(iii) Health financing

Impact of devolution has also been registered on health system change and performance, including assessments that have illustrated positive influence on equity and efficiency in terms of financing and delivery of health services (Jeppsson & Okuonzi, 2000; Bossert & Beauvais, 2002; Bossert, Chitah, & Bowser, 2003; Bossert et al., 2003; Atkinson & Haran, 2004). To date, Other Recurrent Transaction (ORT), budgets, planning, recruitment, payroll, short-term training, and monitoring and evaluation functions have all been devolved to district councils (Ministry of Health, 2018b). Parliament allocates health funds directly to district councils, which in the long term will be able to mobilize resources and control the wage bill (Government of Malawi,

2014; O'Neil et al., 2014). One major implication of the devolution of human resources, however, has been centralization of accounting at the council secretariat (Chiweza, 2018). This centralization is also reflected in the integrated financial management information systems (IFMIS) where budgets are only disaggregated at the sector level (O'Neil et al., 2014). Thus far, the MoH has devolved more than 80% of all sector funds to districts (Tambulasi & Mlalazi, 2015). It has also devolved about 40% of its budgetary resources and staff devolution is being considered, with ongoing consultations (Tambulasi & Mlalazi, 2015). Furthermore, fiscal decentralization has been limited and local government mostly relies on ringfenced sector budgets, with few discretionary funds (Government of Malawi, 2005; O'Neil et al., 2014).

Demonstrating the links between finance, leadership and governance, and human resources, salary payments have now moved to the Ministry of Local Government and Rural Development, while the Local Government Services Commission is responsible for the recruitment and deployment of council health workers (Government of Malawi, 2018; Ministry of Health, 2018a). Overall, the devolution of payroll has been touted as a key achievement in 2016 (Chiweza, 2018), providing more accountability at district level. The empowerment of the District Commissioner to recruit, promote, and transfer staff in the primary healthcare level in consultation with the DHSS, provides further ownership and has potentially increased decision-making capacity. Nevertheless, the extent to which devolution of power translates to full autonomy in decision-making and health spending by local authorities remains to be seen in certain contexts and requires further exploration (Roman, Cleary, & McIntyre, 2017).

(iv) Information systems

The process of moving records management and disciplinary function in Malawi is still in transition (Government of Malawi, 2017a) and serves to demonstrate some of the negative evaluations of the decentralization process (Muñoz et al., 2017: 2). For example, it has been argued that due to the lack of adequate and accurate empirical data, it is difficult to reach firm conclusions on the extent to which health sector decentralization reforms shape health system changes and performance for the better (Munga, Songstad, Blystad, & Mæstad, 2009). Similarly, in Malawi, and although Human Resources Management Information System (HRMIS) is being used, only four of the nine components of the HRMIS are fully functional. These include Employee Records, Payroll, Establishment, and Terminal Benefits. HRMIS is therefore primarily being used as a payroll system, which limits its usefulness, in particular as it cannot effectively be linked to the Government's integrated financial management systems (IFMIS) (Government of Malawi, 2017a).

(v) Service delivery

Earlier sections of the chapter outlined how large demand for service delivery impacted on health workforce. Under decentralization, including the devolution of managerial powers to district health offices, the local authorities are now seen as instruments of service delivery, granting them greater control and authority over service delivery (Tambulasi & Common, 2011). However, health service delivery issues for district councils and city assemblies are not homogenous as there are wide variations in the challenges to service delivery under decentralization in Malawi (Government of Malawi, 2017a). The newly established position of DHSS, with the responsibility for managing health centers and facilities within the district and with a need for his/her own budget and vote (Government of Malawi, 2017a), therefore provides some window of hope as it is envisaged that the DHSS will have jurisdiction over the district. It is not clear, however, whether there shall be another director of health at city assembly level or whether the DHSS will suffice. In the long run, Malawi will need to come up with proper guidelines in terms of coverage of service delivery for the city/urban and rural directorates.

Considerations Going Forward within the Context of Systems Thinking

With all the above-mentioned issues, it is evident that in some cases, devolution in Malawi is a case of one step forward and two steps back. There are inconsistencies, duplications and lapses that need to be harmonized and the systems-thinking lens employed in this chapter has attempted to illustrate how the relationships existing among the building blocks of the health system can help us improve our understanding of the process of decentralization.

Decentralization is about enhancing governance, leadership, and accountability at local level. To increase efficiency and competency, all elements of the system need to be decentralized. Seeing the system as a series of inter-relationships and patterns, as conceptualized by Senge (1990) above, we have explored both successful and incomplete aspects of the process of decentralization in relation to human resources for health, leadership and governance, service delivery, health information systems, and financing. Decentralization in Malawi has, to date, provoked some positive changes, primarily under the building blocks of leadership and governance and health financing, though challenges remain, primarily in relation to the health workforce. But also, one block not covered has been access to essential medicines. There are sparse data on this, and we recommend that this block is taken into consideration in the context of understanding the processes of decentralization.

The 2030 SDGs offer inspiration for countries such as Malawi to ensure that the Agenda for Sustainable Development, and its vision to leave no-one behind is embraced and embedded within the country's policy documents and reforms. Within the context of health care, this puts people at the center of the system. Employment, decent work, and inclusive economic growth as espoused within the spirit of decentralization link to good health and well-being. If properly implemented, decentralization and HR management policies have the capacity to increase investments in human capital, leading to a healthy workforce and population (World Health Organization, 2016). The SDGs challenge government and international partners to align their programs and policy decisions with optimum health outcomes. This is coherent with systems thinking, prioritizing inter-relationships and patterns.

The health workforce gap in low-income countries is substantial, with the need to train and deploy 18 million additional health workers globally by 2030 (World Health Organization, 2016). In this context, the Malawian government needs to be cognizant that as the process of reorientation of the health workforce toward people-centered and integrated healthcare unfolds, new demands on the skills of the existing workforce will arise. It is important to note that the adoption of the National Community Health Workers Strategy in Malawi has offered a first step toward satisfactorily adapting the competencies and skills of health workers to the evolving health needs of communities and populations (Ministry of Health, 2017b). This needs to be implemented across all modes of decentralization—something that is conspicuously missing in the present context of devolution.

The uneven geographical distribution of the health workforce at national and district levels in Malawi reinforces unequal access to healthcare, and a lack of inclusiveness, restricting numbers and limiting the diversity of potential health workers (Dussault & Franceschini, 2006). This is exacerbated by complex decisions on recruitment, selection, appointment, performance assessment, subject to the influence of a central civil service agency (Government of Malawi, 2017a). Embracing an analytical approach that integrates economic growth, social equity, and sustainability in a balanced and strategic manner could assist decentralization to respond effectively to evolving health needs and changes in health labor market demands.

Conclusion

The environment in Malawi can be described as one where reforms or policies such as decentralization and human resource management are not aligned with other overarching policies and national planning systems such as the Malawi Growth Development Strategy. The core purpose of the Development Strategy is to achieve "sustainable poverty reduction through socio-economic and political empowerment of the poor," with good governance at the pinnacle of its implementation (Government of Malawi, 2017c). Connecting decentralization and the health systems building blocks to this structure, as systems thinking conceptualizes, would mean that the strengths of each framework could be integrated.

The extent to which systems thinking can contribute to solving some of the key issues raised in this chapter is very much dependent on the context. Progress on decentralization in Malawi has been greater in some areas than others. Thus, a well-coordinated plan and a realistic application of a systems-thinking approach is imperative to avoid the risk of conflict in situations where decentralization calls for a design of new organizational structures for health service delivery in the country (Kolehmainen-Aitken, 2004).

References

Abimbola, S., Baatiema, L., & Bigdeli, M. (2019). The impacts of decentralization on health system equity, efficiency and resilience: A realist synthesis of the evidence. *Health Policy and Planning, 34*(8), 605–617.

Atkinson, S., & Haran, D. (2004). Back to basics: Does decentralization improve health system performance? Evidence from Ceará in north-east Brazil. *Bulletin of the World Health Organization, 82*, 822–827.

Bossert, T. J., & Beauvais, J. C. (2002). Decentralization of health systems in Ghana, Zambia, Uganda and the Philippines: A comparative analysis of decision space. *Health Policy and Planning, 17*(1), 14–31.

Bossert, T., Chitah, M. B., & Bowser, D. (2003). Decentralization in Zambia: Resource allocation and district performance. *Health Policy and Planning, 18*(4), 357–369.

Bossert, T. J., Larranaga, O., Giedion, U., Arbelaez, J. J., & Bowser, D. M. (2003). Decentralization and equity of resource allocation: Evidence from Colombia and Chile. *Bulletin of the World Health Organization, 81*, 95–100.

Chimwaza, W., Chipeta, E., Ngwira, A., Kamwendo, F., Taulo, F., Bradley, S., & McAuliffe, E. (2014). What makes staff consider leaving the health service in Malawi? *Human Resources for Health, 12*(1), 17. https://doi.org/10.1186/1478-4491-12-17

Chinsinga, B. (2008). Decentralization in Malawi. Acritical appraisal. *In Decentralization in Africa, a pathway out of poverty and conflict?* (pp 73–106). Amsterdam University Press.

Chiweza, A. L. (2010). A review of the Malawi decentralisation process: Lessons from selected districts. Joint Study. Lilongwe: Ministry of Local Governance and Rural Development and Concern Universal.

Chiweza, A. L. (2016). The political economy of fiscal decentralisation: Implications on local governance and public service delivery. In *Political Transition and Inclusive Development in Malawi* (pp. 95–111). Routledge.

Chiweza, A. L. (2018). *Decentralisation roadmap for Malawi*. Lilongwe: Malawi.

Dulani, B. (2004). *The status of decentralisation in Malawi: Report*. University of Malawi. Zomba, Malawi.

Dussault, G., & Franceschini, M. C. (2006). Not enough there, too many here: Understanding geographical imbalances in the distribution of the health workforce. *Human Resources for Health, 4*(1), 1–16.

Government of Malawi. (2005). *A strategy for capacity development for decentralization in Malawi: A report on phase one capacity assessment 2005*. Lilongwe, Malawi: Ministry of Local Government and Rural Development.

Government of Malawi. (2014). Public service reform commission: A look at the future making Malawi work transforming Malawi's public service. Government of Malawi: Lilongwe.

Government of Malawi. (2017a). Decentralisation and human resource devolution. Issues Paper. Presented at Interface Meeting on HR Devolution. Capital Hotel, Lilongwe, May 29, 2017. Government of Malawi.

Government of Malawi. (2017b). *Malawi national quality management policy for the health sector*. January 2017 Draft—v4. Lilongwe: Government of Malawi.

Government of Malawi. (2017c). *The Malawi Growth and Development Strategy (MGDS) III (2017–2022)*. Lilongwe: Government Printing Press.

Government of Malawi. (2018). *Guidelines for human resource management and development in councils*. Lilongwe, Malawi: Government of Malawi.

Jagero, N., Kwandayi, H. H., & Longwe, A. (2014). Challenges of decentralization in Malawi. *International Journal of Management Sciences, 2*(7), 315–322.

Jeppsson, A., & Okuonzi, S. A. (2000). Vertical or holistic decentralization of the health sector? Experiences from Zambia and Uganda. *The International Journal of Health Planning and Management, 15*(4), 273–289.

Kaplan, A. D., Dominis, S., Palen, J. G. H., & Quain, E. E. (2013). Human resource governance: What does governance mean for the health workforce in low- and middle-income countries? *Human Resources for Health, 11*(1), 1–12.

Kolehmainen-Aitken, R.-L. (2004). Decentralization's impact on the health workforce: Perspectives of managers, workers and national leaders. *Human Resources for Health, 2*(1), 5.

Kutengule, M., Kampanje, R., Chiweza, A., & Chunga, D. (2014). *Review of the National Decentralisation Programme II. Joint Review*. Lilongwe: Ministry of Local Government and Ministry of Rural Development.

Liwanag, H. J., & Wyss, K. (2018). What conditions enable decentralization to improve the health system? Qualitative analysis of perspectives on decision space after 25 years of devolution in the Philippines. *PLoS One, 13*(11), e0206809.

Ministry of Health. (2017a). *Malawi health sector strategic plan 2017–2022*. Lilongwe: Ministry of Health.

Ministry of Health. (2017b). *National Community Health Strategy 2017–2022: Integrating health services and engaging communities for the next generation*. Lilongwe: Ministry of Health.

Ministry of Health. (2018a). *Malawi Human Resources for Health Strategic Plan, 2018–2022*. Lilongew: Ministry of Health and Population.

Ministry of Health. (2018b). *Report on the assessment on the current state of district health system decentralisation carried out from 21st to 31st May, 2018*. Lilongwe: Ministry of Health.

Mohammed, J., North, N., & Ashton, T. (2016). Decentralisation of health services in Fiji: A decision space analysis. *International Journal of Health Policy and Management, 5*(3), 173.

Munga, M. A., Songstad, N. G., Blystad, A., & Mæstad, O. (2009). The decentralisation-centralisation dilemma: Recruitment and distribution of health workers in remote districts of Tanzania. *BMC International Health and Human Rights, 9*(1), 9.

Muñoz, D. C., Amador, P. M., Llamas, L. M., Hernandez, D. M., & Sancho, J. M. S. (2017). Decentralization of health systems in low and middle income countries: A systematic review. *International Journal of Public Health, 62*(2), 219–229.

National Statistics Office. (2018). *National Statistical Office. 2018 Malawi Population and Housing Census. Preliminary report*. NSO Zomba, Zomba, Malawi.

Ostrom, E., Gibson, C., Shivakumar, S., & Andersson, K. (2001). *Aid, incentives and sustainability: An institutional analysis of development cooperation*. Stockholm: SIDA.

O'Neil, T., Cammack, D., Kanyongolo, E., Mkandawire, M. W., Mwalyambwire, T., Welham, B., & Wild, L. (2014). *Fragmented governance and local service delivery in Malawi*. London: Overseas Development Institute.

O'Neil, M., Jarrah, Z., Nkosi, L., Collins, D., Perry, C., Jackson, J., … Mlambala, A. (2010). *Evaluation of Malawi's emergency human resources programme*.

President's Emergency Plan for AIDS Relief. (2017). *Malawi country operational plan: 2017 Strategic direction summary*. April 16, 2017. https://www.state.gov/wp-content/uploads/2019/08/Malawi-18.pdf

Roman, T. E., Cleary, S., & McIntyre, D. (2017). Exploring the functioning of decision space: A review of the available health systems literature. *International Journal of Health Policy and Management, 6*(7), 365. doi:10.15171/ijhpm.2017.26

Senge, P. M. (1990). *The Fifth Discipline: the Art and Practice of the Learning Organization*. New York: Doubleday/Currency.

Tambulasi, R. I. C., & Common, R. (2011). Policy transfer and service delivery transformation in developing countries: The case of Malawi health sector reforms. Thesis. Available from: https://www.research.manchester.ac.uk/portal/files/54507466/FULL_TEXT.PDF

Tambulasi, R., & Mlalazi, B. (2015). *Decentralisation of the health sector—Presentation to the Mid-year review MHSP-TA 27 April 2015*. Retrieved from https://www.slideshare.net/mohmalawi/mo-h-myr-2014-2015-decentralisation

Van Lerberghe, W., Adams, O., & Ferrinho, P. (2002). Human resources impact assessment. *Bulletin of The World Health Organization, 80*(7), 525–525.

Wemos Foundation. (2018). *Mind the funding gap: Who is paying the health Workers? Achieving an adequate, fair funding level for a strong health workforce in Malawi.* Country report. Retrieved from https://www.wemos.nl/en/who-is-paying-malawis-health-workers/

World Bank Group. (2018). Malawi Systematic Country Diagnostic: Breaking the Cycle of Low Growth and Slow Poverty Reduction. World Bank, Washington, DC. © World Bank. https://openknowledge.worldbank.org/handle/10986/31131 License: CC BY 3.0 IGO.

World Health Organization. (2007). *Strengthening health systems to improve health outcomes: WHO's framework for action*. Geneva: World Health Organization.

World Health Organization. (2010). *World Health Report, 2010: Health systems financing the path to universal coverage*. Geneva: World Health Organization.

World Health Organization. (2016). *Global strategy on human resource for health workforce 2030*. Geneva: World Health Organization.

Zere, E., Moeti, M., Kirigia, J., Mwase, T., & Kataika, E. (2007). Equity in health and healthcare in Malawi: Analysis of trends. *BMC Public Health, 7*(1), 78. https://doi.org/10.1186/1471-2458-7-78

6
A Systems-Thinking Approach to the Training and Supervision of Community Healthcare Workers in Kenya

Niall Winters, Anne Geniets, and Alice Lakati

Introduction

This chapter promotes a systems-based approach when considering the use of mobile technologies to enhance the supervision and training of community health workers (CHWs). Health systems strengthening is recognized as one of the best ways to bring about change in order to provide socially just (Powers & Faden, 2006) and sustainable healthcare to those in need. Technology has been positioned as a means to help achieve this change, as evidenced by the emergence of mobile health (mHealth) initiatives (Källander et al., 2013). In low- and middle-income countries (LMICs), the term "CHW" usually refers to lay people working within their own community in a health promotion, prevention and delivery capacity (Turinawe et al., 2015). However, the work they undertake is wide ranging and their exact roles, responsibilities, recruitment, remuneration, and training vary from country to country (Haines et al., 2007; Oliver, Theobald, MacPherson, McCollum, & Tolhurst, 2014; Geniets, Winters, Rega, & Mbae, 2015). What is clear is that they play a pivotal role in providing equitable health access in support of poverty alleviation among the most vulnerable and hard to reach (Gilroy & Winch, 2006).

While much worthwhile research has been undertaken in this area (Labrique et al., 2013), the role of mobile technology in supporting the training and supervision of CHWs remains dynamic and complex (Winters, Langer, & Geniets, 2018). Thus, a systems-thinking approach is beneficial. As de Savigny and Adam's (2009) report for the World Health Organization (WHO) noted, the more complex an intervention, the higher the need for systems thinking in order to achieve system-wide effects. In more detail, this report proposed a "framework of health system building blocks [that] effectively describes six sub-systems of an overall health system architecture" (p. 19). In this chapter, we focus on the interlinkages between four components of the system, information, human resources, service delivery, and medical technologies, to develop a mobile training and supervision intervention for CHWs in Kenya. We reflect on the implications of taking this approach and discuss the challenges of integrating mobile-based training and supervision across the community–formal health system divide in support of enhancing CHWs' service delivery. A systems view is particularly

Niall Winters, Anne Geniets, and Alice Lakati, *A Systems-Thinking Approach to the Training and Supervision of Community Healthcare Workers in Kenya* In: *Systems Thinking for Global Health.* Edited by: Fiona Larkan, Frédérique Vallières, Hasheem Mannan, and Naonori Kodate, Oxford University Press.
DOI: 10.1093/oso/9780198799498.003.0006

important here as we know that contextual factors can place significant constraints on health worker performance (Rowe et al., 2005).

The mCHW Project

The mobile community health worker (mCHW) project ran from 2012 to 2015 and was a collaboration between the University of Oxford, University College London, and Amref Health Africa. It was funded by The Economic and Social Research Council (ESRC) and the Department for International Development (DFID). The project aimed to advance the training and supervision of CHWs in Kenya, resulting in improved access to primary healthcare for the marginalized communities of Makueni County and the Kibera informal settlement. The project worked closely with CHWs and their supervisors to collaboratively design, develop implement and evaluate a mobile learning intervention that better connects CHWs and supervisors. The innovative nature of this intervention meant that for the first time CHWs had a mobile portfolio of their practice, easily accessible reference material on their phone and the ability to share practice-related questions and resources with their colleagues through activities which promote peer learning and reflection. Through the use of the mobile intervention, the project aimed to inform supervisors of CHWs' training needs and to provide Amref Health Africa with a better insight into the nature and frequency of their two-way interaction as well as the specifics of on-the-ground support structures needed for intervention implementation. This improved mobile-based supervision and training and linked CHWs more closely to the local primary healthcare system so they could work to improve the access of local communities to healthcare.

(i) Methodology

Project data were gathered through a series of steps. First, meetings were held with groups of five to ten CHWs at which they were invited to talk through a routine day of healthcare practice in the context of their community; these accounts were used to prompt mind-mapping activities that generated overviews of CHW providers' practice. Next, the CHWs were given disposable cameras and asked to take photos of their work and the places in which this took place. This photo elicitation exercise helped to ground the accounts of practice that CHWs gave. Additional notes and observations of community forums and monthly CHW meetings contributed to a better understanding of the relationships between the community health workers as well as their supervisors in the context of the wider community and the formal healthcare system, as well as the training needs and challenges identified by the CHWs. Based on analysis of these data, a mobile application was designed and implemented in an iterative manner with fifteen CHWs and their supervisors (known as community health extension workers (CHEWs) in Kenya). After using the application for eleven months, the CHWs were interviewed and, alongside observations of practice, an assessment of the changes in CHWs' practice and integration of the app into the formal health system was undertaken.

(ii) Ethics

This study was approved by the Ethics Committees of University College London and the University of Oxford, in line with the guidance provided by the British Educational Research Association (BERA) and of Amref Health Africa, conforming to Kenyan Ministry of Health guidelines. All participants read and signed an information sheet and a consent form.

A Systems-Thinking Approach to Mobile Application Design and Implementation

An innovative practice-based tool, termed the REFER app, was co-developed with participants (CHWs, supervisors, and community leaders). The core aim of the mobile intervention was to improve the links between CHWs and the formal health system through improvements in ongoing training and supervision. We opted for a participatory approach (Rogers, 1994) that enabled detailed investigation of CHWs' training needs, thereby attending to the process of integrating mobile-based training and supervision into community programs. Accordingly, our work seeks to move beyond the "what health workers need to know about technology" to reposition health workers as core participants in the development process. A key of their practice that CHWs wanted to address was the assessment of the stages of child development of children under five years old in their communities. To support this process, the REFER app utilized the Malawi Developmental Assessment Tool (MDAT), which was developed by the College of Medicine, Blantyre, Malawi and UK partners "for use in African settings and shows good reliability, validity, and sensitivity for identification of children with neurodisabilities" (Gladstone et al., 2010), a significantly under-research area in global health, particularly in contexts of abuse (Winters, Langer, & Geniets, 2017).

When using the REFER app on the ground, CHWs were engaged in conversation-stimulating questions between CHWs and caregivers. The caregiver is able to respond to the questions and, where possible, the child is engaged in activities to identify potential delays/advances in the child's development. At the end of each assessment, depending on its outcome, the CHW has to decide whether or not to refer the child to the nearest facility. The app generates a report from the assessment undertaken and records the CHW's referral decision, which is automatically sent to their supervisor for review and feedback. The aim was to improve the means to provide ongoing supervision to the CHWs with respect to their practice of assessing the stages of child development. Significantly, the learning design was underpinned by the Conversational Framework (Laurillard, 2002), and using this approach to learning, CHWs were positioned as producers of knowledge for the community. We argue that smartphone technology allows CHWs and their supervisors to engage mutually in learning, training, and supervision that fit with their specific needs and thus ultimately also leads to a better integration of their work with the formal health system. We now discuss this point in more detail.

(iii) A systems-thinking approach

From a systemsthinking perspective, the REFER app used to support the training and supervision of community health workers can be conceptualized through four (of the six) building blocks of the WHO's health system architecture: medical technology, information, human resources, and service delivery. In practical "on-the-ground" terms, as shown in Figure 6.1, this meant that a mobile web app (*medical technology*) was used to help CHW make—and reflect upon—decisions based on the data they collected (*information and service delivery*) when assessing children. Having these data and the decision-making choices around the information enabled supervisors to provide more supportive supervision and training (*human resources*) than they would have been able to without access to the collected data.

The interlinkages here are absolutely critical and take two forms: (i) interlinkages between the subsystems of the health system architecture, shown in light grey on the right in Figure 6.1; (ii) improved communication between CHWs (who are primarily based on the community) and their supervisors (who are primarily based at district health centres), shown in dark grey on the left in Figure 6.1. These can be summarized as follows:

- CHWs are provided with training on how to use the REFER app, including on undertaking child assessments using the MDAT.

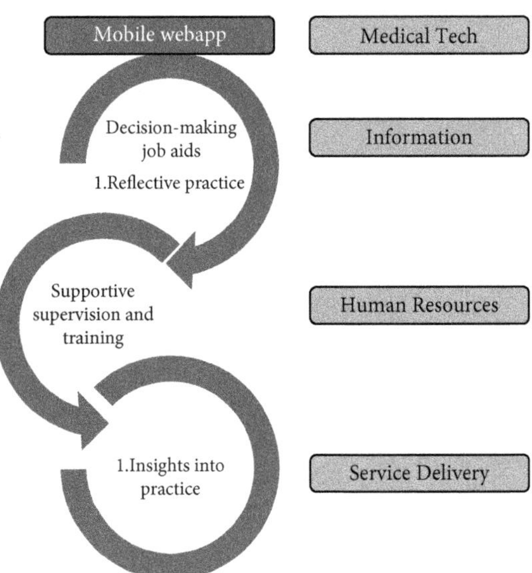

Figure 6.1 A systems-thinking approach to using mobile technologies in on-going training and supervision

- CHWs then go to their communities and assess stages of childhood development using the REFER app. The app provides decision support where necessary to the CHWs. CHW combine this with their existing knowledge to decide what to do, for example whether or not to refer a child for more specialist care. The decision-making process is recorded on the app and shared with their supervisor.
- Using the data collected related to the CHWs' decision-making process, the supervisor can provide tailored and ongoing supportive supervision either through the app, via phone, or face-to-face. Supervisors can also collectively decide, based on data analysis across the cohort of CHWs, whether further training is necessary.
- The combined approach allows supervisors to determine how well training and supervision are (or are not) having an impact on CHWs' day-to-day practice and becomes the basis for improved service delivery through better oversight via the use of mobile technology.

Findings and Discussion

(iv) What are the challenges of integrating mobile technology supported training into the community-based health system?

While there are many issues that could be addressed with respect to the integration of mobile interventions in health systems, given the focus of our mobile webapp on training and supervision, we will concentrate on this aspect of integration. Outside of a limited number of studies (Winters, Oliver, & Langer, 2017; O'Donovan et al., 2018), the ongoing supervision of CHWs' practice using mobile technologies has not been sufficiently addressed in the literature but interestingly has been shown to be very valuable in our project. In our experience, the ongoing nature of supervision helps improve the relationships between CHWs and their supervisors and thus may lead to a higher quality of CHWs' practice. As noted by a public health officer (PHO) in Nairobi, the real-time information on CHW provided by the app enables supervisors to respond directly and specifically to the challenges faced by CHWs:

> It helps me in my supervision because I can know whatever they have done, yeah? Because the system is going to give me feedback actually real-time and if they are undergoing challenges I can be able to respond in the same application on what is their next course of action. (PHO and supervisor from an informal settlement in Nairobi)

A second clear benefit for supervisors is that the information access provided by smartphones enabled them to engage in the continuous development of their expertise. This gave them extra confidence in responding to some of the new questions raised by CHWs:

> What I would say is that it has changed my life as a supervisor because even for me, if I'm asked a question, because sometimes you may not be doing everything at once, so

> when somebody calls you and challenges you with a question then it also gives you an opportunity to go search the information from the internet or possible call another senior person elsewhere, so that it has also improved my skills .... So I have to give very accurate information. I don't have to give any information because it has stuck in my mind, yeah, I have to research well, yes. (Supervisor from an informal settlement in Nairobi)

This was very interesting from an integration perspective because one of the key challenges CHWs face is the fact that their supervisors (as well as the public health officers with whom they work) are part of the formal healthcare system, while the CHWs themselves are not. CHWs in Kenya are largely unpaid health volunteers selected by members of their communities to become their health volunteers. In other words, CHWs can often find themselves at the margins of formal healthcare systems, and so, across the activities of the health system, ways need to be found to develop vital links between communities and the formal health system. The above quotation illustrates how supervisors valued the expertise of CHWs and used it to improve their own knowledge acquisition processes. This centrality of CHWs within a systems-based approaches was fundamental to the mCHW project. Our starting point for designing training was to perceive CHWs as critical to health systems and as experts in their area who know the cultural context and settings and who know what health expertise is needed in their specific areas. In view of that, the mobile intervention used a participatory action research approach to involve CHWs from the outset in the design and development of the mobile phone application. The result was that both communities took ownership of the project and saw it as their project, which in turn resulted in a significant impact on their practice and the relationship between CHWs and their supervisors. Importantly, this meant that both CHWs and supervisors were working in pragmatic solidarity (Gutiérrez, 1983; Farmer, 2003) with their communities health needs—a clear interlinking across the health system that led to better integration between CHWs and the formal health system in terms of improved knowledge, training and supervision, assessment, and informed referrals.

(v) How does mobile technology support service delivery?

A legitimate question to ask is why the REFER app was developed to run on smartphones. Would it not have been better to focus on technologies that are already widely available locally, in most cases, low-end, low-priced phones? Another way to think about this is to examine the relationships between the building blocks and the interactions between them. Are these interactions the same when using smartphones as when using low-end, low-priced phones? We contend that they are not: the possible synergies that emerges from interactions—specifically across information, medical technology, and service delivery—between CHWs and their supervisors are fundamentally different when mediated by smartphones. Based on this status quo, many community-focused health projects start with the premise to build content around what technology is currently available, that is content that runs on low-end phones. (Indeed, this line of reasoning has been additionally supported by increasing pressure to the impact, sustainability, and the cost-effectiveness of intervention designs—see Winters et al., 2020.) We took an alternative approach and started by asking what technology would best support high-quality supervision of CHWs using a systems-thinking approach? It was from here that we examined how to work across the four subsystems to achieve this goal. What become clear from our analysis is that the role of smartphones is critical. Using low-end phones for this purpose would mean making unwarranted concessions in terms of the quality of the intervention. To take just one example that provides an insight into practice and service delivery, supervisors felt that the REFER app gave them evidence of CHWs' home visits, which allows for improved mentoring and tailored follow-up.

> I believe that [the CHWs'] performance has really increased in the sense that the homes that we are able to visit, you have that tangible evidence, that these community health volunteers, they were at those houses. You could also see the people in the community, they are established with them, so that is an indication that the community health volunteers are there for the community and they are working in the community. And now this phone also makes us to have evidence (of that) because somebody not using the phone can work on anything, but we as supervisors, we also go out and follow up and see the kind of homes that have been visited by community health volunteers. (Supervisor from an informal settlement in Nairobi)

Such findings from our empirical work would not have been possible with low-end phones as the "tangible evidence" of CHW visits, that is the data collected by the REFER app, would not have been available. Analysis of the data suggests that CHWs' practices often entail attending to and caring for households within their community through diagnosis, referral, and education, as well as the representation of the households to others, often to those with greater economic reach. In their practices, the CHWs have to overcome many material and organizational challenges, including long distances between households and a pronounced scarcity of resources and training. In addition, we found that the training needs of supervisors are often under-resourced, leading to their supervisory activities being poorly defined and limited to occasional supervisory outreach visits. Given the shortage of qualified supervisors, supervisors often have to work under considerable time constraints, and the costs of travel can mean that CHWs have difficulties in accessing training centers.

Conclusion

This chapter presented a systems-thinking approach to the use of mobile technologies for the training and supervision of CHWs in LMICs. We suggest that mobile technologies are most useful as practice-based tools to enable a bridge between community practice and the formal health system. Mobile technologies can thus support new kinds of practice that enable CHWs to support their communities in ways that were not possible before the introduction of this technology. In summary, if appropriately designed from a systems perspective, a mobile application can be a practice-based tool, much like a stethoscope to a doctor, but with the enhanced ability to scaffold practice. To affect improved intervention design, mobile technologies must address a clear need in the community but also have a benefit to those working in the formal health system. We believe this systems approach aids take-up, although a balance is needed here, particularly when working with vulnerable and marginalized communities who have previously been systematically excluded from care.

However, a note of caution is need here: the use of mobile technologies is definitely not a panacea. In the context of increasing within-country inequalities (Lakner & Milanovic, 2013), it is even more important that equal treatment is available to all. Mobile technologies most definitely have a role to play in this process, by supporting improved CHW practice. Unfortunately, it is clear that this can only go so far if universal health coverage (UHC), through wider health systems strengthening, is not available. This remains a significant challenge. However, as Sacks (2002) has argued, information technologies by nature can potentially have not only a localized, but a systemic impact, in that they change the ways we record and transmit information. Sacks notes that such changes could alter "the most fundamental structures of society" (p. 125), helping to combat structural health inequalities. In the context of healthcare in low-resource settings, it is our hope that future mobile technologies, if appropriately designed and embedded with the formal health system, will ultimately not only support CHWs' practice but will also contribute to strengthening and transforming the nature of UHC. Our work is a first step in this direction.

Acknowledgments

This research was supported by an The Economic and Social Research Council (ESRC) and the Department for International Development (DFID) grant ES/J018619/2. The authors would like to thank the CHWs and their supervisors who took part in the mCHW project and also our colleagues and collaborators Simon Murithi, Hannah Wanjiru, Caroline Mbindyo, Diane Mukami, Isabella Rega, Martin Oliver, and Jade Vu Henry for their contributions to the research.

References

de Savigny, D., & Adam, T. (2009). *Systems thinking for health systems strengthening.* Geneva: World Health Organization.

Farmer, P. (2003). *Pathologies of power: Health, human rights and the new war on the poor.* Berkley, CA: University of California Press.

Gladstone, M., Lancaster, G. A., Umar, E., Nyirenda, M., Kayira, E., van den Broek, N. R., & Smyth, R. L. (2010). The Malawi Developmental Assessment Tool (MDAT): The creation, validation, and reliability of a tool to assess child development in rural African settings. *PLoS Medicine, 7*(5), e1000273. Retrieved from https://doi.org/10.1371/journal.pmed.1000273

Gilroy, K., & Winch, P. (2006). Management of sick children by community health workers: Intervention models and programme examples (2006). Geneva: United Nations Childrens' Fund/World Health Organization. Retrieved from https://apps.who.int/iris/bitstream/handle/10665/44226/9789280639858_eng.pdf?sequence=1&isAllowed=y Gutiérrez, G. (1983). *The power of the poor in history.* Maryknoll: Orbis.

Haines, A., Sanders, D., Lehmann, U., Rowe, A. K., Lawn, J., Jan, S., ... Bhutta, Z. (2007). Achieving child survival goals: Potential contribution of community health workers. *The Lancet, 369,* 2121–2123.

Källander, K., Tibenderana, J. K., Akpogheneta, O. J., Strachan, D. L., Hill, Z., ten Asbroek, A. H. A., ... Meek, S. R. (2013). Mobile health (mHealth) approaches and lessons for increased performance and retention of community health workers in low- and middle-income countries: A review, *Journal of Medical Internet Research, 15*(1), e17. doi:10.2196/jmir.2130

Labrique, A. B., Vasudevan, L., Kochi, E., Fabricant, R., & Mehl, G. (2013). mHealth innovations as health system strengthening tools: 12 common applications and a visual framework. *Global Health: Science and Practice, 1,* 160–171.

Lakner, C., & Milanovic, B. (2013). Global income distribution: From the fall of the Berlin Wall to the great recession, the World Bank Development Research Group Poverty and Inequality Team. Working Paper 6719. World Bank, Washington, DC.

Laurillard, D. (2002). *Rethinking university teaching: A conversational framework for the effective use of learning technologies* (2nd ed.). London: Routledge.

O'Donovan, J., O'Donovan, C., Kuhn, I., Sachs, S. E., & Winters, N. (2018). Ongoing training of community health workers in low-income and middle-income countries: A systematic scoping review of the literature, *BMJ Open, 8,* e021467. doi:10.1136/ bmjopen-2017-021467

Oliver, M., Geniets, A., Winters, N., Rega, I., & Mbae, S. (2015). What do Community Health Workers do? A case study of practice within Kenya, *Global Health Action, 8,* 1. Retrieved from https://doi.org/10.3402/gha.v8.27168

Powers, M., & Faden, R. (2006). *Social justice: The moral foundations of public health and health policy.* Oxford: Oxford University Press.

Rogers, E. S., & Palmer-Erbs, V. (1994). Participatory action research: implications for research and evaluation in psychiatric evaluation. *Psychosocial Rehabilitation Journal, 18,* 3–12.

Rowe A. K. De Savigny, D., Lanata, C. F., & Victora, C. G. (2005). How can we achieve and maintain high-quality performance of health workers in low-resource settings? *The Lancet, 366,* 1026–1035.

Sacks, J. (2002). *The dignity of difference—How to avoid a clash of civilizations.* London: Continuum.

Theobald, S., MacPherson, E., McCollum, R., & Tolhurst, R. (2015, December). Close to community health providers post 2015: Realising their role in responsive health systems and addressing gendered social determinants of health. In *BMC proceedings* (Vol. 9, No. 10, pp. 1–11). BioMed Central.

Turinawe, E. B., Rwemisisi, J. T., Musinguzi, L. K., de Groot, M., Muhangi, D., de Vries, D. H., et al. (2015). Selection and performance of village health teams (VHTs) in Uganda: Lessons from the natural helper model of health promotion. *Human Resources for Health, 13,* 73.

Winters, N., Langer, L., & Geniets, A. (2017). Physical, psychological, sexual, and systemic abuse of children with disabilities in East Africa: Mapping the evidence. *PLoS ONE 12*(9), e0184541. Retrieved from https://doi.org/10.1371/journal.pone.0184541

Winters, N., Oliver, M., & Langer, L. (2017). Can mobile health training meet the challenge of "measuring better?" *Comparative Education, 52,* 4, 115–131. Retrieved from https://doi.org/10.1080/03050068.2017.1254983

Winters, N., Langer, L., & Geniets, A. (2018). Scoping review assessing the evidence used to support the adoption of mobile health (mHealth) technologies for the education and training of community health workers (CHWs) in low-income & middle-income countries. *BMJ Open, 8,* e019827. Retrieved from http://dx.doi.org/10.1136/bmjopen-2017-019827

Winters, N., Venkatapuram, S., & Geniets, A., & Wynne-Bannister, E. (2020). Prioritarian principles for digital health in low resource settings. *Journal of Medical Ethics, 46*(4), 259–264. doi:10.1136/medethics-2019-105468

7
Unpacking Complexity
Systems Thinking for Communities

Brynne Gilmore, Henry Mollel, Nazarius Mbona Tumwesigye, and Eilish McAuliffe

Introduction

The importance of community involvement in health-promoting activities, combined with the need to target more vulnerable populations directly, has resulted in a strong focus on health activities at the community level. However, while strongly advocated for and widely implemented, communities and their health-related actions and activities are often poorly understood and documented.

This chapter aims to contribute to the development of a more in-depth understanding of "the community" as an integral part of all health systems. Specifically, we argue that implementing community health initiatives and community systems strengthening efforts requires two main considerations: (i) seeing community health as part of the overall health system, including ensuring its appropriate incorporation within policies and programing, and (ii) recognizing that communities are complex, with different communities having diverse and distinct characteristics, needs, and priorities. By exploring what we consider to be critical concepts in community health and systems strengthening, and presenting examples from practice, we demonstrate the value of utilizing a systems lens to define, design, understand, and evaluate the place of communities within health systems.

In doing so, we hope that this chapter will encourage the use of systems thinking to strengthen health services at the community level while ensuring that the complexities and uniqueness of communities are also considered.

The Importance of Communities

The importance of working with communities in global health efforts cannot be understated. Strongly endorsed during Alma-Ata and Primary Health Care (PHC) for All, putting people at the center of healthcare through the decentralization of services to communities, a greater investment in hard-to-reach populations, and a focus on participation, has been a key focus to increase coverage over last several decades (Green, 2007). Community health activities often utilize existing community resources, mainly people, to increase participation with the formal health sector and improve access to services. Given that building strong health systems that respond to

Brynne Gilmore, Henry Mollel, Nazarius Mbona Tumwesigye, and Eilish McAuliffe, *Unpacking Complexity* In: *Systems Thinking for Global Health*. Edited by: Fiona Larkan, Frédérique Vallières, Hasheem Mannan, and Naonori Kodate, Oxford University Press.
 DOI: 10.1093/oso/9780198799498.003.0007

citizens' needs is recognized as the most sustainable and effective way to achieve improved health outcomes (Travis et al., 2004; Richard et al., 2011; Hafner & Shiffman, 2013), such efforts should be widely endorsed and strengthened.

Community health strategies are thought to work to reduce the barriers to health and health inequities in several ways. Specifically, they work toward addressing issues of availability, accessibility, acceptability, and affordability of health services by addressing the absolute number of health workers and/or programs in contexts with the greatest shortages and reducing inaccessibility of services in hard-to-reach locations. Additionally, because community health strategies aim to link communities with existing, formalized services, they may result in more affordable basic care for community members. As community-based initiatives are often predicated on providing culturally relevant and accessible health services and information to communities, they may also improve acceptability and quality of programming (Gilmore, Vallières, Mcauliffe, Tumwesigye, & Muyambi, 2014).

While evidence suggests that community care and community interventions are important tools to address health inequality (Gilson, Doherty, Loewenson, & Francis, 2007; Barros et al., 2012), in practice, community health faces many implementation challenges. Specifically, the retention of health workers, lack of political and organizational ability to incorporate the principles of Alma Ata fully, limited connectivity to more formalized services, disconnected understanding and involvement between communities and implementers, and limited community capacity to further engage with, utilize, and take ownership of community health initiatives limits the sustainability and long-term impact of these programs (Lehmann, Dieleman, & Martineau, 2008; Gilmore et al., 2014). The above challenges further imply that weak health systems often act as the biggest rate-limiting factor toward the successful implementation of community health initiatives. Consequently, the contexts in which community health are initiated may fail to support its long-term implementation and thus fail to capitalize on the many benefits community health can bring.

Defining Communities and their Health Systems

Communities are intrinsically heterogeneous, resulting in multiple classifications of community (Rodriguez-Garcia, Bonnel, Wilson, & N'jie, 2013). While Rodriguez-Garcia et al. (2011) place cultural identity at the epicenter of communities, Laverack (2004) provides several guides for defining communities as:

- Communities can have a shared a spatial dimension, (i.e., a place or location);
- Communities can also have non-spatial dimensions (interests, issues, identities) that involve people who otherwise make up heterogeneous and disparate groups;
- Communities can have social interactions that are dynamic and bind people into relationships with each other;
- Communities can have identification of shared needs and concerns that can be achieved through a process of collective action.

Defining "community health" however remains a challenge despite its regular use within the field of global health. Several scholars have offered their own definitions of "community health" (e.g., Goodman, Bunnell, & Posner, 2014), though many definitions fall short of encompassing and capturing the ethos of community health work. We note, however, that "community health" tends to be characterized by *location* (i.e., decentralized, lower levels of implementation), *actors* (lay volunteers or minimally trained workers, often utilizing task-shifting techniques), *integration* (of existing community structures like committees, or existing initiatives), *focus* (often multi-sectoral actions, with elements of primary care activities) and the *involvement* of community members (participation and engagement of community members). Taken together, the above suggests that "community health" cannot merely be defined in terms of where services are located, or how policies are enacted, but rather that community health can have several connotations depending on context. As such, we define community health as "an effort to improve health and reduce health inequities through systematically involving community stakeholders in the administration of multi-sectoral and multi-level health activities aimed at a community level, and through increasing community's participation and control over health."

Communities are Complex

Evident from this discussion is that community health and community systems are complex. Plsek and Greenhalgh (2001) offer basic concepts and key characteristics of a complex health system: they have fuzzy boundaries, as opposed to strict and rigid ones; the agents within systems have internalized (implicit or explicit) non-fixed rules that drive action; the agents within the system are adaptive and often changing; the systems are embedded and co-evolve with (influence and are influenced by) other systems; and they are non-linear and unpredictable, despite it being possible to discern inherent patterns of behavior of the systems (Plsek & Greenhalgh, 2001). Within the field of public health, complex systems are not considered controlled but rather self-organizing, typically by agents following locally applied rules (Cabrera, 2002; Trochim, Cabrera, Milstein, Gallagher, & Leischow, 2006).

Given that they are set within complex health systems and are directed toward complex communities, community health interventions are often categorized as complex health interventions (CHIs). What makes an intervention "complex" has been described in various ways, with a common description compiled by the Medical Research Council (Craig et al., 2008). The MRC's description states that in order to be complex, interventions must have interacting components, a number of different behaviors required to deliver or receive the intervention, a number of groups or organizational levels targeted, a variability of outcomes and a degree of flexibility required.

CHIs are self-organizing systems that are constantly changing and are inextricable from the context in which they operate. Complex health interventions work with the understanding that they comprise a collection of individual agents or components that are connected, but also can act in unpredictable ways, thereby impacting the other components (Plsek & Greenhalgh, 2001). A system is therefore deemed complex not by the number of components within it but by the pattern and density of interaction or inter-dependence between these components.

Community health activities work within open, complex, and dynamic systems that do not operate in predictable ways (Dooris et al., 2007) and function at the interface of the social and individual (Kazi, 2003). Owing to the variety and number of stakeholders involved—including, but not limited to, potential patients, actual patients, the health workforce, suppliers, educators, insurers—and the varying objectives and strategies, linear models for the study, implementation, and understanding of community health should be applied with caution. Indeed, recent advances in community programming have resulted in a paradigm shift to more ecological models that recognize this interdependence of context and individuals within health programming.

Systems Thinking for Communities

Consideration for community systems involves taking a holistic approach to understand the whole system and interactions within it, as opposed to focusing on specific components (Trochim et al., 2006; de Savigny & Adam, 2009). "Systems thinking," defined by Senge as "a discipline for seeing wholes ... a framework for seeing interrelationships rather than things, for seeing patterns of change rather than static snapshots" (Senge, 2006:. 68), emphasizes this holistic approach.

Without such an approach, the complexity of community health, including the interconnected components and partnerships which operate in multifaceted and unpredictable ways, can go unnoticed, resulting in incomplete and possibly a biased understanding of community health and CHIs. Dooris (2007) compiled a list of reasons for the importance of taking a systems perspective in health, which we contend are especially relevant within communities. These reasons include:

- Health issues do not respect boundaries; an issue that manifests in one setting may have its roots in a different setting;
- People's lives cross different settings, concurrently and consecutively;
- There are micro-environments within each setting that offer different experiences to different people, on different days;
- Settings function at multiple levels, with shared and separate domains, and as "elemental" or "contextual" settings may be located within the context of another, consisting of nested settings within interconnected spatial and temporal layers.

Drawing on our earlier discussion of community characteristics, we propose to expand on this list for communities by adding that:

- Communities are often both the receivers and implementers of health initiatives, and therefore transcend traditional unidirectional "patient/provider" relationships found within health.
- Community health initiatives are commonly related to health promotion and behavior change. We therefore need to understand the wider cultural, social, and

personal influences on communities' behavior, going beyond the typical scope of more reductionist explorations.

Using a systems-thinking approach may also support identifying powerful levers, or entry points, that should be factored into the design and evaluation of health interventions (Checkland, 1981; McPake, Blaauw, & Sheaff, 2006; Swanson et al., 2012).

Trochim et al. note that using systems thinking is considered most applicable for public health systems as "they [public health] consist of many interacting stakeholders with often different and competing interests" (Trochim et al., 2006: 539) and are self-organizing. In this, each stakeholder (or agent) within the system has a specific role and an implicit (or sometimes explicit) set of rules to follow. The roles of stakeholders are interconnected and link together to help form the overall system. In community health, for example, this may take the form of a health committee or organization that has internalized roles and rules that they follow, interacting with other members to form a whole group. It may be assumed, for example, that the eldest man will be the chairman of the group, and be responsible for the agenda, or communication, with community leaders outside of the committee. Similarly, all other members will implicitly know that the community health worker (CHW) will coordinate activities within the wider health system, without this role ever being officially ascribed. Similarly, the committee itself can be seen as an actor, with a specific role to play within the wider community health system. How the committee links with the health facility, CHWs, community members, politicians, and leaders contributes to and factors in the functioning of the system.

In sum, systems thinking works to understand complex real-world problems, while also aiming to identify context-specific solutions to such problems. Hence the value of taking a systems-thinking approach to both programming (i.e., design and implementation) and research on community health and community health systems.

Applying Systems Thinking to Community Health

Though a systems approach is frequently advocated for, there are limited explicit examples of systems thinking in community health. And while many researchers or programmers may inherently work to understand contexts or ensure a thorough understanding of the systems and individuals in the design or conducting of research, the absence from the literature of more explicit accounts of the use of this approach hinders its advancement within global health.

Likewise, clear guidance on utilizing systems thinking and lessons learned from others engaging with this topic are scarce. The World Health Organization-based Alliance for Health Policy and Systems Research's (HPSR) 2009 publication entitled *Systems thinking for health systems strengthening* focused mainly on systems thinking within low- and middle-income countries (LMICs). Noting the lack of use of systems thinking in LMICs, the authors attempted to provide concrete recommendations for how to use this approach, drawing from theories or examples from HICs (de Savigny & Adam, 2009). A review of Health Systems Strengthening frameworks by Hoffman et al. (2012), for example, identified forty-one different frameworks, however most had no reference to communities or community health aspects. Building on this, a study by Sacks et al. (2017) identified several recent frameworks that aim to bring communities into the dialogue, albeit to varying degrees. These include Global Fund Community Systems Strengthening (CSS) Framework, Future Health Systems "Unlocking Community Capabilities," WHO's People-centered Health model, USAID's Community Health Framework, and CORE Group's model for community/household integrated management of childhood illness.

One criticism of current systems thinking and strengthening in global health, including the health systems strengthening framework (World Health Organization, 2007), however, is their failure comprehensively to incorporate these critical social aspects of health systems, which, as previously described, are inescapable components of complex health systems (Biesma et al., 2009). While some proponents note that "community engagement" is considered within the governance building block, the lack of explicit and thorough incorporation of communities translates into a lack of importance placed on this essential resource, context, and population. In response to this, the Global Fund's CSS Framework, derived from a systems approach to healthcare, claims to allow for more focused efforts and facilitation at the community level (Terpstra, Coleman, Simon, & Nebeker, 2011). The CSS Framework is not meant to replace the WHO's proposed Health Systems Strengthening Framework but to complement existing efforts by providing a specific focus on strengthening health systems at the community level. The CSS Framework identifies six core components necessary for strengthening communities for health, which work to increase the quality and equitability of services, increase coverage, and improve health outcomes. The six core components include: enabling environments and advocacy; community networks, linkages, partnerships and coordination; resources and capacity building; community activities and service delivery; organizational and leadership strengthening; and monitoring and evaluation and planning (The Global Fund, 2010).

USAID's Maternal and Child Survival Programme (MCSP), in collaboration with the CORE Group, has been investigating how communities and community systems fit within the health system building blocks, identifying the following key components as missing in HSS: community, community-based health services, health production, and civil society engagement (Maternal and Child Survival Programme, 2015). This, in combination with a literature review of existing HSS (Sacks et al., 2017), resulted in an integrated model of community health and HSS, titled "Beyond the Building Blocks," which demonstrates using systems-thinking approaches.

While community health systems frameworks are relatively new, they have been used in a number of limited primary studies. Notably, Mburu et al.'s (2013) study of community groups for HIV palliative care support in Uganda and Bradley et al.'s (2012) study on rural primary healthcare units in Ethiopia both used HSS in combination with community-level factors as part of their study design.

More recently, Gilmore et al. (forthcoming) utilized a systems-thinking approach within a realist evaluation of a community health program in Tanzania and Uganda to identify the contextual conditions which facilitate, or inhibit, the success of community health committees for maternal and child health. This unique approach specifically sought to integrate systems thinking within realist evaluation methodology, which the authors argue have strong theoretical and practical alignment. This enabled

Box 7.1 The Community Health Committees within AIM-Health Programme—The CSS Framework

World Vision's Access to Infant and Maternal Health (AIM-Health) Program (FARST Africa Ltd., 2016) relies on a combination of CHWs, Community Health Committees, and Citizen Voice in Action Teams, to reduce maternal and child mortality in their countries of implementation.

Acting as a fundamental link between communities, CHWs, and the health system, Community Committees (COMMs) aim to empower and strengthen community systems, through three outcomes: community systems strengthening, health systems strengthening, and health worker (CHW) support.

Implementation of COMMs were designed with support from the Global Fund's CSS Framework (International, 2014), to ensure essential components at the community level, and their connectivity to the wider health system, were implemented into programing. In that, the AIM-Health program, and specifically COMMs, worked to strengthen the six CSS building blocks for improved quality and availability of services at the community level.

In their evaluation of the COMMs, Gilmore and colleagues further relied on the CSS Framework to guide their understanding of "how, why and for whom" CHCs contribute to systems strengthening. Aligned to both programmatic and theoretical conceptions of the COMMs, the authors explored how CHCs contributed to each of the building blocks (if they do), across the socio-ecological systems model of the individual, organizational (COMM), community, and wider societal/health systems level. Incorporating a framework for understanding health at the community (CSSF), and with an explicit aim to explore these interactions across the level of the system (beyond just the "community"), enabled the authors to gain a holistic understanding of the operationalization of the COMMs and their wider contribution to systems strengthening.

the research to capture important contextual information at multiple levels of program interactions and present findings across various social, cultural, environmental, and political domains which can work to improve overall implementation (See Box 7.1; Gilmore et al., forthcoming).

As a result of this work, the authors present several considerations for systems thinking at the community level, including:

- While the CSS Framework and other similar resources can be useful to assist researchers and implementers, it is difficult to pinpoint what to look for within systems thinking without having prior knowledge of "the system" itself. This demonstrates the importance of having community members, or those well-versed with the context, be part of program or evaluation designs, allocating sufficient time prior to designing projects for understanding the systems and context, and/or using methodologies that build in such approaches

- Due to the dynamic nature of these systems, change will occur over time. Programs and studies require flexibility of design and protocols that best reflect the evolving nature of communities.
- Systems thinking applied to whole communities is a demanding and complex undertaking, and it is likely to be impossible to address or understand completely the entirety of the community system. Research may therefore require a balance of specificity and sensitivity when addressing systems thinking.
- Community and "formalized" health systems are not separate systems but together comprise a whole health system, each having an important influence on the health of the population. While different considerations for study may be required at different levels, gaining a full understanding of community health requires not just looking at community-level aspects but also integrating conditions for wider health system factors, policies, and systems.

While these new models for how to integrate communities into the wider health system are important, they are still in their infancy. With limited studies examining how they work in practice, there remain many questions on how to best utilize them for evaluations and implementation.

Conclusion

This chapter has argued for the use of systems thinking within community health and services. As community health systems are complex and have interacting, unpredictable components across multifaceted layers within society, research and programming need to ensure a holistic approach which aims to take value from—rather than try to control for—these factors. Frequently, community health systems are either examined as a part of the wider health sphere or as a unique social sphere, not concurrently as both. Existing tools, guidance, frameworks, and approaches need to incorporate these interacting spheres to best understand and plan for community systems. Though there are limited examples of a systems-thinking approach to accommodate and inform how to apply systems thinking for communities, there is growing support for its use. Accordingly, academics and practitioners alike should endeavor to employ systems-thinking approaches when working within community health to improve service delivery in such a way that results in the application of more relevant and contextually aligned actions for communities.

References

Barros, A. J., Ronsmans, C., Axelson, H., Loaiza, E., Bertoldi, A. D., França, G. V., … Victora, C. G. (2012). Equity in maternal, newborn, and child health interventions in Countdown to 2015: A retrospective review of survey data from 54 countries. *The Lancet, 379*, 1225–1233.

Biesma, R. G., Brugha, R., Harmer, A., Walsh, A., Spicer, N., & Walt, G. (2009). The effects of global health initiatives on country health systems: A review of the evidence from HIV/AIDS control. *Health Policy and Planning, 24*, 239–252.

Bradley, E. H., Byam, P., Alpern, R., Thompson, J. W., Zerihun, A., Abeb, Y., & Curry, L. A. (2012). A systems approach to improving rural care in Ethiopia. *PLoS One, 7*(4), e35042.

Cabrera, D. (2002). Patterns of knowledge: Knowledge as a complex, evolutionary system, an educational imperative. In R. Miller (Ed.), *Creating learning communities*. Solomon Press.

Checkland, P. (1981). *Systems Thinking, Systems Practice*. New York, NY: Sons.

Craig, P., Dieppe, P., Macintyre, S., Michie, S., Nazareth, I., & Petticrew, M. (2008). Developing and evaluating complex interventions: the new Medical Research Council guidance. *British Medical Journal, 337*, a1655.

de Savigny, D., & Adam, T. (2009). *Systems thinking for health systems strengthening*. Geneva: World Health Organization.

Dooris, M., Poland, B., Kolbe, L., De Leeuw, E., Mccall, D. S., & Wharf-Higgins, J. (2007). Healthy settings: Building evidence for the effectiveness of whole system health promotion—Challenges and future directions. In D. V. McQueen & C. M. Jones (Eds.), *Global Perspectives on Health Promotion Effectiveness* (pp. 327–352). New York, NY: Springer.

FARST Africa Ltd. (2016). Access—Infant and Maternal Health (AIM) health programme. January 2011–December 2015. Endl Line Programme Evaluation Report. World Vision Ireland. Dublin, Ireland.

Gilmore, B., Vallières, F., Mcauliffe, E., Tumwesigye, N., & Muyambi, G. (2014). The last one heard: The importance of an early-stage participatory evaluation for programme implementation. *Implementation Science, 9*(1), 1–12.

Gilson, L., Doherty, J., Loewenson, R., & Francis, V. (2007). *Challenging inequity through health systems. Final report of the Knowledge Network on health systems*. Geneva: World Health Organization.

Goodman, R. A., Bunnell, R., & Posner, S. F. (2014). What is "community health"? Examining the meaning of an evolving field in public health. *Preventive Medicine, 67*, S58–S61.

Green, A. (2007). *An introduction to health planning for developing health systems*. Oxford: Oxford University Press.

Hafner, T., & Shiffman, J. (2013). The emergence of global attention to health systems strengthening. *Health Policy and Planning, 28*(1), 41–50.

Hoffman, S. J., Røttingen, J.-A., Bennett, S., Lavis, J. N., Edge, J. S., & Frenk, J. (2012). Background paper on conceptual issues related to health systems research to inform a WHO global strategy on health systems research. *Health Systems Alliance*. https://www.who.int/alliance-hpsr/alliancehpsr_backgroundpaperhsrstrat1.pdf

Kazi, M. A. F. (2003). Realist evaluation for practice. *British Journal of Social Work, 33*, 803–818.

Laverack, G. (2004). *Health promotion practice: Power and empowerment*. London: Sage Publications Ltd.

Lehmann, U., Dieleman, M., & Martineau, T. (2008). Staffing remote rural areas in middle-and low-income countries: A literature review of attraction and retention. *BMC Health Services Research, 8*, 19.

Maternal and Child Survival Programme. (2015). WHO building blocks platform for health systems strengthening: Adding communities to the mix. CORE Group Global Health Practitioner Conference: Advancing Community Health Across the Continuum of Care, 2015 Alexandria, Virginia. Maternal and Child Survival Programme (MSCP), USAID.

Mburu, G., Oxenham, D., Hodgson, I., Nakiyemba, A., Seeley, J., & Bermejo, A. (2013). Community systems strengthening for HIV care: Experiences from Uganda. *Journal of Social Work in End-of-Life & Palliative Care, 9*(4), 343–368.

McPake, B., Blaauw, D., & Sheaff, R. (2006). Recognising patterns: Health systems research beyond controlled trials. Meeting of the London School of Hygiene and Tropical Medicine Health Systems Discussion Group.

Plsek, P. E., & Greenhalgh, T. (2001). Complexity science: The challenge of complexity in health care. *British Medical Journal, 323*(7313), 625–628.

Richard, F., Hercot, D., Ouédraogo, C., Delvaux, T., Samaké, S., van Olmen, J., Conombo, G., Hammonds, R., & Vandemoortele, J. (2011). Sub-Saharan Africa and the health MDGs: The need to move beyond the "quick impact" model. *Reproductive Health Matters, 19*(38), 42–55.

Rodriguez-García, R., Bonnel, R., N'jie, N. D., Olivier, J., Pascual, F. B., & Wodon, Q. T. (2011). Analyzing community responses to HIV and AIDS: Operational framework and typology. *World Bank Policy Research Working Paper*, 5532.

Rodriguez-Garcia, R., Bonnel, R., Wilson, D., & N'jie, N. (2013). Investing in communities achieves results. Findings from an evaluation of community responses to HIV and AIDS. In World Bank (Ed.), *Directions in development: Human development.* Washington, DC: World Bank. doi:10.1596/978-0-8213-9741-1. License: Creative Commons Attribution CC BY 3.0.

Sacks, E., Swanson, R. C., Schensul, J. J., Gleave, A., Shelley, K. D., Were, M. K., ... Perry, H. B. (2017). Community involvement in health systems strengthening to improve global health outcomes: A review of guidelines and potential roles. *International Quarterly of Community Health Education, 37*, 139–149.

Senge, P. M. (2006). *The fifth discipline: The art and practice of the learning organization.* New York, NY: Currency Doubleday.

Swanson, R. C., Cattaneo, A., Bradley, E., Chunharas, S., Atun, R., Abbas, K. M., ... Best, A. (2012). Rethinking health systems strengthening: Key systems thinking tools and strategies for transformational change. *Health Policy and Planning*, 27, iv54–iv61.

Terpstra, J., Coleman, K. J., Simon, G., & Nebeker, C. (2011). The role of community health workers (CHWS) in health promotion research: ethical challenges and practical solutions. *Health Promotion Practice, 12*, 86–93.

The Global Fund. (2010). Community systems strengthening framework. In T. A. M. (Ed.), *The Global Fund to Fight Aids.* Geneva. https://www.theglobalfund.org/media/6428/core_css_framework_en.pdf

Travis, P., Bennett, S., Haines, A., Pang, T., Bhutta, Z., Hyder, A. A., Pielemeier, N. R., Mills, A., & Evans, T. (2004). Overcoming health-systems constraints to achieve the Millennium Development Goals. *The Lancet, 364*(9437), 900–906.

Trochim, W. M., Cabrera, D. A., Milstein, B., Gallagher, R. S., & Leischow, S. J. (2006). Practical challenges of systems thinking and modeling in public health. *American Journal of Public Health, 96*, 538–546.

World Health Organization. (2007). *Everybody's business—Strengthening health systems to improve health outcomes: WHO's framework for action.* Geneva: World Health Organization.

World Vision International (2014). COMM project model: Description and guidance for design. Global Health and WASH.

8
Applying Systems Thinking to Health Information Systems
Lessons from South Africa and Tanzania

Annariina Koivu, Margunn Aanestad, and Nima Shidende

Introduction

Health information systems (HIS) provide the underpinnings for decision-making via data (i) generation, (ii) compilation, (iii) analysis and synthesis, as well as (iv) communication and use (World Health Organization, 2010). Through the use of paper-based and electronic HIS, data are collected from health and other relevant sectors, analyzed, and converted into meaningful information for health-related decision-making. HIS are therefore complex, multi-component systems that need to be able to work together at and exchange information with different levels of a health system (Mwanyika et al., 2011).

"Information" is one of the World Health Organization's (WHO) six core health system building blocks. While none of the building blocks should be considered in isolation, this notion is particularly important for the "information" building block, since reliable and fit-for-purpose data are essential for informed decision-making across all other health system building blocks. Both paper-based and electronic HIS are meant to produce information to aid clinical decisions and patient care, managerial and operational decisions, such as resource allocation, detecting and responding to infectious diseases, epidemiological modelling, and monitoring progress toward set goals. Therefore, an approach that fosters better understanding of linkages, relationships, and interactions is fundamental in creating such systems and learning from them. Systems thinking ticks these boxes yet reports on the applications of systems thinking in the design, use, or research of HIS are scarce, particularly in the context of low- and middle-income countries (LMIC) (Kumar, Gotz, Nutley, & Smith, 2018).

The insights on the usefulness of applying systems-thinking approach in HIS are drawn from the authors' in-depth experience of researching and developing HIS in LMIC from 2003 to date. Annariina Koivu, though based in the global north, has a considerable understanding of South Africa's and Tanzania's HIS. Margunn Aanestad has researched HIS in a number of LMIC countries. Being affiliated with the Health Information System program (HISP), she has supervised PhD

Annariina Koivu, Margunn Aanestad, and Nima Shidende, *Applying Systems Thinking to Health Information Systems* In: *Systems Thinking for Global Health.* Edited by: Fiona Larkan, Frédérique Vallières, Hasheem Mannan, and Naonori Kodate, Oxford University Press. DOI: 10.1093/oso/9780198799498.003.0008

and Masters' students from Ethiopia, Mozambique, Tanzania, India, and Malawi. Nima Shidende has studied the Tanzanian HIS in the context of maternal and child health services for about ten years. The data informing this chapter have been collected within multiple studies by using primarily qualitative approaches, such as case studies, ethnographic inspired approaches, and action research, including observation of healthcare services, interviewing health workers and clients, as well as reviewing data collection tools and policy documents.

(For more, see Chilundo & Aanestad, 2005; Shidende, 2005; Shidende, Grisot, Aanestad, 2014; Koivu, 2015; Shidende 2015; Koivu, Mavengere, Ruohonen, Hederman, & Grimson, 2017)

HIS are prone to inconsistent data quality, fragmentation into multiple partially overlapping systems that lead to duplication of efforts, and varying use value for health workers. These challenges are exacerbated in LMICs, where unreliable infrastructure, issues in retention of skilled human resources, and scarcity of material resources are common. As a result, HIS implementations are at risk of failure and unsustainability.

Unsustainability is often caused by a mismatch between the design of technological systems and the existing work context (e.g., Heeks, 2002; Pan, Hackney, & Pan, 2008; Kumar et al., 2018). For instance, data collection tools may have been designed to serve the central health authority's needs and may omit data fields that are crucial to inform local decision-making. Likewise, systems designed in other contexts may have differing requirements for technical infrastructure, such as the need for power supply and connectivity that cannot be met in all settings.

HIS research has documented various efforts for tackling these challenges, such as standardization of information systems (Nyella, 2009; Abdusamadovich, 2013; Poppe, Jolliffe, Adaletey, Braa, & Manya, 2013); using a data warehouse approach (Kossie, Sæbø, Braa, Jalloh, & Manya, 2011; Sæbø, Kossi, Titlestad, Tohouri, & Braa, 2011); training health workers at the district and national levels of health system (e.g., Mphatswe et al., 2012); and, more recently using blockchain technology (Agbo, 2019). However, these strategies have often focused on the needs of health managers or specific programs (Shidende, 2015) or certain technological aspects of HIS, rather than the needs related to the daily work of health professionals. Consequently, many HIS challenges remain unsolved.

We argue that applying systems thinking will yield more holistic approaches to these challenges. In support of our argument, we present case examples which build on our experiences of HIS in South Africa, Tanzania, and other countries. We aim to show how systems thinking could be used to understand the challenges prevalent within HIS and how it could be applied to derive solutions to address these challenges. First, we propose that the multifaceted and often political processes of acquiring HIS may sometimes stem from decision-making processes informed by *static thinking*. Static thinking in HIS acquisition focuses on particular, current diseases, or problems, and stands in contrast to *dynamic thinking* as understood in systems thinking. Second, we show how the structure of the HIS entity, often driven by funding-related factors, may be consistent with *tree-by-tree thinking* (i.e., focusing on details of particular health programs), whereas *forest thinking*—stepping back and understanding the context of relationships—might contribute to better service and more sustainable health outcomes. Third, we explore how data quality issues, frequent within LMICs, could be better analyzed using *operational thinking* rather than *factors thinking*. While theory and models are helpful, operational thinking means putting them aside and thinking in terms of how things really work in their real-life context (Richmond, 1993). Finally, we provide conclusion and lessons learned from applying a systems-thinking approach to HIS challenges.[1]

Seeking New Approaches to HIS Implementations: From Static to Dynamic Thinking

Requiring consideration of various organizational, technical, and socio-political factors, acquiring and implementing HIS are complex undertakings that range from developing an HIS from scratch to the procurement of ready-made systems with limited tailoring options. According to Richmond (2010), in applying a *static line of thinking*, perspectives tend to get caught up in specific events or points at the expense of seeing larger patterns that may evolve over time. We argue that HIS acquisition is often marked by a static approach, in other words responding to particular needs in terms of there "being a problem that needs to be dealt with." The response to such problems is often to implement an information system. However, this response may lead to a number of poorly integrated, disease-specific information systems. While this is a common response globally, this challenge is particularly prevalent in the instance of donor-driven and project-based procurement.

In South Africa, the number of new HIV infections reached epidemic proportions in the 1990s, making HIV/AIDS an unprecedented public health crisis. When antiretroviral treatment (ART) became publicly available in 2004–2008, receiving amplified global and local attention and funding, it prompted increased reporting requirements for the actors involved in treatment provision. Originally, the required data were collected through a plethora of local registers and monitoring and evaluation (M&E) systems at sites where donors had invested in them. In 2010, a nationwide M&E system for ART was adopted by the National Department of Health to manage the information in the world's largest ART program. However, HIV counselling and testing (HCT) and prevention of mother-to-child transmission of HIV (PMTCT) have largely been managed as their own programs, with reports generated through different paper-based and electronic channels.

Fueled by the HIV/AIDS epidemic, South Africa has also become a global tuberculosis (TB) hotspot. An information system called ETR.Net has been used to provide accurate data about confirmed TB cases since 2003. The recognition of the multidrug-resistant (MDR)-TB epidemic has brought about its own electronic TB register called

[1] Action research project based at the Department of Informatics at the University of Oslo, aiming at strengthening HIS in the southern hemisphere through development and implementation of District Health Information Software and capacity development—http://www.dhis2.org.

EDRWeb. Malaria, another globally high-profile disease, also has its own program and information system. In addition to these program-specific information systems, South African health professionals further utilize an integrated district health information system to report a set of standardized key indicators. Finally, several registers, HIS, and electronic medical record (EMR) systems have been created either with a particular information need in mind or in order to link existing data. Currently, increasing availability of patient-level data linkages has led to improved opportunities for integration and consolidation of data in the Western Cape (Boulle et al., 2019), however the situation is less favorable in other provinces in South Africa, as well as in other Sub-Saharan countries.

In addition to disease-specific approaches, HIS planning often fails to account for changing and evolving disease patterns. As this description of the South African HIS landscape illustrates, a common approach to HIS development is to react to emerging, novel information and reporting needs by implementing a HIS that responds to these needs. This strategy ensures that there at least *exist* data on the health problems, however the resulting HIS landscape may become fragmented and expensive to sustain, as has happened in many high-income countries. This fragmentation hinders the performance of HIS overall, creating a duplication of work and data, lack of information sharing, and poor use of information systems (Sauerborn & Lippeveld, 2000; Chilundo, 2004; Meribole et al., 2018). In South Africa and Tanzania, duplicative data collection efforts are particularly prevalent at the clinic (i.e., primary healthcare) level, where staff are already over-burdened and time and material resources limited.

In contrast to these static approaches, systems thinking emphasizes dynamic approaches. In this context, this translates to an emphasis on formulating a long-term strategy with continuous evolution due to new information needs emerging from new disease patterns and new treatments options. In the dynamic real-world, epidemics mature and epidemiological and pharmacological situations change; some drugs gradually lose their effect while others became available; health paradigms change and new issues arise on the global agenda while other lose their significance. As a result, there will always be new information needs. Therefore, more dynamic thinking is necessary to address the existing static approaches to HIS implementation. More recently, dynamic thinking for HIS is represented through an increased emphasis on HIS architectures and eHealth ecosystems, both of which are welcome. Thus, applying systems thinking for HIS would not only help us recognize the particular crisis or problem as such, but also the "pattern of which they are a part" (Richmond 2010). An approach inspired by such dynamic, rather than static thinking for the implementation of HIS would therefore be more responsive to the evolving nature of the global health sector.

Analyzing HIS Components: Tree-by-Tree Thinking versus Forest Thinking

In systems thinking, *forest* thinking invites us to "rise above functional silos and view the system of relationships that link the component parts" (Richmond, 1997). However, in many LMIC contexts, and as demonstrated in the above South African example, the structure of HIS is often characterized by a collection of "siloed systems" or systems designed for a specific disease or a particular health program. As a result, there is sometimes too little consideration given to social context within which HIS are used. Specifically, the work situation of the health workers is rarely taken into consideration in the design or decision-making process for HIS. The consequence of such a lack of forest thinking (attention to the relationships that link the component parts) is that the actual provision of health service and the flow of information may be hindered, rather than facilitated, by the HIS. This point is best illustrated using an example from the care for HIV-positive expecting mothers in Tanzania.

Like South Africa, Tanzania is among the sub-Saharan countries heavily affected by the HIV-AIDS pandemic. Approximately 72,000 new cases of HIV occur annually among adults ages 15 to 64 years (Ministry of Health, Community Development, Gender, Elderly and Children, Tanzania and Ministry of Health, Zanzibar, 2018). The PMTCT program, implemented in public facilities from 2000 to 2004, offers a range of healthcare services that reduce the risks of mother-to-child transmission of HIV during pregnancy, delivery, and breastfeeding periods. The specific services include HIV testing and counseling for pregnant women (and their partners), delivery of ARV prophylaxis or treatment, safer delivery practices, counseling and support related to breastfeeding of the infant, testing of the infant, as well as treatment for mothers and children living with HIV. However, a number of issues were associated with the implementation of PMTCT in Tanzania.

First, the information system was built on the assumption that a patient would attend her nearest clinic regularly, and therefore it did not have the functionality to transfer patient information between clinics. This assumption did not hold, however, for a number of reasons. For instance, patients feared the social stigma associated with an HIV diagnosis and either avoided seeking healthcare or sought treatment in other facilities where they would not be recognized. Sometimes the patient's nearest clinic did not have test kits or drugs, nor did it offer a complete maternity service (i.e., including delivery services), and women would have to be referred to another clinic. Additionally, and while the PMTCT program is usually offered under the umbrella of maternal and child health, an HIV-positive patient would also receive health services from home-based care services, and other clinics such as HIV/AIDS clinics' Care and Treatment Centers (CTC), as well as the occasional TB clinic. As it is rare, especially in rural areas, that care facilities provide comprehensive services for CTC, TB care, antenatal and postnatal care, vaccinations and dispensation of ARV drugs, an HIV-positive pregnant woman would often have to travel to access use of different services.

Secondly, our empirical studies indicate that the PMTCT program was launched with information systems tools that did not adequately take into account the social context of the patients and the real-life working conditions of the health workers (Shidende et al., 2014). For example, in the absence of an HIS that connected the clinics, pregnant women had to carry referral forms, test results, and personal cards with them, and thus were given the primary responsibility for the coordination of their care trajectories. Managerial information needs were prioritized such that they primarily covered data elements necessary to report on the number of clients who had been tested, who were found to be HIV positive, or who enrolled into the PMTCT program. As a result, the existing information tools provided did not support the identification and tracking of clients who did not seek services or who dropped out. In order to be able to track patients who dropped out and follow up patients across services and facilities, a multitude of local and informal documentation practices emerged in the PMTCT clinics (Shidende, 2005; Shidende et al., 2014). For example, health workers would communicate by mobile phone with their peers located in other facilities to learn about certain patients' attendance or seek to trace patients who had stopped attending PMTCT services. *Ad-hoc* registers were created in ordinary exercise books bought in local markets. While these informal systems may have helped health workers address their urgent needs for information to support the health service delivery, these also contributed to fragmentation of the overall HIS, as these differed across clinics.

In South Africa, the health system and HIS entity can also be viewed as reflecting tree-by-tree thinking. For instance, a TB manager is responsible for knowing all about his/her particular area and to demonstrate that knowledge by reporting on TB statistics, collected by the TB nurse in the TB information system. While there are forums for cooperation and sharing information, many managerial positions are accountable for progress toward certain disease-specific indicators. Consequently, managers are compelled to dedicate the majority of their working hours to validating and reporting these data. However, program-specific data often reflect the health issue (i.e., TB) rather than the patients who suffer from that illness (Koivu, 2015).

Drawing more attention to the context of use of an HIS, as well as the need for interaction and coordination between different parts of the healthcare system, has the potential to avoid some of the problems we have illustrated here. Moreover, these examples serve to demonstrate the importance of applying a forest thinking, rather than a tree-by-tree thinking approach for HIS.

Improving Data Quality—With Factors or Operational Thinking?

We next contrast *factors thinking* with *operational thinking*. Factors thinking refers to the notion that people often think in terms of lists of factors that influence some outcome. However, those lists do not usually explain how each factor brings about causality. Operational thinking, on the other hand, aims to capture the nature and structure of the investigated process and understand how behaviors are generated (Richmond, 1997).

As a practical example, let us consider the issue of HIS data quality. Data quality issues can be found around the world, but data quality is of particular concern in LMIC contexts, where many HIS are newly initiated or can be paper based. The quality of data is important, not only for patient care but also for monitoring the performance of health services. Data collected and presented should be accurate, complete, reliable, legible, and accessible to those who are authorized to use it (World Health Organization, 2008).

Traditional evaluations of data quality focus on particular attributes of data, such as the dimensions of accuracy and completeness. These evaluations may list factors that are associated or correlate with limited data quality, such as insufficient supervision and feedback, or inadequate investments in human resources or infrastructure. Consistent with a factors-thinking approach, these assessments may provide measurable information that can be used to make recommendations for improving data quality (e.g., increasing training or paying attention to the appropriate design of HIS tools), operational thinking invites us to look around at the real-world process and ask "is this how it really works?" (Richmond, 1993).

In virtually all health systems there exist several data flow processes that transfer information from the community to national levels. We argue that insightful analysis into these processes may add value to "traditional" factor thinking-based investigations when trying to improve the quality of data with those flows. A factor-thinking approach may focus for instance on attributes related to data capturers and other health professionals, such as their education level or their attitudes. Further, a factor-thinking approach might identify these attributes as potential causes of data quality problems, and to mitigate this, offer as a response the raising of awareness through education, or introducing sanctions and incentives to stimulate the desired behavior. On the other hand, operational thinking would seek to find out more about the true nature of the reporting process in that particular work environment.

Our example comes from the PMTCT program in Tanzania, where incomplete recording and inaccurate reports are common. The health workers routinely reported information such as the total number of children registered in the PMTCT service in the current month, the number of children confirmed as HIV-positive during the first testing (at four to six weeks), second testing (at eighteen months), and third testing (when breastfeeding ends), and the number of children referred to HIV clinics. This type of information gathering required that the health workers go through their register books to aggregate figures to enter into the monthly report. The use of varying formats for patient identification (IDs) used across the various information collection tools impacted on the work burden and subsequent data quality. For example, nurses might immunize a child or provide nevirapine syrup to a child born from an HIV-positive mother without recording these actions on the labor and delivery card. Consequently, inaccurate reports were found to have been forwarded to the higher levels of the health system (Shidende, 2014). Further, it was noted that health workers had multiple roles to fulfil including those related to patient well-being, information management, and medical equipment and supplies resource management. Strategies and guidelines to address data quality, however, tend to focus on information related logic (e.g., data generation cycle points) without taking into account the aforementioned practical challenges.

The reasons for incomplete recording and reporting, however, may also stem from what is happening in the community. Some of our study areas, such as the underprivileged townships of South Africa, are among the most disadvantaged places in world, with high population density and large proportions of sick and otherwise vulnerable people. A limited number of health staff and the busy and crowded public health clinics mean that often only the sickest will attend, waiting all day to be treated. Persistent resource constraints may lead to diminished attention to prevention and health promotion, which in turn increases the number of seriously ill patients in the long term. In South Africa, many health workers are exhausted and experience the pressure of these work challenges while simultaneously struggling in their own personal lives. Moreover, the health workers may be suffering largely the same illnesses and hardships as the community they serve.

Consider, for instance, a data capturer, whose duties consist largely of manually capturing data from sheets and transferring these to registers or to a computer. Having a low education and income level, he or she is also living in a township where most of the residents do not feel safe in their homes. Given these circumstances, it is unsurprising that our study found a lack of "buy-in" across various health worker cadres toward reporting tasks, as well as limitations in the ability to appreciate the importance of accurate data and the rationale of HIS. We argue that this is not merely an attitude or motivation issue but that the difficulties in people's daily life further impact on their ability to buy in and commit to, and concentrate on the tasks at hand. In other words, the environment that health workers live and work in every day does not support the full use of their capacities. How the hardships of township life may affect the data capturers' buy-in to reporting duties is a step toward operational thinking approach, as it is aimed toward understanding how behavior is generated. Understanding this may lead to more effective interventions rather than merely implementing strict accountability lines, sanctions, and incentives.

Conclusion and Lesson Learned

New analytical methods are necessary to tackle the chronic problems facing HIS where the resources are at their most scarce. This chapter offers a number of case examples of the challenges facing HIS in LMIC settings. These include the practice of implementing disease-specific subsystems, which risk evolving into a fragmented, expensive HIS architecture; the focus on individual HIS components rather than the relationships between them and contexts around them, often resulting in inefficiencies; and limitations to the traditional responses to the persistent data quality issues that impede data usage for health improvement. Indeed, while the traditional evaluations of HIS often have a strong technological or managerial focus, they may fail to illuminate the contexts that determine interventions' acceptability, sustainability, and ultimately their success or failure.

In this chapter, we have shown that systems thinking can and should be applied to these challenges. HIS design and implementation processes are costly and complicated. However, if HIS developers, architects, and those who make decisions to implement them are informed by systems-thinking approaches, there is a better chance of reaping the benefits expected from the system. Additionally, and while there is value in understanding the components and the context of HIS, applying systems thinking may add a further layer of knowledge by approaching problems in a way that takes into account technical, social, historical contexts, while acknowledging the various influence of stakeholders. Moreover, systems-thinking approaches call on us to reflect on dynamic and holistic approaches (causes and solutions) that take into account HIS' multifaceted interconnections between its various components (Adam & de Savigny, 2012) such as the actors at different levels of the health system, work practices, IT, and infrastructure.

To summarize, in this chapter we have shown that systems thinking may help HIS researchers, health workers, managers, and policy-makers to design better strategies for resolving health information challenges. A systems-thinking approach, which guides its users to consider interconnections among sub-components, allows us to see the relationships between HIS and the socio-economic context. While we argue that systems-thinking approaches cannot replace the use of other theories within the HIS field, it offers a layer of complementarity to tackle challenges and provide solutions. Given the "information" building block's effects on other health system building blocks, the implementation of HIS requires a systems-thinking approach, and further studies should be conducted to understand how this approach should be used to inform the design, implementation, and study of HIS in LMIC settings.

References

Abdusamadovich, L. M. (2013). *Global standards and local health information system applications: Understanding their interplay in the context of Tajikistan.* (PhD, Faculty of Mathematics and Natural Sciences, University of Oslo, Norway).

Adam, T., & de Savigny, D. (2012). Systems thinking for strengthening health systems in LMICs: Need for a paradigm shift. *Health Policy and Planning, 27*(suppl 4), iv1–iv3.

Agbo, C. C., Mahmoud, Q. H., & Eklund, J. M. (2019). Blockchain technology in healthcare: A systematic review. *Healthcare (Basel, Switzerland), 7*(2), 56. https://doi.org/10.3390/healthcare7020056

Boulle, A., Heekes, A., Tiffin, N., Smith, M., Mutemaringa, T., Zinyakatira, N., ... Vallabhjee, K. (2019). Data centre profile: The provincial health data centre of the Western Cape province, South Africa. *International Journal of Population Data Science*, 4. https://doi.org/10.23889/ijpds.v4i2.1143

Chilundo, B. (2004). *Integrating information systems of disease-specific health programs in low income countries: The case study of Mozambique.* (PhD thesis, Faculty of Medicine, University of Oslo, Oslo).

Chilundo, B., & Aanestad, M. (2005). Negotiating multiple rationalities in the process of integrating the information systems of disease specific health programmes. *The Electronic Journal of Information Systems in Developing Countries, 20*(2), 1–28.

Heeks, R. (2002). Information systems and developing countries: Failure, success and local improvisations. *The Information Society, 18*(2), 101–112.

Koivu, A. (2015). *Key challenges in the current TB & HIV information system in South Africa. A case study in Khayelitsha, Western Cape.* (Doctoral dissertation. Trinity College, Dublin, 2015).

Koivu, A., Mavengere, N., Ruohonen, M. J., Hederman, L., & Grimson, J. (2017). Exploring the information and ICT skills of health professionals in low- and middle-income countries. In T. Brinda, N. Mavengere, I. Haukijärvi, C. Lewin, & D. Passey (Eds.), *Stakeholders and information technology in education. SaITE 2016. IFIP Advances in Information and Communication Technology* (pp. 152–162). Cham: Springer.

Kossi, E. K., Sæbø, J. I., Braa, J., Jalloh, M. M., & Manya, A. (2012). Developing decentralised health information systems in developing countries—Cases from Sierra Leone and Kenya. *The Journal of Community Informatics, 9*(2). https://doi.org/10.15353/joci.v9i2.3164

Kumar, M., Gotz, D., Nutley, T., & Smith, J. B. (2018). Research gaps in routine health information system design barriers to data quality and use in low- and middle-income countries: A literature review. *International Journal of Health Planning and Management, 33,* e1–e9.

Meribole, E. C., Makinde, O. A., Oyemakinde, A., Oyediran, K. A., Atobatele, A., Fadeyibi, F. A., ... Orobaton, N. (2018). The Nigerian health information system policy review of 2014: The need, content, expectations and progress. *Health Information Libraries Journal, 35*(4), 285–297.

Ministry of Health, Community Development, Gender, Elderly and Children, Tanzania and Ministry of Health, Zanzibar. (2018). *Tanzania HIV Impact Survey (THIS) 2016–2017: Final report.* Dar es Salaam, Tanzania: Ministry of Health, Community Development, Gender, Elderly and Children, Tanzania.

Mphatswe, W., Mate, K. S., Bennett, B., Ngidi, H., Reddy, J., Barker, P. M., & Rollins, N. (2012). Improving public health information: A data quality intervention in KwaZulu-Natal, South Africa. *Bulletin of the World Health Organization, 90*(3), 176–182.

Mwanyika, H., Lubinski, D., Anderson, R., Chester, K., Makame, M., Steele, M., & de Savigny, D. (2011). Rational systems design for health information systems in low-income countries: An enterprise architecture approach. *Journal of Enterprise Architecture, 7*(4), 60–69.

Nyella, E. (2009). Challenges in health information systems integration: Zanzibar Experience. *2009 International Conference on Information and Communication Technologies and Development (ICTD)*, pp. 243–251. doi:10.1109/ICTD.2009.5426679

Pan, G., Hackney, R., & Pan, S. L. (2008). Information systems implementation failure: Insights from prism. *International Journal of Information Management, 28*(4), 259–269.

Poppe, O., Jolliffe, B., Adaletey, D. L., Braa, J., & Manya, A. S. (2013). Cloud computing for health information in Africa? Comparing the case of Ghana to Kenya. *Journal of Health Informatics in Africa, 1*(1). https://doi.org/10.12856/JHIA-2013-v1-i1-45

Richmond, B. (1993). Systems thinking: Critical thinking skills for the 1990s and beyond. *System Dynamics Review, 9*(2), 113–133.

Richmond, B. (1997). Forest thinking. *Systems Thinking, 8*(10), 6–7.

Richmond, B. (1997). The "thinking" in systems thinking: How can we make it easier to master. *Systems Thinking, 8*(2), 1–5.

Richmond, B. (2010). The thinking in systems thinking: eight critical skills. In J. Richmond, L., Stuntz, K. Richmond, & J. Egner (Eds.), *Tracing connections: Voices of systems thinkers.* Lebanon, NH: ISEE Systems and Acton, MA: The Critical Learning Exchange.

Sæbø, J. I., Kossi, E. K., Titlestad, O. H., Tohouri, R. R., & Braa, J. (2011). Comparing strategies to integrate health information systems following a data warehouse approach in four countries. *Information Technology for Development, 17*(1), 42–60.

Sauerborn, R., & Lippeveld, T. (2000). Introduction. In T. Lippeveld, R., Sauerborn, & C. Bodart (Eds.), *Design and implementation of health information systems* (pp. 1–14). Geneva: World Health Organization.

Shidende, N. H., Grisot, M., & Aanestad, M. (2014). Coordination challenges in collaborative practices in the prevention of mother to child transmission of HIV in Tanzania. *Journal of Health Informatics in Africa, 2*(1), 1–17. https://doi.org/10.12856/JHIA-2014-v2-i1-88

Shidende, N. H. (2005). *Challenges and approaches to the integration of HIS: Case studies from Tanzania.* (Masters' thesis, University of Oslo, 2005).

Shidende, N. H. (2014). Challenges in implementing patient-centred information systems in Tanzania: An activity theory perspective. *The Electronic Journal of Information Systems in Developing Countries, 64*(1), 1–20.

Shidende, N. H. (2015). *Distributed collaborative practices in resource restricted settings. Ethnographic studies from the Tanzanian primary healthcare information system.* (Faculty of Mathematics and Natural Science, PhD dissertation, University of Oslo, 2015).

World Health Organization. (2008). *Health Information Systems: Toolkit on monitoring health systems strengthening.* Geneva: World Health Organization. Available from: https://www.who.int/healthinfo/statistics/toolkit_hss/EN_PDF_Toolkit_HSS_InformationSystems.pdf

World Health Organization. (2010). *Monitoring the building blocks of health systems: A handbook of indicators and their measurement strategies*. Geneva: World Health Organization.

9
Assistive Technology
The Importance of a Systems-Thinking Approach

Jessica Power, Emma M. Smith, Ikenna D. Ebuenyi, and Malcolm MacLachlan

Introduction

Functional difficulties in daily life can be attributable to long- and short-term disability, changes associated with aging, or illnesses and injuries which prevent an individual from maintaining independence. For those individuals, assistive products (APs) (e.g., glasses, communication aids, walking sticks, prosthetics, hearing aids) can improve quality of life, allowing them to minimize or remove functional limitations and barriers to participation in society. However, the World Health Organization estimates that only one in ten of these individuals receives the APs they need, with an estimated 1 billion people in need of assistive products globally (World Health Organization, 2016b). For example, 360 million people live with moderate to profound hearing loss while only 10% receive products, and 70 million people require a wheelchair but only 5–15% of those in need receive one (World Health Organization, 2016a). This low level of coverage on a global scale is partially attributable to complexities in the needs, supply, and provision of APs. A systems-thinking approach is required to address the complexity of how APs are perceived, designed, produced, manufactured, distributed, serviced, and financed (World Health Organization, 2014; Khasnabis, Mirza, & MacLachlan, 2015).

What is Assistive Technology?

Assistive technology (AT) is a generic term that may refer to different types of APs and may incorporate various aspects of assistive technology systems.

An AP is any product (including equipment, instruments, and software), either "specially designed and produced or generally available, whose primary purpose is to maintain or improve an individual's functioning and independence and thereby promote their wellbeing" (Khasnabis et al., 2015). APs are different from medical devices in that they are outside or on the body, while medical devices are inside or inserted to the body. Common APs include wheelchairs, hearing aids, spectacles, canes, low vision products, and products which assist with communication.

Assistive Technology Systems (ATS) refer to "the development and application of organised knowledge, skills, procedures, and policies relevant to the provision, use,

Jessica Power, Emma M. Smith, Ikenna D. Ebuenyi, and Malcolm MacLachlan, *Assistive Technology* In: *Systems Thinking for Global Health*. Edited by: Fiona Larkan, Frédérique Vallières, Hasheem Mannan, and Naonori Kodate, Oxford University Press.
 DOI: 10.1093/oso/9780198799498.003.0009

and assessment of assistive products" (Khasnabis et al., 2015). ATS may therefore include aspects of ICT (information, communication, and technology) that are not specific to assistive products but which may facilitate them.

Why is Systems Thinking Critical for Assistive Technology?

MacLachlan and Scherer suggest there are a range of interrelated factors involved in the AT system and that these form interlocking components that require a systems-thinking approach (MacLachlan & Scherer, 2018). These components may be described as the "10 Ps." The first of these is *People*; that is, the service or assistive technology users who are intended to be the primary beneficiaries of assistive technology. They note that the World Health Organization has identified four additional strategic drivers for supporting an AT system. These are *Policy, Products, Personnel* (meaning those who have skills relevant to the assessment, training and supporting of AT users), and *Provision*, which concerns the broader organizational context through which AT is provided. However, MacLachlan and Scherer argue that these factors sit within a broader ecosystem, where a range of situational factors are also critical to the extent to which, and the ways in which an AT system does or doesn't work. These situational factors include *Procurement* (where products come from or are acquired), *Place* (referring to distinctive geographical, cultural, or social issues related to AT), *Pace* (how rapidly a health or social system can change its practices), *Promotion* (the need to promote positive images of AT users), and *Partnership* (the collaborative working of different stakeholders throughout the system). An additional P might be the role of *Power* relationships, particularly where AT is provided in the context of international aid; and thus, how power influence other Ps, such as Procurement, Pace, or which sort of Products are prioritized. Addressing these complexities regarding assistive technology is critical for ensuring access to quality and affordable products and services for all who require them. Here we provide a different, but we believe very complementary way of conceptualizing systems thinking for assistive technology. We conceptualize embedded layers of an interconnected system where each layer is, in fact, a system in its own right. Figure 9.1 shows embedded and interconnected layers which are relevant to AT.

As seen in Figure 9.1, each level is embedded within the next and represents a system of its own, each with different stakeholders and complexity. In this respect, our model represents a *holon*, something that is simultaneously a whole and a part (Koestler, 1968). For Koestler, the holon concept allows integration of individual-level analysis with more collective, macro-level analysis. Koestler also used the term *holarchy* to describe a series of linked but independent wholes, organized hierarchically, such as cell–tissue–organ–organism. To describe an organism as just a bunch of cells, or cells as just divisions of an organism overlooks their intrinsic wholeness and their connectedness, that which gives meaning to the overall system in which they operate.

When discussing AT, it is critical to begin at the individual level or the person who requires the use of AT. The AT needs of individuals are unique, and in many cases complex, as they are dependent on the person's functional abilities, activity, and participation needs, and the context and environment around them. Therefore, even at

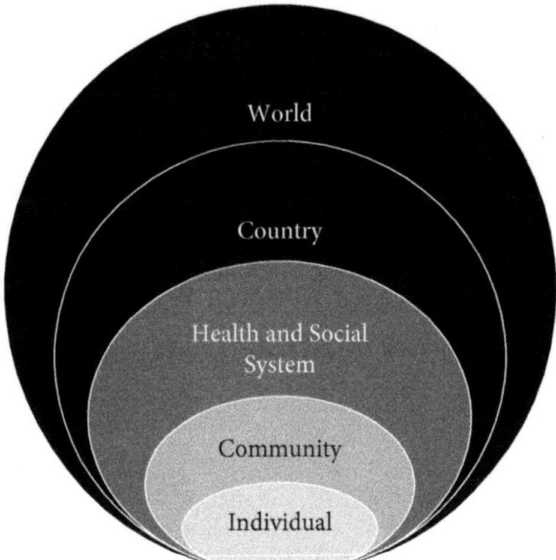

Figure 9.1 The Assistive Technology Embedded Systems Thinking (ATEST) Model

the individual level, a systems approach is necessary to deliver the right AT to meet their needs. Individuals are embedded within communities and complex social structures. Each of these communities is also a complex system as it is a collection of individuals who may each play a distinct role within the community. Communities may take the form of family units, school or work communities, or the broader community where an individual lives. Regardless of the form of community, the provision of AT must be considered within this broader system.

Individuals and communities operate within a health and social system which typically determines the mechanisms available for the provision and procurement of AT. These health and social systems are often governed by complex institutional regulations, which must consider the needs of all the individuals within the community while also balancing public interest, financial considerations, supply of APs, and the role of service providers, including health workers. These health and social systems are typically embedded within government and policy systems at the national or country level. A country is itself a complex system which must consider the resources available to fulfil the needs of its citizens, the competing interests and requirements of different stakeholders, such as government, civil society, and industry, as well as the political priorities of whatever political party or individual is in power.

Finally, at the global level, cooperation between countries provides opportunities for larger-scale approaches to meeting global supply and demand for APs. This may involve countries collaborating on the procurement of APs, perhaps from a market-shaping perspective (MacLachlan et al., 2018), that tries to entice but control the activities of multinationals, to ensure that social and health needs are met by industry rather than cherry-picking the well-off and neglecting those with little purchasing power. At the global level it is key that the systemic approach to AT coincides with internationally agreed global system targets, such as the Sustainable Development Goals (SDG) (Tebbutt et al., 2016). Table 9.1 illustrates how AT may be addressed at each level of the embedded system shown earlier.

Table 9.1 Considerations and examples of systems in assistive technology

Level	Considerations	Example
Individual	Personal capabilities, activity, and participation, personal context	An individual with a cervical spinal cord injury may require multiple APs in a coordinated system, with associated professional and social support, to promote participation in their community.
Community	Inclusion of persons who use AT, social structures, supports	A classroom may have multiple students using AT, which requires support from teachers, educational assistants, and engagement of all students in the class.
Health and Social System	Provision processes, access to and supply of APs, human resources to deliver services, budget	Community health centers may have a clinic which provides AT services to multiple individuals within one or more communities, and must balance the human resources, costs, and products to deliver services equitably, effectively, and ethically.
Country	Legislation, policies, and strategies, import and export regulation, health and social system funding, meeting global responsibilities	A country may have an ATP which stipulates how services are to be provided within health and social systems, meeting the obligations in the United Nations Convention on the Rights of Persons with Disabilities (UNCRPD), while providing assistance to countries with fewer resources to obtain necessary APs.
World	International conventions, import and export regulations, meeting global supply and demand	The WHO's GATE initiative provides global leadership to meet national obligations to the CRPD and promotes cooperation on mass-market production of APs to reduce cost on a global scale and facilitate meeting the SDGs in an inclusive manner.

Source: data from Tebbutt, E., et al. (2016). Assistive products and the Sustainable Development Goals (SDGs). *Globalization and Health*, *12*(1), 1–6. Retrieved from https://doi.org/10.1186/s12992-016-0220-6.

Specific Systems Challenges in Assistive Technology

(i) Unique socio-economic contexts

AT presents specific systems challenges that need to be considered. For example, AT is delivered in diverse contexts. High-income country (HIC) and low- and middle-income country (LMIC) settings have very different population needs, resources, and existing health and social system structures.

(ii) Diverse stakeholders

AT has multiple stakeholder groups including user groups, professional groups, donor agencies, United Nation agencies, member states, researchers, and private industry.

With such diverse stakeholders come differing priorities. While keeping the AP user at the center of the process, consideration also needs to be given to what actors are present and how they may interconnect, both with overlapping and with differing agendas.

(iii) Estimating and meeting national and global need and demand

Estimating need at the national and global level relies on data collection systems which specifically address APs. In addition to seeking information on functional limitations which may be indicative of AP need, data collection systems at the national and global level ideally collect comparable data on current AP use and unmet need (Smith et al., 2019). There may also be a difference between unmet need (those who require APs but do not have them) and demand (those who are seeking access to APs). Understanding the factors which differentiate unmet need from demand (such as awareness, affordability, or geographical proximity) is critical to ensuring that global supply of APs meets the need for them.

The supply of APs is clearly not meeting demand. In addition, the type of products in development are not affordable, particularly for LMICs. There is a bias in research and development toward high-tech AP focused on HIC, with less emphasis on low-cost, high-quality solutions, and those appropriate for LMIC settings (Borg, Lindström, & Larsson, 2009; Iacono, Lyon, & West, 2011). Economies of scale are not being utilized in many cases. There are also issues around suitability of products for differing contexts; for example hearing aids that need specialized skills for molding, which may not be feasible at community level; or hearing aids that do not function well in humid climates (McPherson, 2011, 2014).

Systems Thinking Applied to AT

(iv) Global leadership

Recognizing the challenge of addressing AT on a global scale, the World Health Organization (WHO) developed the Global Cooperation on Assistive Technology (GATE). This partnership is led by the WHO, and includes key stakeholders in AT including user groups, donor agencies, international organizations, academia, and professional groups. GATE has one clear aim: to improve access to high-quality, affordable AT on a global scale. An example of a global initiative to achieve this can be seen in Box 9.1.

(v) A framework for policy guidance

Currently, there is a lack of a structured AT-system framework. Most countries do not have national policies or actions plans on AT and they have little guidance or support

Box 9.1 AT2030—Providing Global and National Leadership in AT Innovation

AT2030 is a project funded by the UK Department for International Development which is addressing access to AT on a global scale through research, partnership, and innovation. AT2030 is supporting innovative technologies and approaches to AT delivery, working with governments, UN agencies, and key global partners—such as the Clinton Health Access Initiative (CHAI)—to address the need for global procurement, the challenge in estimating and meeting AT supply and demand, and working to reduce stigma associated with disability and AT use. AT2030 is an example of addressing different levels of systems simultaneously, understanding the interconnected links between systems.

on what elements to include in AT planning. In order to achieve national integrated AT systems, including human resource needs and service pathways, supportive national policies for AT are needed (MacLachlan et al., 2018). These national policies should indicate how such a system might be developed. A framework is currently under development to provide guidance to policy-makers who are developing these structures. This framework will not aim to be prescriptive but will identify key components for inclusion that could be adapted to suit local settings and needs. At the national level, this will be modified to fit the unique context and/or incorporate aspects of the framework into existing policies (e.g., national disability policy, national rehabilitative policy).

A framework must place emphasis on the inter-sectoral nature of AT. Relevant policy requires action from a variety of sectors in addition to health and social services, (e.g., labor, finance, social security, housing, transportation, justice, and rural and urban development sectors). Where there are inter-sectoral links, it is critical that key components of the policy are explicit so that the roles of all sectors are clear (World Health Organization, 2016a). This inter-sectoral approach stresses the importance of a clear, strong governance structure across sectors (Hussey, MacLachlan, Mji, 2016; McVeigh et al., 2016). For example, in Afghanistan, given the persistent conflict in the country, laws have historically defined disability within the category of war-related injuries, and have called for material provision for them including medical, financial, and economic reintegration, thus contributing to the inter-sectoral nature of the policy (The Comprehensive National Disability Policy in Afghanistan, 2003).

While a policy framework can offer guidance on relevant policy content and policy process issues, the development of national policies should also incorporate other examples of best practice in terms of policy development and implementation. This is particularly important regarding the need to ensure that vulnerable and/or marginalized groups are full participants in the process and are equitable beneficiaries of its outcomes (Amin et al., 2011; Huss & MacLachlan, 2016). An example of a national systems approach to AT provision can be seen in Box 9.2.

Box 9.2 APPLICABLE: A Systems Approach to Developing an AT Policy for Malawi

The APPLICABLE (Assistive Product List Implementation Creating Enablement of inclusive SDGs) Project, funded by the Irish Research Council, is working with a diverse group of stakeholders representing government ministries, civil service and disabled people's organizations, international non-governmental organizations (NGOs), and the private sector, to develop an AT policy for Malawi. This approach addresses the contextual barriers to accessing APs, service provision, and human resources, to develop a sustainable, equitable, and context-relevant policy, which considers each systems layer of individual, community, health and social systems, the country, and participation in the global AT dialog and marketplace, while assisting Malawi to achieve the SDGs in an inclusive manner.

(vi) Alternative service delivery models

The optimum service delivery model for AT is likely to vary depending on context, resources, and the existing systems infrastructure. AT, where possible, should be available at community level. Some products should be relatively easy to provide in the community, while others will require more specialist skills. It will be important to identify which AT fall into which of these categories. With this information a network of specialist referral centers connected to a community context, such as a primary health care infrastructure, will be needed (Smith et al., 2018). This will require a fluid system of communications where there is easy and appropriate referral between the two.

Service provision will be reliant on production of products at the scale necessary to meet the country's needs, the supply chain, and the resourcing of products, as well as their maintenance. One possibility for this is a system of large-scale production at the *global level*, with fabrication at the *country level*, with oversight of demand and supply at the level of the *health and social care system*, while fitting, maintenance, and continued support occur at the *community level*. However, there would be a need to ensure the necessary standards were met at each level. It is also important to build on the skills, experience, and ingenuity of those who may have been involved for many years in smaller-scale provision and/or customization at the community level.

It is important to again emphasize the need for inter-sectoralism, where AT is seen as relevant and empowering across all domains of life and not in a health or rehabilitation silo. This forms part of the tremendous challenge of systems thinking, not just the interdependence of different elements within a system but also for different systems to themselves interplay in a constructive, coordinated, and empowering way.

(vii) Human resources models for AT provision

Provision of AT currently relies heavily on specialized professionals, often with a professional group addressing a single, specific functional domain. For example, if a person requires AT relating to mobility, they often need access to a physiotherapist; for AT relating to continence, they may need referral to a nurse; for AT relating to dressing, access to an occupational therapist. Such a service model only works under certain assumptions (i.e., specialized professionals present at all the places where such services may be needed). Many persons using APs have multiple functional impairments and require multiple products. Obtaining separate referrals and attending separate professionals, often at different centers, is an inefficient and costly method of delivery, especially in resource-poor settings. The number of APs needed, on average, increases as a person ages; thus with the aging population the need for multiple products across multiple functional domains will dramatically increase (Dahlin-Ivanoff & Sonn, 2004; Dahlin Ivanoff & Sonn, 2005; Eide & Oderud, 2009; Kylberg, Löfqvist, Horstmann, & Iwarsson, 2013).

Conventional—default—approaches to AT provision assume that the skill sets of certain professions are necessary to provide all types of APs (including even basic APs). They also often assume that a person may only need one type of AT or have one functional limitation at a time. In most parts of the world, these assumptions are not met. The current human resources for health (HRH) crisis arises from a severe lack of health professionals in LMIC (Samb et al., 2009). This is particularly the case for allied health professionals, many of whom are traditional AP providers (Smith et al., 2018).

Task-shifting to professionals who require shorter training periods has been shown to be effective across maternal and child health and HIV (Callaghan, Ford, & Schneider, 2010; Fulton et al., 2011; Joshi et al., 2014). Task-shifting within community-based rehabilitation (CBR) settings is also developing (MacLachlan et al., 2011) and while there has not yet been enough evidence generated to make definitive conclusions on effectiveness in this setting, its use is encouraged by the WHO CBR guidelines (Mannan, MacLachlan, & McAuliffe, 2012). In systems thinking for HRH and AT, the shortage of health professionals in addition to availability of professionals at community level calls for much greater attention to task-shifting as a mechanism to optimize provision of AT. One way of addressing this need is to explore the tasks that are most commonly undertaken by personnel involved in AT provision; this method of job task analysis has been used to identify core skills used by physiotherapists and occupational therapist working at community level in similar settings, and the skills used by AT professionals (O'Dowd, MacLachlan, Khasnabis, & Geiser, 2015; Oggero & MacLachlan, 2019; Smith et al., 2018).

Inter-connectedness of Elements

In considering the constraints and enablers for access to APs, the inter-connectedness of these elements becomes clear. For example, to ensure suitable high-quality

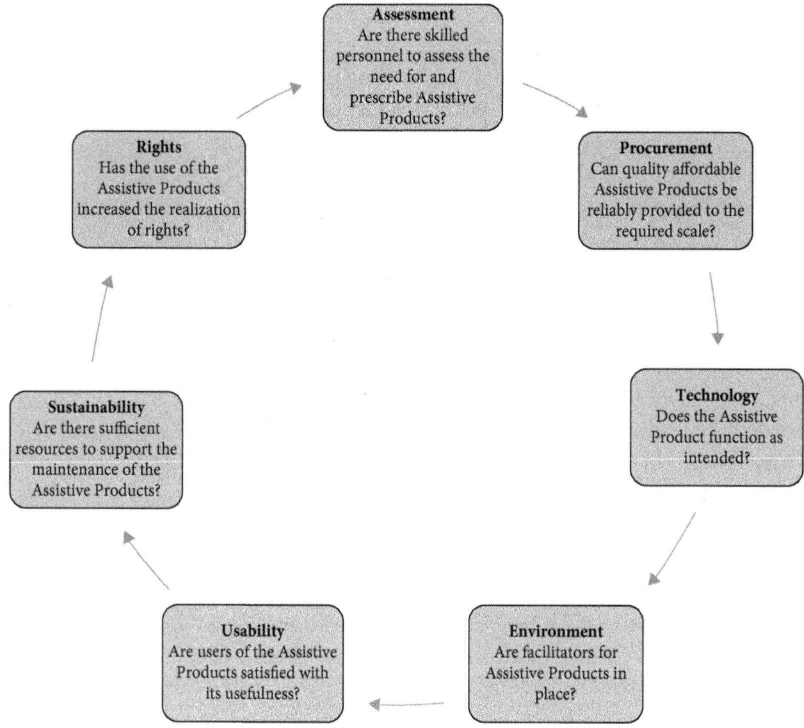

Figure 9.2 Some key questions for assistive technology systems

Adapted with permission from Khasnabis, C., Mirza, Z., & MacLachlan, M. (2015). Opening the GATE to inclusion for people with disabilities. *The Lancet*, *386*(10010), 2229–2230. Retrieved from https://doi.org/10.1016/S0140-6736(15)01093-4

affordable products are available, multiple stakeholders must be involved (e.g., researchers, developers, private industry, AT users, practitioners, donors). However, even if adequate supply of suitable affordable products became available, that supply would be insufficient without HRH to provide them, referral and delivery systems, policy, partnerships, funding, affordability, and quality (Khasnabis et al., 2015). In addition, the APs themselves must be fit for purpose across their respective contexts, so liaising with local AT users to develop of APs is essential. Some key questions to support AT planning can be seen in Figure 9.2.

Challenges to a Systems-Thinking Approach

The use of a systems-thinking approach has many positive aspects. However, it can also have drawbacks. Assessing complex environments with multiple actors, differing needs, and varying agendas can require substantial resources to initiate the process. Such factors may make it more difficult to achieve consensus among key stakeholders. Thus, rather than "thinking big" it may at times be more prudent to aim for "small wins" (Termeer & Dewulf, 2019), helping local producers to increase the scale of their well-established enterprises incrementally.

From a systems perspective, understanding the need for AT in a given population and ensuring APs are affordable are two key considerations for procurement. Generation of mass demand, guided by the Assistive Product List (APL), may allow for mass production and reduction of costs. Currently there are local providers who have a long history of developing and providing APs in their communities. Through development of the APL and use of economies of scale in the sourcing and production of APs, these local providers may be unable to compete with the costs and scale of demand. This may then drive these local providers out of business and potentially to lose their livelihoods. It is important to consider how to support local suppliers within the context of the system, while retaining the to-scale capabilities of large manufacturers. This allows the system to capitalize on the expertise and ingenuity of local supplies and to provide APs that are contextually appropriate and suitable to the needs of individual users while addressing concerns of cost and availability.

Liaison with multiple stakeholders takes time, has many moral and ethical considerations, and requires consensus, practicality, and expedient actions. Thus, we fully acknowledge that systems thinking for AT is not quick, unproblematic, or an easy approach; however, this approach addresses the complex realities of the AT environment and does so at the population level to enhance equitable access to high-quality, affordable products. Systems thinking aims to form the backdrop to a successful user experience, with the foreground being the person-to-person interaction between user and provider in accessible community locations. It is inevitable that "small wins" may be quicker and not require the inertia of systems change or systems evolution. The local context may therefore at times require a twin track approach of (i) small wins with faster, but modest gains in access to AT, and (ii) systems building and/or evolution with longer-term but substantial gains in access to AT.

Reflections and Conclusions on a Systems-Thinking Approach for AT

Access to high-quality, affordable AT requires complex systemic change involving interactions with many building blocks of the health and other sectoral systems, across diverse contexts and with multiple actors within different levels of the embedded systems. Change is required in how AT is perceived, designed, produced, manufactured, distributed, serviced, and financed (World Health Organization, 2014). Approaching this problem with a systems-thinking outlook is crucial to understanding the realities of the health and social systems, as well as systems in the cognate sector, in which AT is provided and used.

References

Amin, M., Maclachlan, M., Mannan, H., El Tayeb, S., El Khatim, A., Swartz, L., . . . Schneider, M. (2011). Equiframe: A framework for analysis of the inclusion of human rights and vulnerable groups in health policies. *Health and Human Rights*, *13*(2), 82–102.

Borg, J., Lindström, A., & Larsson, S. (2009). Assistive technology in developing countries: national and international responsibilities to implement the Convention on the Rights of Persons with Disabilities. *The Lancet*, 1863–1865. Retrieved from https://doi.org/10.1016/S0140-6736(09)61872-9

Callaghan, M., Ford, N., & Schneider, H. (2010). A systematic review of task-shifting for HIV treatment and care in Africa. *Human Resources for Health*, *8*, 1–9. Retrieved from https://doi.org/10.1186/1478-4491-8-8

Dahlin-Ivanoff, S., & Sonn, U. (2004). Use of assistive devices in daily activities among 85-years-old living at home focusing especially on the visually impaired. *Disability and Rehabilitation*, *26*, 1423–1430. Retrieved from https://doi.org/10.1080/09638280400000906

Dahlin Ivanoff, S., & Sonn, U. (2005). Changes in the use of assistive devices among 90-year-old persons. *Aging Clinical and Experimental Research*, *17*, 246–251. Retrieved from https://doi.org/10.1007/bf03324604

Eide, A., & Oderud, T. (2009). Assistive technology in low-income countries. In M. MacLachlan & L. Schwarts (Eds.), *Disability and international development: Towards inclusive global health* (pp. 149–160). New York: Springer Publishing Company. Retrieved from https://doi.org/10.1007/978-0-387-93840-0_10

Fulton, B. D., Scheffler, R. M., Sparkes, S. P., Auh, E. Y., Vujicic, M., & Soucat, A. (2011). Health workforce skill mix and task shifting in low income countries: A review of recent evidence. *Human Resources for Health*, *9*, 1–11. Retrieved from https://doi.org/10.1186/1478-4491-9-1

The Comprehensive National Disability Policy in Afghanistan. (2003). Transitional Islamic State of Afghanistan and Italian Cooperation. Kabul. Accessed from: https://www.who.int/disabilities/policies/documents/Afghanistan.pdf?ua=1. Accessed date 11th Oct 2021.

Huss, T., & Maclachlan, M. (2016). *Equity and Inclusion in Policy Processes (EquIPP): A framework to support equity & inclusion in the process of policy development, implementation and evaluation*. Dublin: Global Health Press.

Hussey, M., MacLachlan, M., & Mji, G. (2016). Barriers to the implementation of the health and rehabilitation articles of the United Nations convention on the rights of persons with disabilities in South Africa. *International Journal of Health Policy and Management*, *5*, 1–12. Retrieved from https://doi.org/10.15171/ijhpm.2016.117

Iacono, T., Lyon, K., & West, D. (2011). Non-electronic communication aids for people with complex communication needs. *International Journal of Speech-Language Pathology*, *13*(5), 399–410. doi:10.3109/17549507.2011.482162

Joshi, R., Alim, M., Kengne, A. P., Jan, S., Maulik, P. K., Peiris, D., & Patel, A. A. (2014). Task shifting for non-communicable disease management in low and middle income countries—A systematic review. *PloS One*, *9*(8), e103754. Retrieved from https://doi.org/10.1371/journal.pone.0103754

Khasnabis, C., Mirza, Z., & MacLachlan, M. (2015). Opening the GATE to inclusion for people with disabilities. *The Lancet*, *386*(10010), 2229–2230. Retrieved from https://doi.org/10.1016/S0140-6736(15)01093-4

Koestler, A. (1968). The ghost in the machine. Macmillan. New York.

Kylberg, M., Löfqvist, C., Horstmann, V., & Iwarsson, S. (2013). The use of assistive devices and change in use during the ageing process among very old Swedish people. *Disability and Rehabilitation: Assistive Technology*, *8*, 58–66. Retrieved from https://doi.org/10.3109/17483107.2012.699585

MacLachlan, M., Banes, D., Bell, D., Borg, J., Donnelly, B., Fembek, M., … Hooks, H. (2018). Assistive technology policy: A position paper from the first global research, innovation, and education on assistive technology (GREAT) summit. *Disability and Rehabilitation: Assistive Technology*, *13*(5), 454–466.

MacLachlan, M., McVeigh, J., Cooke, M., Ferri, D., Holloway, C., Austin, V., & Javadi, D. (2018). Intersections between systems thinking and market shaping for assistive technology: The SMART (systems-market for assistive and related technologies) thinking matrix. *International Journal of Environmental Research and Public Health, 15*(12), 2627–2642. Retrieved from https://doi.org/10.3390/ijerph15122627

MacLachlan, M., Mannan, H., & McAuliffe, E. (2011). Staff skills not staff types for community-based rehabilitation. *The Lancet, 377*(9782), 1988–1989. Retrieved from https://doi.org/10.1016/S0140-6736(10)61925-3

MacLachlan, M., & Scherer, M. (2018). Systems thinking for assistive technology: A commentary on the GREAT summit. *Disability and Rehabilitation: Assistive Technology, 13*(5), 492–496. Retrieved from https://doi.org/10.1080/17483107.2018.1472306

Mannan, H., MacLachlan, M., & McAuliffe, E. (2012). The human resources challenge to community based rehabilitation: The need for a scientific, systematic and coordinated global response. *Disability, CBR & Inclusive Development, 23*, 6–16.

McPherson, B. (2011). Innovative technology in hearing instruments: Matching needs in the developing world. *Trends in Amplification, 15*(4), 209–213. https://doi.org/10.1177/1084713811424887

McPherson, B. (2014). Hearing assistive technologies in developing countries: Background, achievements and challenges. *Disability and Rehabilitation: Assistive Technology, 9*, 360–364. https://doi.org/10.3109/17483107.2014.907365

McVeigh, J., MacLachlan, M., Gilmore, B., McClean, C., Eide, A. H., Mannan, H., . . . Normand, C. (2016). Promoting good policy for leadership and governance of health related rehabilitation: A realist synthesis. *Globalization and Health, 12*(49), 1–18. https://doi.org/10.1186/s12992-016-0182-8

O'Dowd, J., MacLachlan, M., Khasnabis, C., & Geiser, P. (2015). Towards a core set of clinical skills for health-related community based rehabilitation in low and middle income countries. *Disability, CBR & Inclusive Development, 26*(3), 5–43.

Oggero, G., & MacLachlan, M. (2019). Identifying a set of core skills to enable the provision of priority assistive products. In Natasha Layton & Johan Borg (eds.), *Global perspectives on assistive technology: Proceedings of the GReAT Consultation 2019* (*Vol. 2*, pp. 225–246). Geneva: World Health Organization.

Samb, B., Evans, T., Dybul, M., Atun, R., Moatti, J. P., Nishtar, S., . . . Van Lerberghe, W. (2009). An assessment of interactions between global health initiatives and country health systems. *The Lancet, 373*(9681), 2137–2169. Retrieved from https://doi.org/10.1016/S0140-6736(09)60919-3

Smith, E. M., Gowran, R. J., Mannan, H., Donnelly, B., Alvarez, L., Bell, D., . . . Wu, S. (2018). Enabling appropriate personnel skill-mix for progressive realization of equitable access to assistive technology. *Disability and Rehabilitation: Assistive Technology, 13*(5), 445–453. Retrieved from https://doi.org/10.1080/17483107.2018.1470683

Smith, Emma Maria, Rizzo Battistela, Li., Contepomi, S., Gowran, R. J., Kankipati, P., Layton, N. A., & Toro Hernandez, M. (2019). Measuring met and unmet assistive technology needs at the national level: Comparing national database collection tools across eight case countries. In N. A. Layton & J. Borg (Eds.), *Global perspectives on assistive technology: proceedings of the GReAT Consultation 2019* (*Vol. 1*, pp. 24–35). Geneva: World Health Organization.

Tebbutt, E., Brodmann, R., Borg, J., MacLachlan, M., Khasnabis, C., & Horvath, R. (2016). Assistive products and the Sustainable Development Goals (SDGs). *Globalization and Health, 12*(1), 1–6. Retrieved from https://doi.org/10.1186/s12992-016-0220-6

Termeer, C. J. A. M., & Dewulf, A. (2019). A small wins framework to overcome the evaluation paradox of governing wicked problems. *Policy and Society, 38*(2), 298–314. Retrieved from https://doi.org/10.1080/14494035.2018.1497933

World Health Organization. (2014). *Concept note: Opening the GATE for assistive health technology: Shifting the paradigm*. Geneva: World Health Organization.

World Health Organization. (2016a). *Assistive technology fact sheet*. Geneva: World Health Organization.

World Health Organization. (2016b). *Priority assistive products list: Improving access to assistive technology for everyone, everywhere*. Geneva: World Health Organization.

10
Responding to Health Needs in War and Armed Conflict
What Can Systems Thinking Contribute to Best Practice?

Marion Birch, Maria Kett, and Mike Rowson

Introduction

As has been noted in previous chapters, the uncertainty, complexity, and fluidity of war and armed conflict present both a challenge for systems thinking and a significant opportunity. Health programs are a key aspect of the humanitarian response to armed conflict. Effective health responses need to follow principles of best practice while interacting with an analysis of the needs and background of specific situations and taking into account a range of other actors. Systems thinking has the potential to assist in this analysis and in the design of flexible responses that remain focused while taking complex and changing situations into account.

Following one practical example as an introduction, this chapter considers how the principles of systems thinking—even if not identified as such—have contributed to an effective response to health needs as part of humanitarian programs in the recent past. It goes on to consider some situations which might have had a better outcome if there had been a greater use of the principles and tools of systems thinking. After a brief consideration of some areas where caution might be needed, it finally considers how an increase in the use of the principles and tools of systems thinking could enhance the response to health needs created by war and armed conflict in the future. Case studies and reports of field experience are used as well as academic articles and reports to make this chapter as practical and rooted in reality as possible.

Systems thinking has been described as "a useful framework for communicating about complex issues" (Kim, 2000) and is based on certain principles, including:

1. The need to understand "complex interconnections of circular causality" and
2. The need to understand situations at a variety of levels: events, patterns of events, systemic structure, and shared vision (Kim, 2000).

The relevance of these principles for health responses during armed conflict, and a potential application of systems thinking, can be illustrated by considering the following example of a practical dilemma—one that appears relatively simple—but in fact has "complex interconnections of circular causality."

A convoy carrying humanitarian assistance, including a range of health supplies, is stopped by a group of non-state actors who ask for a small number of bandages and

Marion Birch, Maria Kett, and Mike Rowson, *Responding to Health Needs in War and Armed Conflict* In: *Systems Thinking for Global Health.* Edited by: Fiona Larkan, Frédérique Vallières, Hasheem Mannan, and Naonori Kodate, Oxford University Press.
 DOI: 10.1093/oso/9780198799498.003.0010

dressings. If supplied the convoy will be allowed to continue. It is 4 p.m., there is another hour of travel to arrive at the convoy's destination, and curfew is at 6 p.m. The organization's health officer is travelling with the convoy. She reasons that they want a small amount of relatively cheap items (the convoy is also carrying medicines including antibiotics, saline fluids, and topical disinfectants, among other items in short supply) and she knows it will be risky if they do not arrive before curfew. She decides to give them the bandages and dressings and the convoy is allowed to continue, arriving in time at their destination, where a patient in urgent need of antibiotics is able to be treated.

This seems a straightforward action, resulting in safe arrival before curfew with all other items intact, but it could have various repercussions including:

- an expectation on the part of the non-state actors that if they stop convoys, they will be given supplies in the future.
- information about what happened being passed to government forces who also supply permits to travel in areas affected by the conflict, resulting in distrust and problems with future permits.
- criticism of the health officer as there are strict institutional rules about giving supplies to anyone for whom they are not intended.

All these repercussions may have further consequences.

If trust between the organization and government forces is compromised, they may be delayed at government checkpoints in the future, or not given permits to travel; if they are unable to travel, people may die due to lack of supplies.

There may be different attitudes to what has happened at different levels of the various organizations involved, and—as in systems thinking—the need to understand things at a variety of levels (Kim, 2000). The head office of the organization for which the health officer works may consider it a disciplinary issue; those who are closer to the ground—the health officer's immediate manager, for example—may understand the pressures she was under rather better. Those who are fighting on the ground in the government's armed forces, who have suffered because of the non-state actors, may find it harder to accept what was done than more senior officers who want to maintain an image of good relations with international organizations.

And so it goes on . . . .

Could the health officer be expected to weigh up all those things at the time? They could probably help her decide one way or another, even though the various outcomes are unclear.

Will an awareness of all these issues help those who are judging her to think through all the reasons lying behind her action? Probably.

Will a discussion of all these issues help to modify guidelines (or decide if any modification is needed) for the future? Almost certainly.

Figure 10.1 illustrates just one of the ways a few of these considerations could be illustrated using elements of systems thinking: feedback loops, balancing loops, and delay.

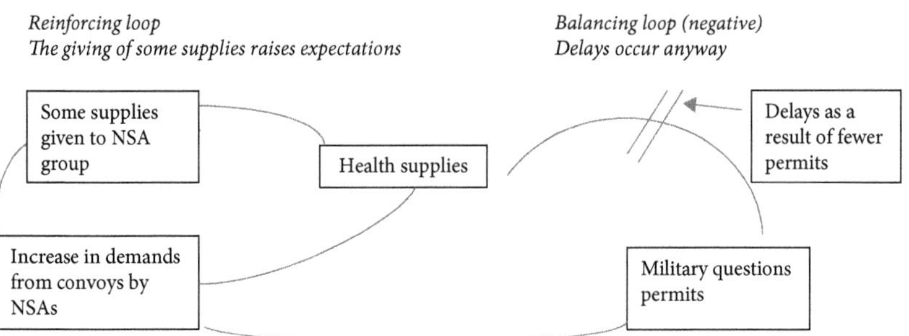

Figure 10.1 Reinforcing loop, balancing loop, and delay

A History of the Use of Systems-Thinking Principles in Responding to Health Needs in War and Armed Conflict

Those wanting to provide healthcare during conflict have always had to negotiate and use systems, which must have necessitated some form of systems thinking in their planning even if not identified as such. While the causal loop diagrams of present systems thinking seem quite recent, it is important to recognize they are just the most recent tools of long-established principles that recognize the importance of systems. When Henry Dunant successfully advocated for a special status for those who were wounded or otherwise "*hors de combat*" (out of the battle) during war, a landmark response to one category of health needs created by war was established (International Committee of the Red Cross, n.d.). While his initial response was to persuade local residents to help care for the wounded in the small town of Castiglione, his next step was to plan a system, aspiring to involve all nations, national relief societies with respected governing boards, and training for volunteers (Dunant, 1947). Dunant also recognized that for the system to be respected the categories of combatant and non-combatant would need to be universally recognized. This resulted in the historically "first" Geneva Convention of 1864 (Harouel, 1999). Although this was never ratified it started the process which led to the inclusion of these definitions in international humanitarian law (IHL) as part of the Geneva Conventions in 1949, with the International Committee of the Red Cross (ICRC) given special status under IHL, and a "right of initiative" to act within states to uphold it (International Committee of the Red Cross, 2010).

From concern for wounded soldiers to the distinction between combatant and non-combatant being given international legal status, this process involved the collective understanding emphasized by systems thinking (Kim, 2000). It encouraged governments and their militaries, and those responding to health needs, to adopt a common purpose; layers of responsibility were established, at least in theory, from the treatment of the individual soldier to the representative of the state of which they were a member.

Situations of armed conflict can often increase demand for healthcare while limiting the ability of health workers to meet that demand. Access to services may be limited, supplies delayed, and health workers themselves may be in danger. Unrealistic expectations of what can be achieved, witnessing suffering to which they cannot respond, and the inability to achieve standards established during training can lead to health workers becoming frustrated and demoralized. The "big picture" approach of systems thinking, with network analysis as one of its tools (Peters, 2014), frames the individual as a player in a system of multiple causes and effects and can help establish what it can be reasonably expected of an individual in those circumstances. The humble flowchart—in manifestations of differing complexity—is one basic tool of systems thinking which can be used to illuminate the relationships in a network as in the following example.

In the mid-1980s, the conflict in then recently independent Mozambique was having a devastating effect on population health (Cliff, 1988); between 1982 and 1990, 48% of the primary healthcare network was destroyed (Cliff, 1993). Health workers in the newly established primary healthcare system, highly motivated to do the best for their country, were restricted geographically and targeted by the RENAMO opposition fighters. An in-service training program for health workers was established, with the aim of both keeping them up to date with emerging issues and helping them to cope with large numbers of displaced people in very difficult circumstances. At the beginning of each workshop, in response to the question "why is this child malnourished?" participants created a flowchart, which often extended across the whole floor of the training room, to answer this question (from personal experience). The completed flowchart established links between the malnourished child and destabilization of the country by then apartheid South Africa and Mozambique's position in the Cold War. This mapping made "clear current processes" (Peters, 2014) and enabled the health workers to view their situation objectively, including what influence they had and what they could realistically be expected to do in these circumstances. It also provided "a pictorial representation of a sequence of actions and responses" (Peters, 2014) which contributed to thinking realistically about what others could be asked to do to address the situation.

The Food Security Information Network (FSIN) estimated that in 2017 there were almost 74 million food-insecure people in need of urgent assistance globally, and that conflict and insecurity were the major drivers of this insecurity in eighteen countries and territories (Food Security Information Network, 2018). Monitoring food insecurity is an essential activity in trying to address this level of need and many food security activities have systems thinking characteristics. Monitoring and analyzing food prices, the sale of livestock, and other behavior patterns such as reducing daily meals (Food and Agricultural Organisation, 2008) all involve cause, effect, and feedback loops. Combined with macro-economic indicators, nutrition survey results, and other behavioral or anthropological data, they also make up the "big picture" analysis proposed by systems thinking, and the coordination among different sectors necessary to provide it. While food security monitoring has become increasingly sophisticated over recent decades, there is still a suggestion that an increased application of systems thinking could help improve it (Howe, 2010).

A clear example of trying to apply a systems approach to improve the response to health needs in conflict is the many attempts to clarify and improve coordination among international humanitarian actors. What could have stayed as a loose coalition of central and local government, UN agencies, the ICRC, Red Cross, donors, international and national non-governmental organizations (NGOs), and community groups has, over the years, emerged as some sort of a system. In 1991, the United Nations General Assembly (UNGA) passed Resolution 46/182 which specifically addressed coordination (United Nations General Assembly, 1991). Among other measures this established the Department of Humanitarian Affairs (DHA)—formerly the Office of the UN Disaster Relief Coordinator—established the post of Emergency Relief Coordinator and the Inter-Agency Standing Committee (IASC) and processes for coordinated assessment and funding (Davey, 2013). These and subsequent attempts to improve coordination have had to try to ensure communication lines are not too long, complicated, and time-consuming, and that management is sufficiently flexible to respond to specific and sometimes urgent circumstances. More recently the cluster approach, including the health cluster, introduced in 2006 as part of the UN Humanitarian Reform process brings together responders around specific sectors to work together with common objectives according to the needs of particular situations (Humphries, 2013). It is designed to improve coordination, leadership, and accountability, and the "predictability, timeliness, and effectiveness of humanitarian response" (World Health Organization, 2007). However, welcome attempts to improve coordination are vulnerable to one of the dangers of any system: that the system itself takes priority rather than serving the function for which it was created. In Uganda, "their [health clusters'] potential to create an additional layer of bureaucracy into already complex and bureaucratic humanitarian response architecture is a real concern" (Olu, 2015).

Could the Principles and Tools of Systems Thinking Have Contributed to a Better Response to Health Needs in War and Conflict—with the Benefit of Hindsight

The previous section considered areas in which the principles of systems thinking have contributed positively to responses to health needs in situations of armed conflict in the past, even if they were not identified as such.

This section considers areas in which, if systems thinking—or a greater degree of systems thinking—had been employed in the past, processes and outcomes could potentially have been improved. Some related areas are then picked up in the final section which looks to the future. The benefit of hindsight is a marvelous thing; it is also a potential learning tool. The cases considered in this section are not meant to be critical.

External actors may initially have to provide care in parallel to national services for several reasons: national services may have been destroyed or never have existed in some areas, health workers may have been killed, displaced, or already in short supply prior to the conflict, or the urgency of need may initially be too great for attention to be paid to integration. While this may be necessary initially, insufficient effort is sometimes made to liaise with national services in the longer term and support them in a sustainable way. This is particularly important in chronic and recurring conflict situations, when collaboration can assist national services with longer-term planning. The need for more effective support of national health staff is recognized (Mowafi, 2007).

One of the problems that may arise is in relation to renumeration: if the external actor pays a living wage to some health workers this may undermine what the government can pay to the majority, set an unsustainable precedent (Onyango, 2008), and limit the capacity of the national services. Systems-thinking tools which can draw out the conflicting and reinforcing links between different actors and layers of responsibility (e.g., Figure 10.2) could perhaps have helped discussion and mutual understanding of these issues.

National or regional guidelines can also be a difficult issue if external actors do not follow them or do not consider that they provide the best therapeutic response (Inbaraj, 2003). Conflict and disaster situations can present opportunities to "build back better" (Fan, 2013) which have not always been taken, despite general agreement on the advantages. In the case of treatment regimes, systems-thinking tools could help collaboration and facilitate discussion about the many factors involved, including the cost of implementing new treatment protocols nationally, and patent issues, the long-term benefits, the consequences for other budgets, and the reliability of donor support. This would help clarify what actions were reinforcing, balancing, or undermining of immediate and longer-term health needs.

Setting priorities is a key part of "building back better" and of planning the reconstruction of health services in the post-conflict period. The government may feel under pressure to reconstruct things the way they were before the conflict, for example by giving priority to the rebuilding of tertiary care hospitals (Pavignani & Colombo, 2001). Donors may also find this useful as a clear illustration for their domestic audience of what they are supporting. While these influences may not be directly related to health needs, they may nevertheless exist and need to be acknowledged and discussed, alongside the knowledge that more children could potentially be saved and treated by prioritizing the primary healthcare services. The potential for systems thinking to represent these issues objectively, and to illustrate their eventual positive or negative implications for health, including potential leverage points, could perhaps have helped in these situations. There has been considerable work on planning reconstruction and

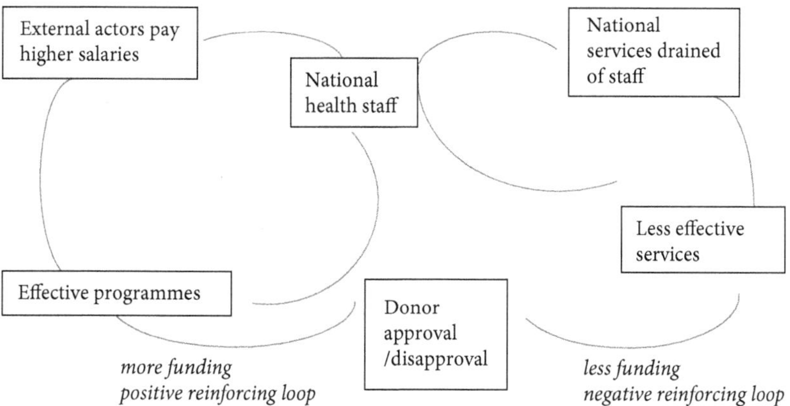

Figure 10.2 Possible consequences of higher salaries paid to national health staff by external actors

providing effective support for the health sector (Kruk, 2010; Shakarishvili, 2011), however discussion of possible wider influences at an early stage could help common understanding.

A Few Notes of Caution

Systems thinking has underlying principles, many of them based on intuitive thought processes and a diverse range of tools and models. It seeks to promote mutual understanding of processes and outcomes of different courses of action and create some commonality of vision about the future. As with all process models, a negative outcome could be that in the desire to find clarity, the model becomes more important than the reality of what is being considered, which it then lacks the sensitivity to reflect.

Systems thinking needs time for collaboration: time for meetings, discussions, working together on mapping, and using the various tools. This may be difficult to prioritize for health workers keen to respond to the increased health needs frequently created by conflict. Systems thinking could be practiced out of context as a way of considering issues that are likely to arise to try to get around this.

Systems thinking promotes strategic thinking and its models are designed to facilitate the mutual understanding and collaborative development of plans. Different actors will have, or be perceived to have, different levels of influence and power depending on their role and background. In theory, systems thinking can give all actors a more equal voice by making issues more transparent; however, transparency will mean that all actors, including those who will work together in the future, will be encouraged to "show their hand." In situations of conflict people can be theoretically on the same "side" but have different views about the conflict and different affiliations that could, if not managed sensitively, pitch them against each other if they were to be revealed.

Those who could be encouraged to improve their coordination around health responses through systems thinking include donors, UN agencies, national government representatives, community groups, NGOs, and military actors, among others. Different norms may exist in relation to what should and shouldn't be communicated and how communication should take place. Some actors may be quite at ease with interrogating how they think and testing assumptions; for others, this may not be an easy process. While this sort of issue can perhaps be overcome with carefully selected discussion groups and assurances of anonymity where appropriate, this will mean the process needs more time and resources which may be difficult to find when planning health responses during times of conflict.

How Could an Increase in the Use of Systems Thinking Principles and Tools Enhance the Response to Health Needs Created by War and Armed Conflict in the Future?

(i) Conflict preparedness

Disaster preparedness for extreme weather events and other "natural" disasters, and the integral preparations for an effective health response are far more developed than preparedness for armed conflict. Systems thinking has been proposed for some aspects of disaster preparedness (e.g., Khyrina, 2012). Conflict preparedness can bring complications because preparing for the consequences of conflict before it breaks out can be perceived as fanning the flames of a dispute when there is still a possibility of peaceful resolution. Nevertheless, during times of heightened tension, systems thinking could inform planning of the response to the anticipated health needs that would be created should conflict occur: how the conflict is likely to unfold, the most likely resulting needs and resource gaps, and potential challenges to physical access and to access to sufficient resources.

This sort of planning would need an estimation of what the health consequences are likely to be, the sort of health impact assessment that is carried out routinely in anticipation of other potentially negative impacts on health (Birch et al., 2014). This would also make the likely consequences of their actions clearer to the potential belligerents. In this way systems thinking applied to conflict preparedness also has the potential to promote peaceful solutions before a resort to violence.

Systems thinking gives importance to explicit accountability in partnership frameworks (Bosmans, 2016b) and, in the face of the likely health consequences should armed conflict occur, could encourage transparency about the motivations of the actors involved. These are things that are unlikely to be discussed openly and include strategic alliances, domestic audiences, economic and natural resource impacts, and the market in arms sales. By providing an objective framework, systems thinking has the potential to encourage transparency or make it harder to obfuscate about these issues.

(ii) Including the potential of all actors

The humanitarian actors who respond to health needs are many and diverse. As well as the need to respond to these needs, they may be under various other pressures to act: international NGOs may want to show their supporters that they are there "on the ground"; military actors may be instructed by their respective governments to show they are "doing something," and military medical personnel may feel a professional need to respond; the expectations and pressures of donor countries will be on UN agencies. These pressures may mean that a clear and objective discussion about the best responders in any given situation—and where it is best for resources to be allocated—is not held. Attempts to address this have been made, for example by improving the allocation of funds (Disasters Emergency Committee, n.d.) and trying to ensure support for the most effective actors (Archer, 2017), but distribution based primarily on need has not been achieved. The application of a systems-thinking approach using stakeholder analysis as part of a logical framework could help address this issue.

A systems-thinking approach also has the potential to promote greater understanding of more clearly contentious issues. Whether military actors should carry out humanitarian work, and are well equipped to do so, has been debated (Jæger, 2009), particularly in conflicts where, as well carrying out "humanitarian" work, the armed forces of a particular country are also engaged in active fighting (Birch & Ratneswaren, 2009). Their status as a party to the conflict makes it impossible for them to adhere to the humanitarian principles of neutrality and independence, and almost certainly that of impartiality. However, this debate has frequently limited itself to who has the best skills for certain tasks, how much it costs different actors to carry them out, and how impartial and independent any actors are (personal experience). A systems-thinking approach would widen the analysis from the skills and resources of various actors to consider wider more systemic issues and the specific situations in which they might apply including the effect of military aid provision on the security of the population, the ability of armed forces to act in any way independently of their government's foreign policy even in matters of health, alternative ways in which services could be delivered, and resources used in situations of insecurity.

(iii) Health workers in danger: analyzing the risks

The risks that health workers take when responding to health needs has received considerable attention because of a tragic increase in the numbers killed over the last fifteen years. This has given rise to some high-profile initiatives such as Healthcare in Danger Project of the International Committee of the Red Cross, and the Safeguarding Health in Conflict Coalition, a group of international NGOS working on the issue who collaborate with the Healthcare in Danger Project. They work toward better documentation and understanding of this increase and to promote international humanitarian law which should protect health workers, their facilities, and transport. There has been significant work on the extent of the problem in Syria (Fouad, 2017). All this has raised the profile of the issue which has also gone up the agenda of the United Nations (Zerrougui, 2016) and donor governments. The World Health Organization (WHO) has said more understanding of the reasons behind the attacks is needed, as is a standard list of motives which could be used for data collection (World Health Organization, 2016). Systems thinking could help this process and draw in the many reasons health workers might be vulnerable, another example of which is given in what follows.

Twenty-one health workers were killed and five wounded in 2014 while immunizing against polio as part of the Global Polio Eradication Initiative in north-east Pakistan (Safeguarding Health in Conflict, 2016), and vaccinators continue to be targeted. One of the main reasons appears to be that the polio vaccine is viewed with suspicion, and by some groups as part of a "Western" plot, particularly after a team of vaccinators (although not against polio) were—many unwittingly—used to confirm the residence of Osama bin Laden (Shah, 2012). The campaign has nevertheless continued, partly due to the understandable pressure to wipe out remaining pockets where the virus is still active as part of the global eradication campaign. However, although immunization has been stopped for short periods due to a lack of security, there appears to have been little analysis of whether this ongoing drive is "worth" the risks to community health workers, and whether a strategic longer-term view of eradication might be more successful. This is a difficult discussion with many feedback loops where systems thinking could be applied at various levels: local, national, and in the WHO, so all perspectives on degrees of risk are taken into account in planning what should occur from now on.

(iv) Data and health information: mapping the wider influences on accuracy and availability

Information and data are key to any effective health response in a conflict situation when it can be difficult and sometimes dangerous to collect such data and other needs may take priority and records can be destroyed or go missing. A lack of baseline data can make it difficult to establish trends, and insufficient coordination may mean agencies collect information using different case definitions and cut-off points (Pavagnani, 2003). Health data, particularly mortality, can become politicized (Taylor, 2016) if it is used to reflect on the conduct of parties to the conflict and may be suppressed, manipulated, or made up to suit the agenda of one side or other. While work in this area has improved the quality of health data collected during conflict (e.g., Checchi & Roberts, 2005), there are still many challenges, including the opportunities created by social media (Baliki, 2014). The emphasis that systems thinking puts on anticipating and mapping challenges in the wider environment, flexibility and addressing issues as they occur to restore equilibrium (Bosmans, 2016a) could help a deeper understanding and a more effective response to the challenge of collecting timely, reliable, and consistent health information and data in the future.

Conclusion

The principles underpinning systems thinking, and some of the tools it uses, could usefully be applied to improve the response to health needs in conflict situations. Systems thinking could help analysis of the larger picture in complex conflict situations, improve transparency in planning, and clarify the effect of multiple influences and whether they are positive or negative. The following points need to be taken into account.

Systems thinking has the potential to bring together and clarify complex and challenging sets of issues; in doing this, there needs to be recognition and inclusion of the work that has already been done in these areas.

The principles behind systems thinking and the tools it uses could be integrated strategically into ongoing processes within institutions and organizational groups, and help these processes be clear, transparent, and constructive; it should not be introduced as an additional layer of process and should recognize where principles are already being applied.

An increased use of the systems-thinking approach could help mutual understanding of issues, reveal motives and increase objectivity in addressing sensitive subjects; in so doing, it could nudge common understanding forward and contribute to a practical conclusion.

In these ways systems thinking could effectively contribute to a better response to health needs during conflict.

References

Archer, D. (2017). *The future of humanitarian crises is urban*. International Institute for Environment and Development. Retrieved from https://www.iied.org/future-humanitarian-crises-urban

Baliki, G. (2014). *Measuring conflict incidence in Syria in aspects of the conflict in Syria. SIPRI Yearbook 2014* (pp. 17–22). Stockholm International Peace Research Institute and Oxford: Oxford University Press.

Birch, M. (2010). Delivering health care in insecure environments: UK foreign policy, military actors and the erosion of humanitarian space. *Medicine, Conflict & Survival, 26*, 80–85. doi.org/10.1080/13623690903553277

Birch, M., & Ratneswaren, S. (2009). From Solferino to Sri Lanka: health workers, health information, and international law. *Medicine, Conflict and Survival, 25*(3), 191–192.

Birch, M., Cave, B., Elmi, F., & Karpf, B. (2014). Predicting the unthinkable: Health impact assessment and violent conflict. *Medicine, Conflict & Survival, 30*(2), 81–90. doi:10.1080/13623699.2014.896174. PMID: 24968516.

Bosmans, M., Bossyns, P., Flahaut, A., Goeman, L., Gyselinck, K., Piraux, J., Van Bastelaere, S., Van Waeyenberge, S., & Verle, P. (2016a). Development cooperation as learning in progress: Dealing with the urge for the fast and easy. *Health Services Organization & Policy, 33.* ©ITGPress, Nationalestraat 155, B-2000 Antwerp, Belgium.

Bosmans, M., Bossyns, P., Flahaut, A., Goeman, L., Gyselinck, K., Piraux, J., Van Bastelaere, S., Van Waeyenberge, S., & Verle, P. (2016b). Development cooperation as learning in progress: Dealing with the urge for the fast and easy. *Studies in Health Services Organization & Policy, 33.*

Checchi, F., & Roberts, L. (2005). *Interpreting and using mortality data in humanitarian emergencies. Humanitarian Practice Network Paper 52.* September 2005. Overseas Development Institute.

Cliff, J., & Noormahommed, A. R. (1988). Health as a target: South Africa's destabilization of Mozambique. *Social Science & Medicine, 17*, 7, 717–722.

Cliff, J., & Noormahommed, A. R. (1993). The impact of war on children's health in Mozambique. *Social Science & Medicine, 36*, 7, 843–848.

Davey, E., Borton, J., & Foley, M. (2013). *A history of the humanitarian system. HPG Working Paper, June 2013.* Overseas Development Institute.

Dunant, H. (1947). *A memory of Solferino*. London, Cassell.

Fan, L. (2013). *Disaster as opportunity? Building back better in Aceh, Myanmar and Haiti. Humanitarian Policy Group, Working Paper November 2013.* Overseas Development Institute.

Food and Agricultural Organisation. (2008). *An introduction to the basic concepts of food security. Food Security Information for Action Practical Guides.* EC—FAO Food Security Programme.

Fouad, F. (2017). Health workers and the weaponisation of health care in Syria: A preliminary inquiry for The Lancet–American University of Beirut Commission on Syria. *The Lancet, 390*, 2516–2526. doi.org/10.1016/S0140-6736(17)30741-9

Food Security Information Network. (2018). *Global report on food crises 2018.* Food Security Information Network. Rome, Italy. Retrieved from http://vam.wfp.org/sites/data/GRFC_2018_Full_Report_EN.pdf?_ga=2.181353895.1010112213.1522081801-1640856075.1522081801

Harouel, V. (1999). Les projets genevois de révision de la Convention de Genève du 22 août 1864 (1868–1898). *International Review of the Red Cross, 81*(834), 365–386.

Howe, P. (2010). Archetypes of famine and response. *Disasters, 34*(1), 30–54. doi.org/10.1111/j.1467-7717.2009.01113.x

Humphries, V. (2013). Improving humanitarian coordination: Common challenges and lessons learned from the cluster approach. *The Journal of Humanitarian Assistance, 30*. Retrieved from http://sites.tufts.edu/jha/archives/1976

International Committee of the Red Cross. (2010). *The ICRC's mandate and mission*. Retrieved from https://www.icrc.org/eng/who-we-are/mandate/overview-icrc-mandate-mission.htm

International Committee of the Red Cross. (n.d.). https://www.icrc.org/en/who-we-are/history/founding

Inbaraj, S. (December 28, 2003). HEALTH: Ethiopia blasts MSF for advocating alternative malaria treatment. Inter Press Service. Retrieved from http://www.ipsnews.net/2003/12/health-ethiopia-blasts-msf-for-advocating-alternative-malaria-treatment/

Jæger, T. (2009). Humanitarian and military action in armed conflict–side by side, not hand in hand. *Nordic Journal of International Law, 78*(4), 567–579.

Khyrina, A., Burairah, H., & Hasan Basari, A. (2012). A systems thinking in natural disaster management: Evacuation preparedness. *Proceedings of the 1st WSEAS International Conference on Risk Management, Assessment and Mitigation (RIMA '12)*, 384–389. Addis Ababa, Ethiopia.

Kim, D. (2000). *Systems thinking tools: A user's reference guide*. Pegasus Communications Inc.

Kruk, M. E., Freedman, L. P., Anglin, G. A., & Waldman, R. J. (2010). Rebuilding health systems to improve health and promote state building in post-conflict countries: A theoretical framework and research agenda. *Social Science & Medicine, 70*, 1, 89–97. doi.org/10.1016/j.socscimed.2009.09.042

Mowafi, H., Nowak, K., & Hein, K. (2007). Human Resources Working Group: Facing the challenges human resources for humanitarian heath. *Prehospital & Disaster Medicine Sept-Oct, 22*, 5, 351–359.

Olu, O., Usman, A., Woldetsadik, S., Chamla, D., & Walker, O. (2015). Lessons learnt from coordinating emergency health response during humanitarian crises: A case study of implementation of the health cluster in northern Uganda. *Conflict and Health, 9*, 1. doi.org/10.1186/1752-1505-9-1

Onyango, M. (2008). Humanitarian responses to complex emergencies. In Harald Kristian (Kris) Heggenhougen (Eds.), *International Encyclopedia of Public Health* (pp. 487–495). Academic Press. https://doi.org/10.1016/B978-012373960-5.00071-X

Pavignani, E., & Colombo, A. (2003). Lost behind desert mirages? Consideration about rationale, aims and flaws of rapid needs assessments in health, as witnessed during the Iraq crisis. https://researchonline.lshtm.ac.uk/id/eprint/4648772/1/EP3-4_214-art1.pdf

Pavignani, E., & Colombo, A. (2001). *Providing health services in countries disrupted by civil wars: A comparative analysis of Mozambique and Angola 1975–2000*. World Health Organization, Department of Emergency and Humanitarian Action. Retrieved from http://apps.who.int/disasters/repo/14052.pdf

Peters, D. (2014). The application of systems thinking in health: Why use systems thinking? *Health Research Policy and Systems, 12*, 51.

Safeguarding Health in Conflict. (2016). *No protection, no respect. Safeguarding health in conflict coalition*. Retrieved from https://www.safeguardinghealth.org/sites/shcc/files/SHCC2016final.pdf

Shakarishvili, G., Lansang, M. A., Mitta, V., Bornemisza, O., Blakley, M., Kley, N., Burgess, C., & Atun, R. (2011). Health systems strengthening: A common classification and framework for investment analysis. *Health Policy & Planning, 26*, 316–326. https://doi.org/10.1093/heapol/czq053

Shah, S. (February 22, 2012). Health workers linked to CIA's Osama bin Laden assassination plot are sacked. *The Guardian*. Retrieved from https://www.theguardian.com/world/2012/feb/22/health-workers-osama-bin-laden-assassination

Taylor, A. (March 5, 2016). The Syrian war's death toll is absolutely staggering. But no-one can agree on the number. *Washington Post*. Retrieved from https://www.washingtonpost.com/news/worldviews/wp/2016/03/15/the-syrian-wars-death-toll-is-absolutely-staggering-but-no-one-can-agree-on-the-number/?utm_term=.b1e00ebd8f79

United Nations General Assembly. (1991). *Strengthening the coordination of humanitarian emergency assistance of the United Nations A/RES/46/182*. Retrieved from http://www.un.org/documents/ga/res/46/a46r182.htm

World Health Organization. (2007). *Humanitarian health action. Annex 7: The cluster approach*. Retrieved from http://www.who.int/hac/techguidance/tools/manuals/who_field_handbook/annex_7/en/

World Health Organization. (2016). *Attacks on healthcare: Protect, prevent. provide*. Geneva: World Health Organization. Retrieved from http://www.who.int/hac/techguidance/attacksreport.pdf

Zerrougui, L. (2016). *Strategies for ending attacks on health workers, facilities and patients. Statement by the Special Representative of the Secretary-General for Children and Armed Conflict*. World Humanitarian Summit, Istanbul, May 24, 2016. Retrieved from https://childrenandarmedconflict.un.org/statement/world-humanitarian-summit-strategies-for-ending-attacks-on-health-workers-facilities-and-patients/

11
Governance in Conflict-affected Fragile States
Systems Thinking for Collaborative Decision-making in Reproductive Health

Khalifa Elmusharaf, Elaine Byrne, and Diarmuid O'Donovan

Introduction

One of the main factors that contributes to the failure of maternal health programs globally is the mismatch between the needs of people and the means by which healthcare is provided (Kanté & Pison, 2010). Globally, there is evidence to suggest a lack of understanding among many health system actors in relation to challenges faced by mothers and their families in accessing their first choice of maternal healthcare, the magnitude of maternal health problems, and the barriers that affect access to maternal care (DCA, 2011; Organisation for Economic Co-operation and Development, 2011; Sabuni, 2011). Indeed, most studies on the utilization of maternal, newborn, and child health (MNCH) services focus on individual characteristics and actions of women and their families (Maine & Larsen, 2004), with considerably less attention given to the features of the health system that shape their choices. Therefore, and while achieving high coverage of essential maternal healthcare services is important, this alone will not translate to reductions to maternal mortality rates (Souza et al., 2013). Just as essential is whether women *access* these services and whether health interventions are designed to reflect the specific needs of women (Elmusharaf, Byrne, Manandhar, Hemmings, & O'Donovan, 2017b). Health systems frameworks are commonly used to describe the health system from a bird's eye perspective, with the World Health Organization (WHO) Building Blocks (2007) being perhaps the most well-known and cited framework. While organizing the health system into its operational building blocks has its practical uses, the tendency of these frameworks is toward health systems as a "supply" issue. Focusing on the supply, however, runs the risk of ignoring the interdependence between the various parts of the health system and the values and the principles of its users.

A common approach to generate knowledge in health research is that researchers collect data from the community, analyze it, communicate the results to providers and policy makers, with the hope and intention that they will utilize this information to influence their practice. This researcher–push approach is common in developing countries. Missing from this approach, however, is the interaction between those who conduct research and those who might be able to use it, generating a wide knowledge-to-action gap (Lomas, 2000; Graham et al., 2006; van Kammen, de Savigny, Sewankambo, 2006).

Khalifa Elmusharaf, Elaine Byrne, and Diarmuid O'Donovan, *Governance in Conflict-affected Fragile States* In: *Systems Thinking for Global Health.* Edited by: Fiona Larkan, Frédérique Vallières, Hasheem Mannan, and Naonori Kodate, Oxford University Press.
 DOI: 10.1093/oso/9780198799498.003.0011

The need for patient involvement in planning and delivery of healthcare originates in the Alma Ata declaration which states: "The people have the right and duty to participate individually and collectively in the planning and implementation of their health care" (World Health Organization, 1978). This sentiment is echoed in the statement from the Third Global Health Systems Symposium on Health Systems Research (Health Systems Global, 2014). Ultimately, public involvement is about change and improving health services and policy. It is about human relationships, networks, and communications. Akin to systems thinking, public involvement means conceptualizing health systems as a social institution that functions "at the interface between people and the structures that shape their broader society" to ensure safe, acceptable and accessible maternal health care globally (Freedman et al., 2005). This chapter examines this interface as an example of systems thinking. Specifically, we demonstrate how multiple-level engagement of different actors enables the planning, development, and implementation of localized and culturally appropriate approaches to health service planning and provision, even in the most resource constrained and complex settings.

Conflict-affected Fragile States

People have the right to a health system that is effective, that encompasses access, availability, affordability, quality, and the underlying determinants of health, and that is responsive to national and local priorities (Hunt, 2007). This right also holds for individuals within conflict-affected fragile states (CAFS), despite the added presence of additional stressors. For example, clinics in CAFS are often damaged and under or unstaffed (Michael et al., 2007; Rubenstein, 2009). Moreover, and while understanding the context is crucial when working in CAFS, there is often little reliable health and contextual information available to aid in decision-making. The dearth of timely and reliable information is further driven by the absence of safe and communal platforms where stakeholders and community members can meet, exchange knowledge, and debate in order to find common ground so that mutually beneficial decisions can be made (Byrne & Gregory, 2006). Finally, the combination of poverty, loss of livelihood, and breakdown of social support systems damages the health of the population (Pedersen, 2002; Waters, Garrett, & Burnham, 2007). Together, the lack of understanding of the local context, the lack of reliable information, limited capacity and experience, and slow responsiveness to new information or research findings have hugely disrupted programs and services in CAFS. Despite these added difficulties however, the health system is still required to deliver services that balance the expectations of the people and the expectations of the state.

In CAFS, women are often hardest to reach and are thus excluded from the health system. Their exclusion can be due to a number of factors including cultural norms, lack of education, and geographic remoteness. Sufficient knowledge exists to inform global action about the strategies required to improve maternal health in CAFS. These include providing access to family planning, antenatal care with provision of misoprostol for prevention of postpartum hemorrhage during home births, availability of skilled birth attendants, and referral systems that include basic and comprehensive emergency obstetric, neonate, and postnatal care (Ronsmans & Graham, 2006; Prata, Sreenivas, Greig, Walsh, & Potts, 2010; Ahmed, Li, Liu, & Tsui, 2012). Despite this, little priority is often given to reaching women in CAFS.

Giving women a platform such that their voices can be incorporated into issues related to their health is essential if the rights of women to safe and accessible care is going to be upheld in CAFS. Specifically, the delivery of reproductive health services within in CAFS should be co-determined by senior government officials and women in the community. The challenge in finding common ground however is that the capacity of women in the community to participate in such forums is often assumed. Additionally, the capacity of decision makers to make informed decisions is equally assumed (Byrne & Sahay, 2007). In order to address this challenge, three main issues need to be considered:

1. The capacity for women in the community to participate in research and action;
2. The capacity of stakeholders to utilize information they have access to; and
3. Platforms where both parties can meet and fruitfully exchange knowledge and to develop trust for action to occur.

Drawing from a case study we conducted in South Sudan (2008–2014), we further detail how applying systems thinking to these three issues resulted in building capacity at multiple levels, generated dynamic platforms for knowledge brokering, and enabled marginalized women to work with senior government officials to co-generate, utilize, and broker knowledge to improve maternal, newborn, and child health.

Setting: Renk County, South Sudan

South Sudan is a nation long afflicted by conflict. The most recent twenty-three-year civil war resulted in large-scale destruction that has left little physical and institutional infrastructure. As in many war-affected areas, communities are still in the process of restoring education services, and the international community continues to support the rebuilding of the healthcare system. The low skills level severely constrains access to and improvement of education, healthcare, water, and sanitation services for South Sudanese in isolated communities.

Priority is not always given to maternal health, services do not usually match the needs of the people, most of the facilities are not functioning, and many healthcare providers lack necessary skills. The voices of hard-to-reach populations are usually excluded or not heard. Social issues hugely influence access. Women usually do not take informed decisions and even if they do, they either do not act on them or only do so at a very late stage.

Improvements in access to maternal health in South Sudan will remain slow unless we take care of women in local communities, and unless women are empowered to make decisions about their care at the right time, without waiting for others to make the decision for them. An enabling environment for this decision-making process is required.

The Health System of South Sudan is a decentralized system that exists at four main levels: central, state, county, and community. This study was conducted in

Renk County, one of the thirteen counties that constitute the Upper Nile state in South Sudan.

Methodology

A brief overview of the approach adopted in this study is provided here, with further details of the methodology available elsewhere (Elmusharaf, Byrne, & O'Donovan, 2015; Elmusharaf et al., 2016; Elmusharaf, Elmusharaf, Byrne, & O'Donovan, 2017a; Elmusharaf et al., 2017b;; Elmusharaf et al., 2017c). Fourteen women in South Sudan were trained in Participatory Ethnographic Evaluation Research (PEER) to design research instruments, appropriate for their literacy level. They collected data through oral interviews and narratives with forty-two local women located across fourteen villages in Renk. Analysis of this data was then conducted jointly through conversation, role plays, and acting. The PEER-trained women were granted certificates for their participation in the PEER.

PEER-trained women then engaged in Innovative Participatory Health Education (IPHE). They utilized the results of the data analysis to develop health action messages, created health education materials, and worked with a local theatrical team to deliver the developed materials to their community in forms of pictograms (Figure 11.1), songs, (Table 11.1) and drama.

In parallel, ten senior officers at the Renk County Department of Health were engaged in a capacity development training course on Reproductive Health Project Management (RHPM). During a four-day workshop, senior officers were given a series of lectures, group exercises, class discussion, and assignments. They identified what they perceived to be the ten most important maternal health problems in the region. Then, in a plenary session, they were introduced to the maternal issues that were identified by PEER trained women. Senior officers commented on issues, compared them with their own list, and reflected on their current practices for developing maternal health services. Senior officers were then asked to write project proposals to

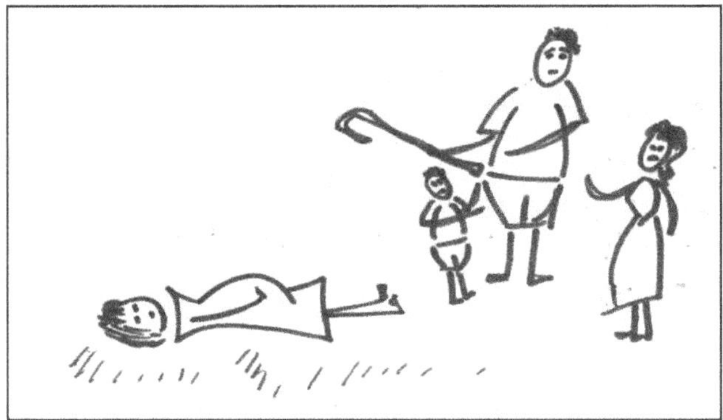

Figure 11.1 Example of a pictogram developed by PEER trained women as part of IPHE
"Don't hit pregnant women and solve all problems without violence"

Table 11.1 Translation of the lyrics of one of the songs developed by PEER-trained women as part of IPHE

1. Oh father, don't hit my mom.
2. My mom is carrying us in the womb.
3. Leave aside all the problems.
4. Mom, and dad too.
5. Don't let problems affect us.
6. Come on mom, go to your check-up in time.
7. Our fathers, follow up with our mothers.
8. When they are pregnant take them for check-up.
9. Our families, let us provide good healthy foods for the pregnant woman.
10. This could help her baby a lot.
11. Mom, foods like vegetables and fruits, eggs, and milk, and your health becomes well.
12. A lot of heavy chores, people, is not good for the pregnant woman.
13. Let her rest, and her baby becomes well too.

improve maternal health based on the priorities identified by PEER-trained women. In the last day of the workshop, the senior officers and the fourteen PEER-trained women all came together in one room. Senior officers were asked to present their project proposals to the fourteen PEER-trained women, seeking their feedback and approval. They all engaged in discussing maternal health issues in the community and how to work together in the future. Once women approved the proposals, we then granted the senior officers certificates for their completion of the course. Figure 11.2 summarizes the process in its entirety.

Capacity Development for Collaborative Decision-Making

The fragility of CAFS arises mainly as a result of a failure to balance the expectations of the people and the expectations of the state adequately and the inability to consider the context when delivering services (Organisation for Economic Co-operation and Development, 2008). While understanding the context (historical, political, sociocultural, and economic) is crucial when working in CAFS, there is often little reliable health and contextual information available to facilitate this understanding. There is no emphasis on reaching excluded women or on creating a platform where stakeholders and women from the community can meet, exchange knowledge, and debate in order to find common ground so that mutually beneficial decisions can be made. (Langer, Horton, & Chalamilla, 2013). This research proposes a novel methodology to address these gaps.

(i) Developing capacity of women to participate in research and action

A common criticism of participatory research is that it ignores potential contextual structures that may leave participants vulnerable to exploitation by the research team (Cleaver, 2001; Francis, 2001). Additionally, participatory approaches have also been criticized for a lack of clear procedures and mechanisms and inadequate

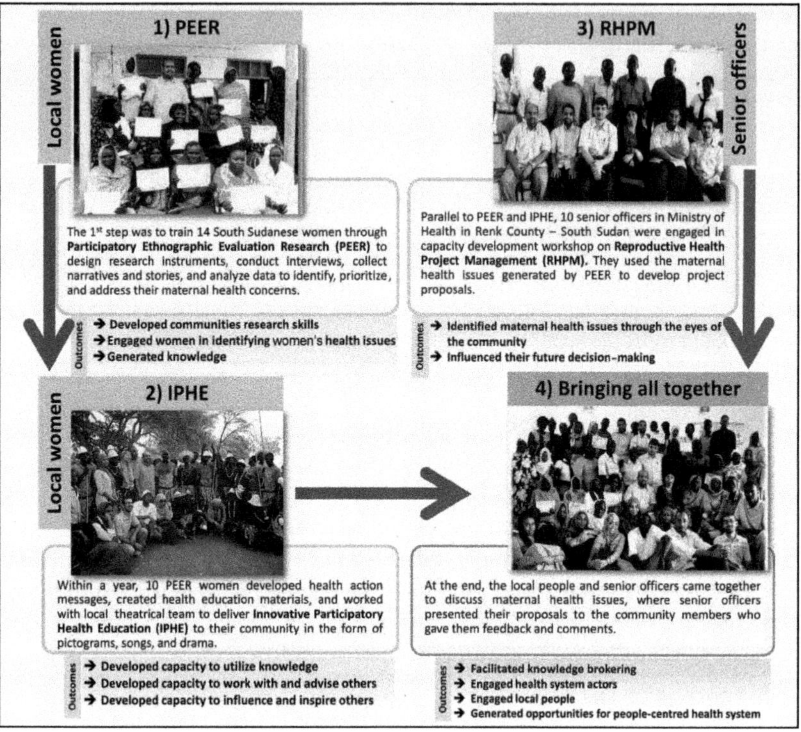

Figure 11.2 Stages in co-development of health system interventions

understanding of power relationships (Kapoor, 2002). Capacity development is required to overcome these constraints and to tackle issues of responsibility, knowledge, and access to resources (Jonsson, 2003). Facilitating community members to share, reflect on, and evaluate their knowledge eventually enables them to plan and act (Chambers, 1994; Byrne & Sahay, 2007).

A major aspect of participatory research is that participants adapt to different forms of communication and that they recognize the value of communication in research. This is not as simple as it seems, with there being many challenges involved in developing genuine listening skills, tools, and techniques (Slim & Thompson, 1993). Key to our approach was therefore adopting culturally appropriate communication styles. Dealing with a largely illiterate population meant designing image-based data collection instruments with role plays and theatre becoming important communication medium for analysis and dissemination. Denzin and Lincoln (2005) highlight the important implications of using practical, progressive approaches to interpretive research that focuses on indigenous participatory theatre. Mda (1993) has long advocated for "theatre-for-development" as a means to enhance "between the center and the periphery, and within the periphery itself."

The empowerment philosophy adopted in this study is based on the fact that women should have the opportunity to make choices (Feste & Anderson, 1995). Thus, if those who have been denied the opportunity to make strategic life choices are to be empowered, they need to be involved in a process that facilitates acquiring such opportunity (Kabeer, 1999). The involvement of women in the process of PEER provided them with a space for dialogue and reflexivity about maternal health issues in their community.

The initial steps in PEER were to build the capacity of PEER researchers to participate and to enhance their reflective practices. PEER did not only give the fourteen women the opportunity to collect and analyze the data, but it built their capacity to do so. While the PEER workshop trained them to be *researchers*, reflecting on and analyzing the data made them *evaluators*. The networks that they established in their community made them *agents of change*. The success of this approach is evidenced by the fact that twelve months after the PEER workshop, ten out of the fourteen PEER researchers were still able to lead work on health communication with employees of local non-governmental organizations (NGOs) and local theatrical band members. PEER researchers also stated that PEER enhanced their credibility. They were more confident about their ability to influence change. When they returned to their social circles, people were more accepting of what they said because they were perceived to know more than others. Women further reported how delighted they were that the maternal health issues that had been identified by them could be used by the senior officers to plan for future services and projects.

People involved in research, particularly in CAFS, need to be able to reflect on the changing context as their needs and situation also change. This level of capacity development is critical because it enables individuals to bring about change not only at an individual level but also at a community level. This is further enhanced by including women in the community as the researchers, whose mode of communication was that of the community under investigation.

(ii) Developing capacity of stakeholders to use information and translate knowledge into action

As part of this study, the reproductive health project management workshop strengthened the capacity of senior officers to be more responsive to and capable of absorbing available knowledge, including using the findings of PEER to link to the local context and reality. Using these findings further sensitized them to the local needs and prepared them to work with community members. Stakeholders bring their accumulated experience, their local knowledge as well as their own desire and intentions to the research process (Taylor, Suarez-Balcazar, Forsyth, & Kielhofner, 2006). However, these capacities can be unproductive unless stakeholders have the appropriate capacity to absorb and utilize the generated knowledge (Deng, Doll, & Cao, 2008), that is the "ability of a stakeholder to recognise the value of new, external information, assimilate it, and apply it" (Cohen & Levinthal, 1990b).

The face-to-face interviews conducted separately with key stakeholders highlighted that many of the senior decision-makers in the Department of Health were unaware of the magnitude of maternal deaths occurring in the region and did not fully realize the sociocultural determinants that might influence access to care.

The senior officers reported that this approach helped them to identify maternal health issues through the lens of the local women, and that this would influence their decision-making process in the future. They stated that most of their existing activities and programs did not match the needs of the community, and that they tended to think about issues from a service provider's point of view. They reported underestimating the difficulties faced by people in reaching facilities such as financial, geographical, and social challenges. They also did not fully understand the reasons for delays in obtaining healthcare including delays in making the decision to seek healthcare, delays in reaching the appropriate facility, and delays within facilities to receive appropriate care. This is consistent with the global literature (DCA, 2011; Organisation for Economic Co-operation and Development, 2011; Sabuni, 2011). The lack of understanding of the local context, the lack of reliable information, and the limited capacity, experience, and responsiveness to research findings have all been found to disrupt programs and services in South Sudan (Sabuni, 2011).

(iii) Developing a platform for knowledge brokering

The approach described in this chapter developed community research skills, engaged women in identifying maternal health issues, developed their capacity to work with and advise others. It also helped senior officers to identify maternal health issues through the eyes of the community members and influenced their future decisions. This approach facilitated knowledge brokering and generated opportunities for people-centered health systems.

The unequal nature of social relationships and positions between different actors and between institutions within the county was recognized from the beginning of this study. Therefore, different forums were established that suited the needs of the various groups. Discussions were also facilitated by people who were familiar with the area and those who also had an understanding of the local norms and values. Interviews and meetings were held in the local language. It was only after this capacity had been developed that the two groups met to share the findings from their research and to discuss the project proposals.

Overall, this study (see Figure 11.3) generated a dynamic platform for knowledge brokering. The PEER approach enabled the participants to be *knowledge generators*. The IPHE project gave them the chance to become *knowledge utilizers* through actions in their community. Involving them in the transfer and exchange of the generated knowledge with the senior officials made them *knowledge brokers*. On the supply side, the reproductive health project management workshop enabled the senior officers to be *knowledge utilizers*.

This method developed capacities to collect and use information for users and suppliers of the health services. To co-develop projects, contextual data were needed that could be used within the existing constraints of the county resources. Enhancing the relationships between stakeholders and local people increases the capacity of health services (Ridley & Jones, 2002). In most health systems, mechanisms for engaging with local people, and particularly marginalized groups who are often socially

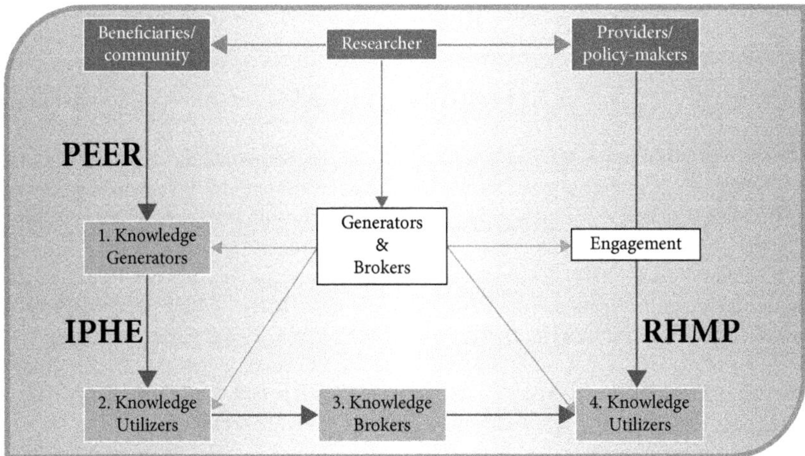

Figure 11.3 Dynamic platform for knowledge brokering

excluded from public debate on policy issues, are often missing. Capacity development can be developed individually but as we can see in this case, capacity also comes about through interaction between actors (Woodhill, 2010).

Conclusion

The approach described in this chapter explained how systems thinking facilitated collaborative decision making in maternal health in complex settings. Systems thinking in our case study was dynamic, holistic, and operational. It provided a framework for creating interrelationships at multiple levels within the broader context and facilitated knowledge creation, retention, transfer, and utilization (Newman & Conrad, 2000). This "knowledge interaction" was an interactive and contextual approach that emphasizes social, dialogical, and interpretative ways of knowing (Davies, Nutley, & Walter, 2008).

Transferring results of research alone will not close the knowledge-to-action gap. There is a need for interactive processes and capacity-strengthening approaches that encourage knowledge users (policy-makers and healthcare providers) to be more responsive and absorptive to research findings (Cohen & Levinthal, 1990a; van Kammen et al., 2006). There is also a need to bring together researchers and healthcare providers in a collaborative, dynamic process to facilitate knowledge translation (Baumbusch et al., 2008).

Systems thinking represented a social process of negotiation between people in order to develop a shared understanding of their own and each other's interests, perceptions, and roles. This was a highly political exercise that addresses issues of equity, power, information sharing and social transformation. The negotiation in itself was empowering and formed an integral part of the system design, development process, and establishing networks at multiple levels.

References

Ahmed, S., Li, Q., Liu, L., & Tsui, A. O. (2012). Maternal deaths averted by contraceptive use: An analysis of 172 countries. *The Lancet, 380*, 111–125.

Baumbusch, J. L., Kirkham, S. R., Khan, K. B., Mcdonald, H., Semeniuk, P., Tan, E., & Anderson, J. M. (2008). Pursuing common agendas: A collaborative model for knowledge translation between research and practice in clinical settings. *Research in Nursing and Health, 31*, 130–140.

Byrne, E., & Gregory, J. (2006). Co-constructing local meanings for child health indicators in community-based information systems: The UThukela District Child Survival Project in KwaZulu-Natal. *International Journal of Medical Informatics, 76*(Suppl 1), S78–88.

Byrne, E., & Sahay, S. (2007). Community-based health information systems: Implications for participation. *Journal of Information Technology for Development, 13*, 71–94.

DCA. (2011). *The listening project. Local perceptions of international engagement in fragile states and situations.* Cambridge, MA: CDA Collaborative Learning Projects. https://www.cdacollaborative.org/publication/local-perceptions-of-international-engagement-in-fragile-states-and-situations/

Chambers, R. (1994). The origins and practice of participatory rural appraisal. *World Development, 22*, 953–969.

Cleaver, F. (2001). Institutions, agency and the limitations of participatory approaches to development. In B. Cooke & U. Kothari (Eds.), *Participation: The new tyranny* (pp. 36–55). New York, NY: Zed Books.

Cohen, W. M., & Levinthal, D. A. (1990a). Absorptive capacity: A new perspective on learning and innovation. *Administrative Science Quarterly, 35*, 128–152.

Cohen, W. M., & Levinthal, D. A. (1990b). Absorptive capacity: A new perspective on learning and innovation. *Administrative Science Quarterly, 35*, 128–152. https://doi.org/10.2307/2393553

Davies, H., Nutley, S., & Walter, I. (2008). Why "knowledge transfer" is misconceived for applied social research. *Journal of Health Services Research and Policy, 13*, 188–190.

Deng, X., Doll, W. J., & Cao, M. 2008. Exploring the absorptive capacity to innovation/productivity link for individual engineers engaged in IT enabled work. *Information & Management, 45*, 75–87.

Denzin, N. K., & Lincoln, Y. (2005). *The Sage handbook of qualitative research* (3rd ed.). Thousand Oaks, CA: Sage.

Elmusharaf, K., Byrne, E., & O'Donovan, D. (2015). Strategies to increase demand for maternal health services in resource-limited settings: Challenges to be addressed. *BMC Public Health*, 15, 870. https://doi.org/10.1186/s12889-015-2222-3

Elmusharaf, K., Byrne, E., & O'Donovan, D. (2017a). Social and traditional practices and their implications for family planning: A participatory ethnographic study in Renk, South Sudan. *Reproductive Health, 14*, 10. https://doi.org/10.1186/s12978-016-0273-2

Elmusharaf, K., Byrne, E., Manandhar, M., Hemmings, J., & O'Donovan, D. (2017b). Participatory ethnographic evaluation and research: Reflections on the research approach used to understand the complexity of maternal health issues in South Sudan. *Qualitative Health Research, 27*, 1345–1358.

Elmusharaf, K., Tahir, H., Donovan, D. O., Brugha, R., Homeida, M., Abbas, A. M. O., & Byrne, E. (2016). From local to global: A qualitative review of the multi-leveled impact of a multi-country health research capacity development partnership on maternal health in Sudan. *Globalization and Health, 12*(1), 20. doi:10.1186/s12992-016-0153-0. PMID: 27184907; PMCID: PMC4869333.

Elmusharaf, K., Byrne, E., Abuagla, A., Abdelrahim, A., Manandhar, M., Sondorp, E., & O'Donovan, D. (2017c). Patterns and determinants of pathways to reach comprehensive emergency obstetric and neonatal care (CEmONC) in South Sudan: qualitative diagrammatic pathway analysis. *BMC Pregnancy Childbirth, 17*, 278. doi:10.1186/s12884-017-1463-9. PMID: 28851308; PMCID: PMC5576292.

Feste, C., & Anderson, R. M. (1995). Empowerment: From philosophy to practice. *Patient Education and Counselling, 26*, 139–44.

Francis, P. (2001). Participatory development at the World Bank: The primacy of process. In B. Cooke & U. Kothari (Eds.), *Participation: The new tyranny* (pp. 72–87). New York, NY: Zed Books.

Freedman, L., Waldman, R., de Pinho, H., Wirth, M., Mustaque, A., Chowdhury, R., & Rosenfield, A. (2005). UN Millennium Project, Task Force on Child Health and Maternal Heath. Who's Got the Power: Transforming Health Systems for Women and Children. London; Sterling, Va.: Earthscan.

Graham, I. D., Logan, J., Harrison, M. B., Straus, S. E., Tetroe, J., Caswell, W. & Robinson, N. (2006). Lost in knowledge translation: Time for a map? *Journal of Continuing Education for Health Professionals, 26*, 13–24.

Health Systems Global. (2014). *Cape Town Statement from the Third Global Symposium on Health Systems Research*. Cape Town, South Africa: Health Systems Global. Retrieved from https://www.healthsystemsglobal.org/upload/other/Cape-Town-Statement.pdf

Hunt, P. (2007). *Report of the Special Rapporteur on the right of everyone to the enjoyment of the highest attainable standard of physical and mental health. Implementation of general assembly resolution 60/251 of 15 March 2006 entitled "Human Rights Council."* Geneva: United Nations.

Jonsson, U. (2003). *Human rights approach to development programming*. Nairobi: UNICEF. https://digitallibrary.un.org/record/525201?ln=en

Kabeer, N. (1999). Resources, agency, achievements: Reflections on the measurement of women's empowerment. *Development and Change, 30*, 435–464.

Kanté, A. M., & Pison, G. (2010). Maternal mortality in rural Senegal. The experience of the new Ninéfescha Hospital. *Population (English edition), Institut national d'études démographiques, 65*, 653–678.

Kapoor, I. (2002). The devil's in the theory: A critical assessment of Robert Chambers' work on participatory development. *Third World Quarterly, 23*, 101–117.

Kruk, M. E., Freedman, L. P., Anglin, G. A., & Waldman, R. J. (2010). Rebuilding health systems to improve health and promote statebuilding in post-conflict countries: A theoretical framework and research agenda. *Social Science and Medicine, 70*, 89–97.

Langer, A., Horton, R., & Chalamilla, G. (2013). A manifesto for maternal health post-2015. *The Lancet, 381*, 601–602.

Lomas, J. (2000). Using "linkage and exchange" to move research into policy at a Canadian foundation. *Health Affairs (Millwood), 19*, 236–240.

Mda, Z. 1993. *When people play people: Development communication through theatre.* Johannesburg: Wits University Press.

Michael, J., Andreini, M., Mojidi, K., Pressman, W., Rajkotia, Y., & Stanton, M. E. (2007). *Southern Sudan maternal and reproductive health rapid assessment.* Juba, South Sudan: Government of Southern Sudan Ministry of Health and USAID.

Newman, B. D., & Conrad, K. W. (2000). A framework for characterizing knowledge management methods, practices, and technologies. In U. Reimer (Ed.), *Third international conference on practical aspects of knowledge management*, 2000 Basel, Switzerland. Swiss Life: 1601–1611.

Organisation for Economic Co-operation and Development. (2008). *Concepts and dilemmas of state building in fragile situations from fragility to resilience. Discussion paper.*

Paris: Organisation for Economic Co-Operation and Development. Retrieved from http://www.oecd.org/dac/incaf/41100930.pdf

Organisation for Economic Co-operation and Development. (2011). *Conflict and fragility international engagement in fragile states: Can't we do better*? Paris: Organisation for Economic Co-operation and Development.

Pedersen, D. (2002). Political violence, ethnic conflict, and contemporary wars: Broad implications for health and social well-being. *Social Science and Medicine, 55,* 175–90.

Prata, N., Sreenivas, A., Greig, F., Walsh, J., & Potts, M. (2010). Setting priorities for safe motherhood interventions in resource-scarce settings. *Health Policy, 94,* 1–13.

Ridley, J., & Jones, L. (2002). *User and public involvement in health services: A literature review.* Edinburgh, UK: Partners in Change [Scottish Human Services Trust. https://www.sehd.scot.nhs.uk/involvingpeople/A%20literature%20review.pdf

Ronsmans, C., & Graham, W. J. (2006). Maternal mortality: Who, when, where, and why. *The Lancet, 368,* 1189–1200.

Rubenstein, L. (2009). *Post-conflict health reconstruction: New foundations for U.S. policy.* Washington, DC: United States Institute of Peace.

Sabuni, A. (2011). *FSP Country scorecard: Republic of South Sudan.* South Sudan: OECD Publishing

Slim, H., & Thompson, P. (1993). *Listening for a change: Oral testimony and development.* London: PANOS.

Souza, J. P., Gulmezoglu, A. M., Vogel, J., Carroli, G., Lumbiganon, P., Qureshi, Z., … Say, L. (2013). Moving beyond essential interventions for reduction of maternal mortality (the WHO Multicountry Survey on Maternal and Newborn Health): A cross-sectional study. *The Lancet, 381,* 1747–1755.

Taylor, R. R., Suarez-Balcazar, Y., Forsyth, K., & Kielhofner, G. (2006). Participatory research Approach. In G. Kielhofner (Ed.), *Research in occupational therapy: Methods of inquiry for enhancing practice* (pp. 424–433). Philadelphia, PA: F. A. Davis Company.

Van Kammen, J., de Savigny, D., & Sewankambo, N. (2006). Using knowledge brokering to promote evidence-based policy-making: The need for support structures. *Bulletin of the World Health Organization, 84,* 608–612.

Waters, H., Garrett, B., & Burnham, G. (2007). *Rehabilitating health systems in post-conflict situations. Paper No. 2007/06.* Helsinki, Finland: United Nations University, World Institute for Development Economics Research.

Woodhill, J. (2010). Multiple Actors. In Ubels, J., Acquaye-Baddoo, N. A., & Fowler, A. (Eds.), *Capacity development in practice* (pp. 25–41). Washington, DC: Earthscan.

World Health Organization. (1978). *Declaration of Alma-Ata International Conference on Primary Health Care, Alma-Ata.* Geneva: World Health Organization.

12

Implementing Systems Thinking for Global Mental Health during Humanitarian Emergencies

Frédérique Vallières, Mohamed Elshazly, Jihane Bou Sleiman, Rony Abou Daher, Caoimhe Nic a Bháird, Ruth Ceannt, Philip Hyland, and Peter Ventevogel

Introduction

Marked by wide-scale destruction, humanitarian emergencies are further characterized by threats to one's livelihood and security, lack of access to basic needs, the loss of friends and family members, mass forced displacement, and severe damage to social and community infrastructure. In light of these experiences, it is unsurprising that those affected are at greater risk of developing mental health conditions including depression, anxiety, post-traumatic stress disorder, bipolar disorder, and schizophrenia (Charlson, van Ommeren, Flaxman, Cornett, Whiteford, & Saxena, 2019). Moreover, those with pre-existing chronic psychiatric conditions are particularly vulnerable to relapse and exacerbation of their condition(s) (Ventevogel, van Ommeren, Schilperoord, & Saxena, 2015).

The term "mental health and psychosocial support" (MHPSS) is commonly employed within humanitarian settings and refers to any support that aims to protect or promote psychosocial well-being or prevent or treat mental conditions. The delivery of MHPSS requires cross-sectoral approaches, with close collaboration between sectors such as health, education, and protection.[1] In practice, however, provision of humanitarian assistance still favors "compartmentalized" approaches, with disjointed interventions delivered across supposedly "separate" domains, and where responsibilities for each domain are spread across different actors, including government ministries and humanitarian organizations. This compartmentalization is problematic for MHPSS, which is, by definition, a cross-sectoral issue, and stands in stark contrast to systems-thinking. Therefore, humanitarian assistance must move away from siloed approaches and reductionistic medical psychiatric interventions toward more interdisciplinary and system-wide approaches (Inter-Agency Standing Committee, 2007). Moreover, essential for effective MHPSS is the active participation of communities to

[1] Here, protection refers to protection within humanitarian work, including within armed conflict, climate change, and natural disasters including four areas of responsibility: child protection; gender-based violence; land, housing and property; and mine action.

Frédérique Vallières, Mohamed Elshazly, Jihane Bou Sleiman, Rony Abou Daher, Caoimhe Nic a Bháird, Ruth Ceannt, Philip Hyland, and Peter Ventevogel, *Implementing Systems Thinking for Global Mental Health during Humanitarian Emergencies* In: *Systems Thinking for Global Health.* Edited by: Fiona Larkan, Frédérique Vallières, Hasheem Mannan, and Naonori Kodate, Oxford University Press. DOI: 10.1093/oso/9780198799498.003.0012

strengthen mutual support within families and other social networks, and to ensure socially and culturally acceptable MHPSS programing.

Effective mental health programs must consider that cultural, physiological, social, and environmental systems interact with each other and jointly affect the well-being of individuals. As such, the current chapter further argues that while thinking across the conventional six building blocks (i.e., leadership and governance, information systems, financing, human resources, essential medical products and technologies, and health service delivery) for the delivery of mental health services in humanitarian emergencies is important, such an approach must further be complemented by the active involvement of communities across each of these building blocks. Using selected international case examples chosen for their relevance to and application of systems thinking under each building block, we demonstrate how systems thinking—with its emphasis on specific parts as well as on the relationships *between* these parts and how these are connected within a health system—serves as a useful analytical tool to develop appropriate mental health responses within humanitarian contexts.

Leadership and Governance for Mental Health in Emergencies

Relief efforts are usually led by a country's governmental bodies, in collaboration with United Nations (UN) agencies, international, and national non-governmental organizations (NGOs). The cross-sectoral nature of MHPSS necessitates the presence of strong leadership to strengthen ties between MHPSS coordination platforms and other sectors such as health, protection, and education (Elshazly, Budosan, Alam, Khan, & Ventevogel, 2019). Within large-scale emergencies, and where governments lack capacity and experience to take on these tasks, the governance of the MHPSS response is often led by UN agencies and NGOs. Often overlooked however, is the importance of including community leaders in this process, whereby a lack of involvement of community leadership for MHPSS in humanitarian responses may lead to under-utilization of services, which are perceived as unacceptable and inappropriate.

Involvement of governments is important, ideally from the early stages of an emergency, to ensure MHPSS sustainability, effectiveness, and credibility. A good example comes from Lebanon where, in 2014, and with support of the World Health Organization (WHO) and the United Nations Children's Fund (UNICEF), and in partnership with International Medical Corps (IMC), the Lebanese Ministry of Public Health (MoPH) established the Lebanese National Mental Health Programme (NMHP) (El Chammay, Karam, & Ammar, 2016). The NMHP, in turn, established a MHPSS taskforce which includes over sixty organizations working in Lebanon, with the aim of harmonizing and mainstreaming MHPSS across all sectors, improving access to care, and acting as a single coordination mechanism (Ministry of Public Health Lebanon, 2016). Due to the strong leadership of the MoPH, the MHPSS taskforce has since developed into a permanent forum where national strategies, policies, interventions, and coordination plans are discussed, evaluated, and set out for implementation. In this case, the emergency therefore further provided an opportunity for important mental health service reform (Pérez-Sales, Férnandez-Liria, Baingana, & Ventevogel, 2011; Epping-Jordan et al., 2015).

Case example—Bangladesh: Leadership and field-level coordination

Background: The aforementioned siloed approach to coordination (i.e., mental health coordinated by the health sector and psychosocial activities coordinated by the protection sector) makes it challenging to coordinate different MHPSS services and to develop referral pathways. Moreover, a lack of consistent quality standards for MHPSS across different sectors, weak inter-sectoral communication, and poor involvement of affected communities in service coordination are key barriers for effective MHPSS service delivery.

Systems-Thinking Approach: Following the influx of hundreds of thousands of Rohingya refugees from Myanmar into Bangladesh in the fall of 2017, an MHPSS working group (MHPSS-WG) was established to discuss and coordinate the MHPSS response. The group included representatives from the government, local and international NGOs, UN agencies, and academics. Structurally, the MHPSS-WG was considered a subgroup of the health sector, but it established close ties to other sectors and sub-sectors including those for protection, gender-based violence, and child protection. Over time, the group provided strong leadership and governance.

Key Outcome(s): Key to the success of the MHPSS-WG was that it functioned as a *technical* working group that was not bound to one sector. Today, over sixty member organizations participate in the MHPSS-WG. Establishing cross-sectoral taskforces or subgroups to address specific issues (e.g., suicide prevention, integration of MHPSS into different sectoral activities) facilitated intersectoral communication and coordination. The MHPSS-WG also initiated "field," or local level, coordination meetings (Elshazly, Alam, & Ventevogel, 2019). These field-level coordination meetings helped to facilitate inter-sectoral communication at the local level, where partner organizations and, in some cases, community leaders, traditional healers, or religious leaders could meet to coordinate around practical issues concerning the same camp or location.

Information Systems for Mental Health in Emergencies

Mental health information systems (MHIS) are systems "for collecting, processing, analyzing, disseminating and using information about a mental health service and the mental health needs of the population it serves" (World Health Organization, 2005). Unfortunately, there is no unified system for data collection for MHPSS in humanitarian settings, with information gathered through multiple systems in different formats. What is more, governmental Health Information Management Systems

(HIMS) in many low- and middle-income countries (LMICs) often do not, or only minimally include, mental health data (Upadhaya et al., 2016). When included, the indicators are often limited to mental health consultations or numbers of occupied psychiatric in-patient beds (Jordans et al., 2016). Moreover, HIMS tend to collect only data for individuals who have met the clinical criteria for a 'mental disorder', thus excluding those with significant psychological distress but still requiring intervention, as well as those with comorbid mental health conditions in addition to a general medical diagnosis. Consequently, service providers in humanitarian contexts often set up their own, organization-specific, databases for internal reporting and reporting to donors. The comprehensiveness of data varies across organizations, ranging from number of clients seen to routine monitoring data on functional outcomes and symptom reduction (e.g., Centers for Victims of Torture (CVTs) use extensive data on symptoms and social functioning before, during, and in the months after treatment in their programs in Africa and the Middle East (personal communication PV with CVT, September 2020)).

Another type of information is mapping of available services. Since MHPSS activities are implemented across different sectors, sectoral mappings do not capture all services. Therefore, a standard mapping exercise, the 4Ws: *Who is Where, When, doing What* (IASC-RG MHPSS, 2012), was established in 2012. The 4Ws exercise offers detailed information on MHPSS services within humanitarian contexts, helping decision-makers plan, implement, and evaluate mental health programs throughout the course of a humanitarian response. It has since been used in a wide range of contexts (O'Connell et al., 2013). A critical feature of the 4Ws is the detailed description of how activities must be coded, which is important because terms such as "counseling" and "psychosocial support" can be understood in different ways by different actors.

Case example—Inclusion of mental health within UNHCR's Integrated Refugee Health Information System

Background: Since 2009, the UNHCR's Refugee Health Information System (RHIS) for humanitarian settings has included seven categories related to mental, neurological, and substance use (MNS) conditions.

Systems-Thinking Approach: In 2018, the RHIS' mental health categories were revised to enhance their utility and compatibility with newer clinical tools, including the mhGAP Humanitarian Intervention Guide (World Health Organization, 2016). The mental health Gap Action Programme (mhGAP) is a WHO program that seeks to address the lack of care for people suffering from mental, neurological and substance use (MNS) conditions. Maintaining a high level of consistency with the earlier case definitions—such that future data could be meaningfully compared with previously collected data and to explore longitudinal patterns and regional variations in service utilization—was considered of utmost importance. The new *integrated* Refugee Health Information System (iRHIS), however, also includes several new features. First, data are now entered through tablets/computers/android phones, with data stored in the cloud. Secondly, the new system allows for multiple categories to be selected for a single patient at a single consultation to register comorbidity, a function lacking in routine HIS systems in LMICs (Kane et al., 2018). Thirdly, the iRHIS differentiates between new cases and revisits. Fourthly, new age categories (under-fives, five to seventeen years, eighteen to fifty-nine, and over sixty years) allow for reporting in line with standards of Ministries of Health in refugee-hosting countries.

Key Outcome(s): Two rounds of consultations involving thirty-four experts in humanitarian mental health led to the addition of separate categories for organic psychiatric conditions such as dementia and delirium, as well as for self-harm and suicide attempts (Ventevogel, Ryan, Kahi, & Kane, 2019). The final set of categories in iRHIS includes nine case definitions for MNS conditions: epilepsy/seizure, alcohol/substance use disorder; intellectual disability/developmental disorder; psychotic disorder (including mania); delirium/dementia; depression or other emotional disorder; other emotional complaint; medically unexplained somatic complaint; and self-harm/suicide. Furthermore, the use of additional specifiers enables dedicated mental health professionals to document a more refined diagnosis, with a total of twenty-two different categories that make the system compatible with the modules of the mhGAP program, without adding too much complexity. For example, whereas the category "psychotic disorder (including mania)" can still be used by general health workers, dedicated mental health workers can further specify its variants, including acute psychosis, chronic psychosis, or manic psychosis. This option to add specifiers, however, is only open to health staff having received specialized training in mental health, such as psychiatric nurses, psychiatric clinical officers.

Mental Health and Psychosocial Support Financing in Emergencies

Most refugees and displaced populations reside in LMICs, where mental health spending as a proportion of total health spending stands well below that of high-income countries. While the inter-sectoral nature of MHPSS means that funding should not be solely reliant on health-sector funding, in practice, it remains challenging to track spending for MHPSS programing across sectors (i.e., child protection and gender-based violence). Finally, financial resources earmarked for developmental projects in recipient countries are sometimes reallocated to refugees, in support of the humanitarian response. The severe lack of funding for MHPSS in emergencies, combined with challenges in tracking funding for MHPSS programing and a divestment of recipient country resources, has prompted calls to define MHPSS indicators in planning documents and to assign specific MHPSS codes within financial tracking systems for humanitarian responses (Inter-Agency Standing Committee, 2019). However, this has yet to materialize.

Case example—Funding for MHPSS in Lebanon

Background: The lack of financial coverage of Mental Health in Lebanon continues to be one of the major factors affecting access to services. Currently, mental health services in Lebanon are incorporated within the budget of the Ministry of Public Health. There is no specific budget allocated for mental health but an estimated 5% of the MoPH healthcare expenditures are directed toward mental health. Of this expenditure, more than half (54%) went to psychiatric hospitals, with very little going toward outpatient care at primary care centers (PHCC) (World Health Organization & Ministry of Health Lebanon, 2015). This affects the availability of mental health services within communities and in peripheral areas, where most Syrian refugees are concentrated.

Systems-Thinking Approach: Funding directed toward Lebanon as part of the Syrian humanitarian response led to several mental health programs implemented by NGOs. International Medical Corps (IMC) Lebanon for example, introduced transportation allowances, allowing service users to reach the PHCC and return home without costs. Mental health and psychosocial support services, including any associated medications, were also offered free of charge for the service user. This increased availability for vulnerable populations. A fixed-fee model was adopted to reduce the cost of MHPSS interventions. As part of this model, psychotherapists are paid per working day rather than by consultation, thereby prioritizing quality of care over the absolute number of clients seen.

Key Outcome(s): Ultimately, further cost reductions occurred when IMC's Mental Health teams were integrated into the governmental PHCCs, whereby the MH teams were remunerated under governmental salary scales, as an example of an opportunity for health system strengthening within humanitarian emergencies.

Human Resources for Mental Health and Psychosocial Support in Emergencies

Of the entire health workforce globally, only 1% works in mental health. Human resources for mental health are particularly scarce in LMICs, as those most affected by humanitarian emergencies (World Health Organization, 2016b). Moreover, most mental health professionals tend to be located in urban centers, far from rural areas and refugee camps. Therefore, in the initial phase of a humanitarian response, non-specialized professionals and lay people are often trained in the delivery of simplified and manual interventions under the supervision of more skilled workers (i.e., "task-shifting" or "task-sharing"). Leveraging existing human resources as well as integrating mental health care into existing community health services improves access to mental health services and also leads to more acceptable and accessible services at community level.

Case example—Nepal: Task-sharing and task-shifting for MHPSS in Emergencies

Background: In 2015, two earthquakes struck Nepal, killing over 8,700 people and injuring more than 22,000. Large parts of Nepal's infrastructure, including over 1,000 health facilities, were destroyed or damaged. At the time of the earthquakes, Nepal registered only sixty psychiatrists (0.22 per 100,000 population), twenty-five psychiatric nurses (0.09 per 100,000), and sixteen clinical psychologists (0.06 per 100,000) for the entire country (International Medical Corps, 2017).

Systems-Thinking Approach: In the immediate aftermath of the earthquake, IMC and Transcultural Psychosocial Organization Nepal (TPO) delivered a program of activities designed to strengthen the capacity of health workers and community members to provide MHPSS; support the delivery of community-based MHPSS services through improving staffing, information systems, and medication supply; and improve access to MHPSS services through awareness-raising initiatives and anti-stigma campaigns. Government health workers in primary health care centers (doctors, health assistants, auxiliary health workers, staff nurses, and auxiliary nurse midwives) were trained and supervised to incorporate MHPSS into their regular healthcare duties through the mhGAP program. Psychological first aid (PFA) training strengthened the skills of community leaders (health workers, teachers, women's group members, youth leaders, and female community health volunteers) to provide basic psychosocial support, recognize psychological needs, and appropriately refer people in need. Finally, psychosocial counselors received advanced training covering counseling for alcohol problems, family counseling, health activities, problem solving, and self-help group formation, using a curriculum designed by TPO Nepal and endorsed by the National Health Training Center. The different staff jointly conducted community outreach activities to raise awareness of MHPSS, reduce stigma, and encourage participation of people with mental health problems in the community. Community-based care workers were hired to support the initial development of a referral network between community and health facility levels, creating a stronger link between government (i.e., health facility) staff and community resources.

Key Outcome(s): In total, 3575 training courses were completed by 1,041 unique participants affiliated with seventy-eight health facilities. Brief mental health orientations were provided to 1,900 community members, and 626 community leaders participated in PFA workshops. Trainees reported significant improvements in knowledge and skills, with 92% reporting improved perceived competency. In interviews, they reported greater confidence in the detection, diagnosis, and treatment of mental disorders. MHPSS services reached 3,422 services users, with trained community members providing home-based support and referrals, and clinical staff providing more intensive care at health facilities. Health workers highlighted how this "joint effort" between multiple cadres working at different levels helped to deliver a holistic and integrated program.

Access to Essential Medical Products and Technologies for Mental Health and Psychosocial Support in Emergencies

The WHO's "Model List of Essential Medicines" contains a small number of psychotropic medications. Specifically for use within acute humanitarian emergencies, the Inter-agency Emergency Health Kit contains an even more restricted range of just five psychotropic drugs (van Ommeren et al., 2011). While effective, with an acceptable side-effect profile and reasonably priced, drugs for mental disorders and other non-communicable diseases are not often routinely available in governmental health systems in LMICs (Barbui & Chattherjee, 2015). Psychotropic medication are further not often prioritized by planners and may be subject to strict regulations for controlled substances (Padmanathan & Rai, 2016). Some psychotropic drugs are sold outside the formal healthcare system, for example by physicians in private practice or by non-authorized prescribers in pharmacies, grocery stores, and in markets (Raja, Kippen Wood, & Reich, 2015). While important however, increasing access to psychotropic drugs alone is insufficient to address the burden of mental health, with a more important resource being access to MHPSS professionals themselves. Emerging technologies, such as the use of tele-mental health, offer promising new ways of service delivery and are increasingly considered to improve access to mental health and psychosocial services for affected communities in emergencies, as well as to reduce stigma related to mental illness and mental health services.

Case example: Delivering MHPSS to Refugees during the COVID-19 Pandemic

Background: Requisite physical distancing measures implemented during the COVID-19 pandemic meant that many organizations had to quickly adapt the delivery of existing MHPSS services, including the discontinuation of group-based and a reduction in face-to-face services. Moreover, facility-based services, often reserved for those with moderate to severe mental health conditions, were, in some cases, replaced with less frequent home-visits and the provision of a longer supply of existing medication. Likewise, large group MHPSS training, which would have typically taken place with all participants traveling to a central location, were instead delivered by trainers traveling to a number of different sites to train smaller groups.

Systems-Thinking Approach: Adaptations of MHPSS programing during the COVID-19 pandemic further included the use of existing technologies, such as popular radio programs in Tanzania and the Kurdistan Region of Iraq, to deliver community messaging around mental health and well-being and how to manage distress. Likewise, telephone helplines were established for those experiencing psychological difficulties in Uganda and Ecuador, whereby listeners were trained to listen to and discuss issues of emotional well-being, and where possible, were used to link individuals to existing MHPSS services. For more moderate to severe cases, psychologists, such as those in Lebanon, were trained in new ways of providing psychotherapy using remote measures, such as through Skype™ or similar solutions. Similarly, psychiatric consultations in the Kurdistan Region of Iraq took place via video between patients and consulting psychiatrists (United Nation High Commissioner for Refugees, 2020).

Key Outcome(s): The rapid and widespread implementation of measures taken to curb the spread of COVID-19 necessitated the use of existing technologies (e.g., telephone, radio, SMS) that made use of programs already familiar to communities and end-users (e.g., WhatsApp, Facebook groups), and which leveraged people's existing capacity, knowledge, and motivation to engage with these familiar technologies. While new technologies offer promising, scalable tools in humanitarian settings (Burchert et al., 2019; Harper Shehadeh et al., 2020; Tol, 2020), consideration must also be given as to whether the technology is culturally acceptable, appropriate for the technological literacy of its users, and takes into account the cost and the availability of existing infra-structure (e.g., Internet connection).

Service Delivery for MHPSS in Emergencies

Guidelines for MHPSS service delivery in humanitarian settings follow a "pyramidal" approach, organized across four levels (see Figure 12.1). This multilayered approach

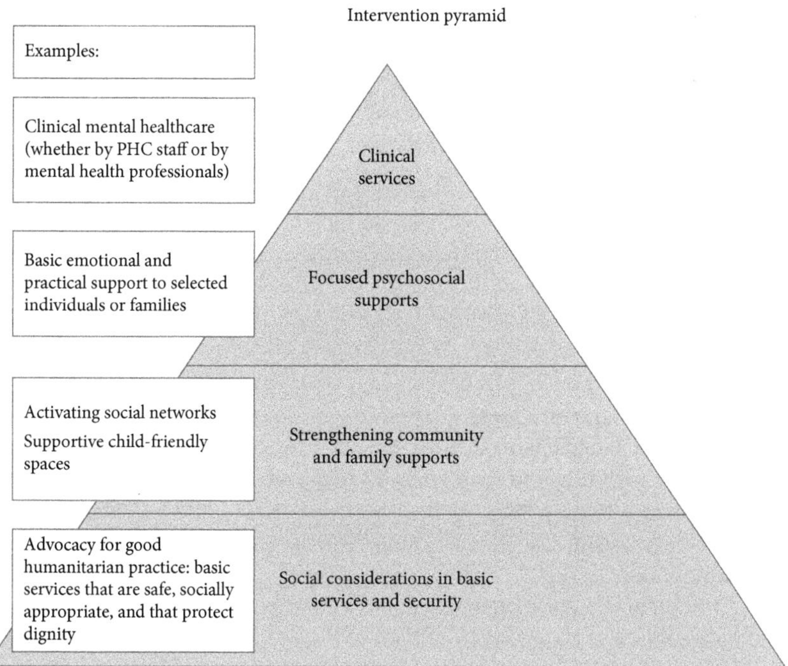

Figure 12.1 The IASC Pyramid. Reproduced with permission from UNHCR (2013) Operational Guidance for MHPSS Programming in Refugee Settings

allows for the design of services and interventions to meet different needs, and to utilize available resources in the best way possible. Critically, the base of the pyramid seeks to strengthen active participation, garnering community and social support to promote mental health and well-being. The upper layers of the pyramid cater to those in need of more specialized case-management support or referral to more specialized care.

Critical to the delivery of community-based approaches is the recognition that cultural backgrounds affect the mental health and psychosocial issues experienced and expressed by affected individuals. Therefore, addressing MHPSS needs within humanitarian emergencies requires cultural competence in order to improve the accessibility, acceptability, and effectiveness of MHPSS interventions. There is however limited empirical evidence around cultural competency guidelines and the cross-cultural validity of existing mental health interventions (Perera et al., 2020). Consequently, the failure to consider community perceptions and expectations of MHPSS programing, as well as the failure to culturally adapt MHPSS interventions, may reduce program effectiveness and undermine existing social support structures.

Case example: Lebanon—Case management approaches for MHPSS service delivery

Background: Aligned to systems thinking, mental health case management (MHCM) is a multidisciplinary, client-centered-based approach, with the goal of responding holistically and thoroughly to each individual's unique set of needs (International Medical Corps, 2017). Within MHCM, a professional case manager (typically a social worker) assesses the needs of the client and the support systems in place, and arranges, coordinates, and monitors a package of multiple services to meet the specific client's complex needs.

Systems-Thinking Approach: In Lebanon, case managers, who participate in both outreach and clinic-based services, were set up and placed within primary health care centers (PHCCs) closest to refugee camps. They conducted assessments to determine beneficiary needs, made referrals within IMC or to other organizations, and involved other mental health staff, such as a psychotherapist (adult and child) or psychiatrist, where necessary. Case managers also provided basic counseling, problem solving, and other psychosocial support, whereby those in need of more intensive case management were referred to psychological or psychiatric services. In addition to case management, investments were made to build competency in psychotherapy, including interpersonal psychotherapy (Verdeli et al., 2003), as well as to strengthen the competency of health workers to identify and manage mental health problems using the WHO's mhGAP Intervention Guide (World Health Organization, 2016).

Key Outcome(s): Case managers offered a continuum of care for those in need of mental health care, acting as the first point of contact and continuously following up with them throughout their treatment. Given that mental health services were available alongside other health services within PHCCs, individuals did not have to worry about being identified as seeking out mental health services, reducing the possibility of stigmatization. Ultimately, 70% of the consultations were delivered by case managers, 20% were referred for psychotherapy intervention and only 10% were referred for psychiatric services, including psychotropic medications.

Conclusion

Armed conflicts and natural disasters cause significant psychological and social suffering. The psychological and social impacts of emergencies may be acute in the short term but can also undermine the long-term mental health and psychosocial well-being of affected populations. As evidenced by the case examples in this chapter, these emergency situations, while presenting challenges, can also provide opportunities to strengthen pre-existing mental health systems. While systems thinking offers an important approach through which to accomplish this, systems-strengthening cannot occur in the absence of the recognition of the important role that communities play in the coordination, delivery, information gathering, accessibility, and acceptability of MHPSS interventions. In emergency responses, MHPSS programing is therefore best conceptualized within the context of existing formal health and social service systems as well as informal systems of diverse cultural and religious traditions, beliefs, and rituals.

References

Barbui, C., & Chattherjee, S. (2015). Improving access to medicines for mental disorders in low-resource settings: Some achievements but still a long road ahead. *Epidemiology and Psychiatric Sciences, 25*(25), 1–3. doi:10.1017/ S2045796015000992

Burchert, S., Alkneme, M. S., Bird, M., Carswell, K., Cuijpers, P., Hansen, P., ... Van't Hof, E. (2019). User-centered app adaptation of a low-intensity e-mental health intervention for Syrian refugees. *Frontiers in Psychiatry, 9*, 663.

Charlson, F., van Ommeren, M., Flaxman, A., Cornett, J., Whiteford, H., & Saxena, S. (2019). New WHO prevalence estimates of mental disorders in conflict settings: A systematic review and meta-analysis. *The Lancet, 394*(10194), 192–194.

El Chammay, R., Karam, E., & Ammar, W. (2016). Mental health reform in Lebanon and the Syrian crisis. *The Lancet Psychiatry, 3*(3), 202–203.

Elshazly, M., Alam, A. M., & Ventevogel, P. (2019). Field-level coordination of mental health and psychosocial support (MHPSS) services for Rohingya refugees in Cox's Bazar. *Intervention, 17*(2), 212–216.

Elshazly, M., Budosan, B., Alam, A. M., Khan, N. T., & Ventevogel, P. (2019). Challenges and opportunities for Rohingya mental health and psychosocial support programming. *Intervention, 17*(2), 197–205.

Epping-Jordan, J. E., van Ommeren, M., Ashour, H. N., Maramis, A., Marini, A., Mohanraj, A., ... Saxena, S. (2015). Beyond the crisis: Building back better mental health care in 10 emergency-affected areas using a longer-term perspective. *International Journal of Mental Health Systems, 9*, 15. doi:10.1186/s13033-015-0007-9

Harper Shehadeh, M. J., Abi Ramia, J., Cuijpers, P., El Chammay, R., Heim, E., Kheir, W., ... Watts, S. (2020). Step-by-step, an e-mental health intervention for depression: A mixed methods pilot study from Lebanon. *Frontiers in Psychiatry, 10*, 986.

Inter-Agency Standing Committee. (2007). *IASC guidelines on mental health and psychosocial support in emergency settings*. Geneva: Inter-Agency Standing Committee.

Inter-Agency Standing Committee-Reference Group for Mental Health and Psychosocial Support. (2012). *Who is where, when, doing what (4Ws) in mental health and psychosocial support: Manual with activity codes (field test-version)*. Geneva: Inter-Agency Standing Committee.

Inter-Agency Standing Committee. (2019). *Summary record, IASC Principals meeting, 5 December 2019*. Geneva: Inter-Agency Standing Committee. Retrieved from https://interagencystandingcommittee.org/inter-agency-standing-committee/summary-record-iasc-principals-meeting-5-december-2019.

International Medical Corps. (2017). *The integration of mental health & psychosocial support services in primary health care facilities in post-earthquake Nepal*. Kathmandu: TPO Nepal and International Medical Corps. Retrieved from https://www.mhinnovation.net/innovations/integrating-mhpss-services-primary-health-care-facilities-post-earthquake-nepal

International Medical Corps. (2017). *Approach to mental health and psychosocial support case management*. Retrieved from https://cdn1.internationalmedicalcorps.org/wp-content/uploads/2017/07/International-Medical-Corps-2012-Our-Approach-to-Mental-Health-Psychosocial-Support.pdf.

International Medical Corps. (2017). *Mental health case management training package*. Retrieved from https://www.mhinnovation.net/sites/default/files/downloads/resource/MHCM%20Modules%20in%20PDF.zip.

Jordans, M. J., Chisholm, D., Semrau, M., Upadhaya, N., Abdulmalik, J., Ahuja, S., ... Mugisha, J. (2016). Indicators for routine monitoring of effective mental healthcare coverage in low- and middle-income settings: A Delphi study. *Health Policy and Planning. 31*(8), 1100–1106. doi:10.1093/heapol/czw040

Kane, J. C., Vinikoor, M. J., Haroz, E. E., Al-Yasiri, M., Bogdanov, S., Mayeya, J., ... Murray, L. K. (2018). Mental health comorbidity in low-income and middle-income countries: a call for improved measurement and treatment. *Lancet Psychiatry, 5*(11), 864–866. doi:http://dx.doi.org/10.1016/S2215-0366(18)30301-8

Ministry of Public Health Lebanon. (2016). *Turning adversity into opportunity: The Syrian crisis and mental health reform in Lebanon*. Beirut, Lebanon: National Mental Health Programme. Retrieved from http://www.mhinnovation.net/sites/default/files/downloads/innovation/reports/NMHP_PolicyBrief_FINAL.pdf.

O'Connell, R., Poudyal, B., Streel, E., Bahgat, F., Tol, W., & Ventevogel, P. (2013). Who is where, when, doing what: Mapping services for mental health and psychosocial support in emergencies. *Intervention, 10*(2), 171–176.

Padmanathan, P., & Rai, D. (2016). Access and rational use of psychotropic medications in low- and middle-income countries. *Epidemiology and Psychiatric Sciences, 25*, 4–8.

Perera, C., Salamanca-Sanabria, A., Caballero-Bernal, J., Feldman, L., Hansen, M., Bird, M., ... Vallières, F. (2020). No implementation without cultural adaptation: A process for culturally adapting low-intensity psychological interventions in humanitarian settings. *Conflict and Health, 14*(1), 46. https://conflictandhealth.biomedcentral.com/articles/10.1186/s13031-020-00290-0

Pérez-Sales, P., Férnandez-Liria, A., Baingana, F., & Ventevogel, P. (2011). Integrating mental health into existing systems of care during and after complex humanitarian emergencies: rethinking the experience. *Intervention, 9*(3), 345–358.

Raja, S., Kippen Wood, S., & Reich, M. R. (2015). Improving access to psychiatric medicines in Africa. In E. Akyeampong, A. G. Hill, & A. Kleinman (Eds.), *The culture of mental illness and psychiatric practice in Africa* (pp. 262–281). Bloomington, IN: Indiana University Press.

Tol, W., Leku, M. R., Lakin, D. P., Carswell, K., Augustinavicius, J., Adaku, A., ... & van Ommeren. (2020). Guided self-help to reduce psychological distress in South Sudanese female refugees in Uganda: A cluster randomized trial. *Lancet Global Health, 8,* e254–e263.

United Nation High Commissioner for Refugees. (2020). *Emerging practices: Mental health and psychosocial support in refugee operations during the COVID-19 pandemic.* Geneva: United Nation High Commissioner for Refugees.

United Nations Office for the Coordination of Humanitarian Affairs. (2019). *Global humanitarian overview 2020.* Retrieved from https://reliefweb.int/sites/reliefweb.int/files/resources/GHO-2020_v9.1.pdf.

Upadhaya, N., Jordans, M. J., Abdulmalik, J., Ahuja, S., Alem, A., Hanlon, C., ... Semrau, M. (2016). Information systems for mental health in six low and middle income countries: Cross country situation analysis. *International Journal of Mental Health Systems, 10*(1), 60. https://ijmhs.biomedcentral.com/articles/10.1186/s13033-016-0094-2

van Ommeren, M., Barbui, C., de Jong, K., Dua, T., Jones, L., Perez-Sales, P., ... Saxena, S. (2011). If you could only choose five psychotropic medicines: Updating the interagency emergency health kit. *PLoS Medicine, 8*(5), e1001030. doi:10.1371/journal.pmed.1001030

Ventevogel, P., Ryan, G. K., Kahi, V., & Kane, J. C. (2019). Capturing the essential: Revising the mental health categories in UNHCR's refugee health information system. *Intervention, 17,* 17–22.

Ventevogel, P., van Ommeren, M., Schilperoord, M., & Saxena, S. (2015). Improving mental health care in humanitarian emergencies. *Bulletin of the World Health Organization, 93*(10), 666–666A.

Verdeli, H., Clougherty, K., Bolton, P., Speelman, L., Lincoln, N., Bass, J., Neugebauer, R., & Weissman, M. M. (2003). Adapting group interpersonal psychotherapy for a developing country: experience in rural Uganda. *World Psychiatry: Official Journal of the World Psychiatric Association (WPA), 2*(2), 114–120.

World Health Organization. (2005). *Mental health information systems.* Geneva: World Health Organization.

World Health Organization, & Ministry of Health Lebanon. (2015). *WHO-AIMS Report on mental health system in Lebanon.* Geneva: World Health Organization. Retrieved from https://www.moph.gov.lb/en/Pages/0/9109/who-aims-report-on-mental-health-system-in-lebanon.

World Health Organization. (2016). *mhGAP Intervention Guide (mhGAP-IG) version 2.0 for mental, neurological and substance use disorders for non-specialist health settings.* Geneva: World Health Organization.

13
Innovative Education Pathways for Refugees to Strengthen Health Systems

Minerva Rivas Velarde

Introduction

The chapters explores how technology-mediated interventions can enable refugee youth to contribute to health care delivery, from a health systems approach (Mutale, 2013; World Health Organization, 2010). It aims to contribute to the call issued by the Alliance for Health Policy and Systems Research and the World Health Organization (WHO) (George, Paina, & Scott, 2017) to understand the human agency of the health workforce in fragile contexts and to understand the social and political contexts that are shaping their workplaces and practices. This chapter builds upon the findings of a larger research study conducted by the University of Geneva looking at strengthening the capacity of the health workforce in Dadaab (Burkardt, Krause, & Rivas Velarde, 2019). In this study, the issue being considered is from the perspective of a junior professional in Dadaab refugee camp.

Using the WHO's health system building blocks this chapter will present the findings from a study examining the development and implementation of a blended program for capacity building on Dadaab refugee camp in Kenya, which was considered the largest refugee camp in the world, and the attempt of the Kenyan government to repatriate its 350,000 Somali refugees. This case study analyses the interaction between human resources, technology, governance, and service delivery.

The following section will provide an overview of the refugee crisis, a review of the available literature, and present key facts about the Dadaab refugee complex. It will continue by assessing the trends and gaps in available knowledge regarding how technology tools and blended learning can enable refugee youth to contribute to healthcare delivery in refugee camps. The findings of this study will shed light on the complexities of the health system in refugee settings. It will use four of the six building blocks of the WHO's health system architecture to examine the interaction of human resources, technology, governance, and service. The findings include a qualitative analysis of the views of refugee youth and health services managers. The conclusion will reflect on how person-centered health systems need to address the social and macro-structural constraints faced by refugees, as well as the human agency of people in this context, as these dynamics are shaping the profile of important aspects of the health workforce and consequently health service delivery in the region.

Minerva Rivas Velarde, *Innovative Education Pathways for Refugees to Strengthen Health Systems* In: *Systems Thinking for Global Health*. Edited by: Fiona Larkan, Frédérique Vallières, Hasheem Mannan, and Naonori Kodate, Oxford University Press. © Oxford University Press 2023. DOI: 10.1093/oso/9780198799498.003.0013

The Refugee Crisis and Dadaab, Kenya

In recent years, the world has been facing a refugee crisis of unprecedented proportions (United Nations High Commissioner for Refugees, 2017). The number of people affected by humanitarian crises and conflicts has almost doubled over the past decade and is expected to keep rising (World Humanitarian Summit, 2015). According to the United Nations High Commissioner for Refugees (UNHCR), 65.6 million people around the world have been forced out of their homes due to conflict, persecution, and acute social crisis.

In 2017, Kenya hosted 490,656 registered refugees and asylum seekers. The large majority of these individuals are Somali nationals, who represent 62% of the total refugee population in Kenya. This chapter reports the findings of a pilot project conducted in the Dadaab refugee camp from February 2017 to February 2018. Dadaab, located in Garissa County, was once considered the largest refugee camp in the world. It was first established in 1991 after the collapse of the Somali government caused civilians to flee the civil war and cross the border into Kenya. A second large influx occurred in 2011, when nearly 130,000 refugees arrived, escaping drought and famine in southern Somalia (United Nations High Commissioner for Refugees, 2014, 2017).

More than twenty years after the camp was first established, it became clear that a solution must be found for the refugees. In 2013, the governments of Somalia and Kenya and the UNHCR signed the Tripartite Agreement designed to promote the voluntary return of Dadaab's 400,000 refugees to Somalia (United Nations High Commissioner for Refugees, 2013). The principle of voluntary return and the right to return in safety and dignity were at the core of the Tripartite Agreement. It also made clear that repatriation was the solution preferred by the Kenyan government. A year later, a permanent encampment policy was put in place. In 2014, Kenya amended the Refugees Act of 2006 to adopt a permanent encampment policy. This provision stated that "[e]very person who has applied for recognition of his status as a refugee and every member of his family shall remain in the designated refugee camp until the processing of their status is concluded."

Later in 2015, Kenya suffered a series of terrorist attacks. As a consequence of this wave of violence, in May 2016 the government of Kenya announced the immediate closure of Dadaab and the repatriation of its 350,000 Somali refugees, as it believed that terrorist organizations had infiltrated the camp (Kenyan Government, 2016). Somalia is not safe, and this forced repatriation put thousands of civilians at risk. The Kenyan Human Rights Commission, alongside other international non-governmental organizations (NGOs), challenged this decision in court. This decision was then overturned in February 2017 by the Kenyan High Court, which ruled that the decision by the government to repatriate all refugees collectively violated the principle of the 1951 United Nations Convention Relating to the Status of Refugees Article 33.

Governance: Its Impact on Human Resources for Health

The High Court ruling means that refugees in Dadaab can stay in the camp at present and thus the encampment policy also remains. Training and capacity-building opportunities for youth living in the camp are very limited. Furthermore, regarding employment, refugees in Kenya can only participate in the workforce at the camp as "incentive staff" or seek employment in the informal sector. "Incentive staff" is a category of employment. "incentive work" only allows refugees to earn an income in the form of incentives as opposed to salaries. Incentives may include cash, vouchers, or in-kind goods as remuneration for work or services. Mbai, Mangeni, & Abuelaish (2017) found that refugees were often present in health services across the refugee complex and made a significant contribution to the healthcare workforce. Thus, however, this study also highlighted that refugees, formally hired in healthcare facilities, tended to hold mostly entry-level jobs, such as nursing assistant, and received limited training or none at all. Their results also demonstrated that incentive work schemes were having a negative impact on building capacity across the health workforce in refugee camps, as health workers in Dadaab often felt demotivated by the lack of payment. Even if refugees happen to be qualified, they cannot achieve the necessary registrations from the relevant national councils for health professionals or obtain a work permit. While the Kenya Citizenship and Immigration Act allows refugees and their spouses to apply for and obtain a "Class M" work permit, the availability and accessibility of this type of work permit seems questionable. According to the Refugee Consortium of Kenya, "it is unclear if these are currently being issued at all." As a result, refugees can either participate in the workforce under the category of incentive workers in the camp or seek employment in the informal sector. There is no formal guidance or standards for incentive work at present (Morris, 2014; Burkardt et al., 2019).

Education, Constraints Faced by Refugees Youth, and Human Resources for Health

In recent years, the lack of professional education for refugees has appeared to be worsening. In 2019, the UNHCR publish that less than 3% of refugees worldwide had access to post-secondary education. While the provision of primary and secondary education showed improvements in access, that to higher education deteriorated. In addition, this publication showed that a number of humanitarian agencies were rolling out programs with the aim of enabling refugees living in camps to access post-secondary education, including professional health education (United Nations High Commissioner for Refugees, 2019). To date, there is very little scientific literature on the implementation and effect of such programs.

Available literature regarding professional health education for refugees and the refugee health workforce in refugee camps will be now presented. The few studies identified focused on technical inputs and the effect which this type of education for refugees could have on population health. Burkardt et al. (2019) found delivering quality professional health education via blended learning in refugee camps could be an efficient way of strengthening human resources for health and service delivery. The authors noted that education gaps, severe scarcity, and infrastructural constraints, alongside the lack of recognition of educational credits and credentials in both countries of origin and countries of resettlement are some of the main barriers to the implementation of such post-secondary health education for refugee youth in refugee camps. Particularly pertaining to Dadaab, Mbai et al. (2017) found that due to infrastructural constraints, professional degrees in areas such as nursing and medicine although needed were not feasible on Dadaab refugee camps. Thus training community health workers could positively contribute to the needs of the health services and strengthening health service delivery in Dadaab and, in the longer term, in Somalia (Mbai et al., 2017).

Khan (2019) found that making prenatal care training available and accessible to refugee women in refugee camps has a positive impact in health services both internally and out in communities. Also in relation to maternal care, Sami (2017) found that delivering high-quality, short professional training to the refugee workforce in refugee camps in South Sudan could have a positive impact on health service delivery. On the Thailand–Burmese border, Minden (1997) and Turner et al. (2013) found that capacity-building training for lay refugees living in refugee camps has a positive impact in supportive care for babies in a neonatal intensive care unit. Furthermore, Chen et al. (2008) analyzed the impact of delivering sexual and reproductive training to lay refugees in forty-eight camps in Guinea. Their results showed a positive impact on the control of sexually transmitted diseases (STDs) and maternal health interventions. In the Americas, Cropley (2004) utilized a controlled post-test, community-based study to evaluate the effects of a health education intervention that involved training up lay refugee health workers to deliver education on child malaria treatment-seeking practices among rural refugee mothers. Their results also showed a positive effect on treatment-seeking behaviors. Ehiri et al. (2014) analyzed the available literature via systematic review and concluded that providing training in basic health services to lay refugees and internally displaced populations could bring about positive outcomes for population health, although evidence remains weak.

As outlined, available research tends to focus on the technical inputs rather than the agency that refugees bring into health services. In contrast, this chapter aims to contribute to understanding the role of refugees as a health workforce. From a systems-thinking perspective, capacity building for refugee youth living in refugee camps and development of effective and sustainable professional training models and pathways can be better analyzed by using four of the six building blocks of the WHO's health system architecture, namely medical technology, information, human resources, and service delivery. This study offers empirical data of the use of technology tools used to deliver high-quality training of international recognition. This promotes empowers of refugee youth and better working conditions and opportunities, addressing governance issues, while solving the human resources shortage in refugee camps and potentially in countries of origin and settlement countries.

Woodward, Sondorp, Witter, & Martineau (2016) stated that health system research in conflict-affected areas and fragile contexts should priorities action toward understanding the health workforce. They considered that investing in building the capacity of a health workforce will improve healthcare delivery and may have a positive impact on rebuilding communities and states. Health systems researchers continue to call for additional research that enables a better understanding of the social agency of health workers and the microstructural relationships that influence them (Schneider & Leman, 2016).

The literature reviewed in this chapter points out gaps and methodological shortcomings but also provides a baseline to expand and explore the profile of the health workforce in the region and the provision of professional health education as part of a complex system.

(i) Blended learning course, technology tools, and its delivery

The "Distance Basic Training of Healthcare Professionals" was a blended training course provided by the University of Geneva to junior healthcare personnel in the Dadaab Refugee complex. The course was designed to address constraints faced by students in the refugee camp and to open career opportunities for them in the health sectors locally and abroad as it credits were internationally recognized. The course materials were delivered using a Moodle platform. Students were able to access a desktop computer with Internet connection at a student hub and at the local health setting which was a partner to the University of Geneva in the delivery of this course. Local transportation fees from campsite to the study sites were covered by the University of Geneva. A universal serial bus (USB) stick provided to all students contained all written materials in order to avoid Internet connectivity issues. Course training materials were complemented by teaching support from medical students of the University of Geneva, via e-tutorials on WhatsApp. Students also received a face-to-face teaching input on site.

The research protocol was submitted to the Swiss Ethics Committees on research involving humans. Information sheets were distributed, participation was voluntary, and confidentiality and anonymity were assured. The research ethics approval was granted by the committee. The assigned protocol number is 2017-00632.

Data Collection and Analysis

A research study accompanied the piloting of a blended learning course on basic medical science, targeted at refugee youths and offering with a certificate of successfully completing secondary education. Those who completed the course were given grades that made them eligible for higher education; it was aimed at those who would like to pursue a career in healthcare or were already active in a junior post in the health sector. The author who was in charge of the scientific validation of this course evaluated the course, its structure, contents, and relevance. Tool used included online surveys, learning analytics data, and exchanges in online forums and student chat groups. Data from all of these sources were used to inform three major research questions pertaining to the overall contribution of such interventions in the refugee context, the questions were how blended learning in refugee camps could be adapted to the refugee camps context, what are the barriers and enablers for higher education in the refugee camp context, and how technology-mediated interventions can enable refugee youth to contribute to healthcare delivery, from a health systems approach.

This study explored the perceptions of refugee youth regarding access to training, higher education, and employment, their experiences with blended learning, using computer and their mobiles phones for training, as well as their perception on pursuing a career in the health sector. It includes a focus group of ten refugee graduates and ten individual semi-structured interviews. Nine of the ten of the participants were active in the health workforce or had held health-related posts within the health setting as incentive staff. This study also includes semi-structured interviews with four managers from the health service who directly supervised the refugees and a fact-finding mission that involved informal information sessions and meetings with several key actors from the health and education sectors, which informed the interpretation of the published literature and the empirical research.

The audio-recorded data from the interviews were transcribed and the transcripts sent by email to the interviewees for validation (Mero-Jaffe, 2011). This process provided the interviewees with the opportunity to verify what was reported, and during this validation process the participants were asked to add more comments, change their replies, and add questions or withdraw from the research if they so wished. Subsequently, all of the information was coded, and thematic analysis techniques were applied. Three interrelated themes emerged, namely: perceptions of a career in the health sector; training and education needs; and governance, mobility, and views on Somalia. These will be outlined in the following section.

Findings

Health workers are the heart of health systems. Their own narratives of their lived experience have been analyzed to gain an understanding of the social norms and structural forces that shape the roles they are currently playing in healthcare. This section centers on three interrelated themes: (i) Entering the health workforce; (ii) Technology tools, training, and education needs; and (iii) Governance, mobility, and migration.

The views of refugees have been compared and contrasted with the views of the health personnel who have supervised junior staff. The analysis was informed by information collected during a mission that included meetings with stakeholders from the education and health sectors in the region. Refugee participants have been assigned a number, and the letters "FG" will be used for quotations from the focus group; managers will be identified by a letter. Given the small sample of participants, no gender or any other types of personal information will be cited.

Entering the Health Workforce

All participants, including health personnel and refugee participants, described their communities as severely underserved and needing an increase in the coverage of their health services. They recalled frequent shortages of health services and health personnel available to them. Refugee alumni referred to their decisions to pursue a career in healthcare as fulfilling a responsibility to serve their communities. This decision was also often linked to their desire to care for sick relatives and for more disadvantaged members of their community. Their narratives about entering often resemble an emancipatory action, as it appeared that being able to care for the family and communities translated into taking action against neglect and negative personal experiences. The following quotes synthesized these thoughts:

> "I would like to have this (professional health worker) as a career because I could help my family." 1
>
> "I would like to help my father with hepatitis." 8
>
> "The community does not get enough medical care—I would like to contribute and help." 5

Nevertheless, their expressed will to enter and move up the ladder within the local health sector was accompanied by a clear account of the limitations attached to their refugee status and the lack of pathways available to them in the camp. In that respect, gaining accredited training was seen as something that could enable them to overcome those barriers. Entering the health sector was seen as being able to facilitate social mobility: refugee graduates also saw a career in the health sectors as entering a prestigious sphere in their community—one that was often unobtainable to them as refugees. They felt that entering this field would gain them the respect of their communities. Furthermore, obtaining an entry-level position and a basic medical science education boosted their self-confidence and made them feel more assertive about gaining the necessary qualifications to be a professional health worker. For females, this feeling was stronger than in males and was evident to others. Managers who supervised junior staff who were also graduates narrated how these young female refugees seemed more confident, curious, and independent after accessing accredited training. The young women were also described as champions in their communities and the managers believed that they had inspired other young females to pursue further education and enter the health workforce. They stated:

> "If you know medical [science], you will be respected in the society. I believe I can be even a doctor." 2
>
> "She [is] motivating other youths [and] other women to study. This training gives them respect in [their] community." M

Furthermore, entering the health workforce was often associated with gaining control over one's destiny; participants believed that entering this field would also open doors that would enable them to access opportunities that could help them to be self-sufficient, to leave the camp, to enter further training, or to gain employment elsewhere, particularly in Somalia. The following quotations capture these ideas:

> "I need more practical skills. I would like to get outside the camps if it's possible." 10
>
> "If I got the chance, I will go [to work] alone, if my family come [it] is OK, but I might go alone." 7

> "I know the theory [but] this certificate delayed me. But, I just need to get it ... My friend told me when you get a certificate come [to Somalia] immediately [and] you will get a job." 2

The data collected corroborated what the literature outlines: that pursuing professional health education is very difficult for young refugees due to the policies of their encampments and the legal restrictions that prohibit them from leaving their camp, accessing further training, and having previous training recognized (Burkardt et al., 2019). The refugees interviewed mentioned these limitation and stated that they find it to be demotivating and devaluing their contribution:

> "If you see your friends making 1,000 dollars and compare it what we [are] making here, I [would] prefer a job in Somalia." 7

Refugees employed in health services in Dadaab are hired under the "non-skilled" workers category, according to managers. The managers interviewed claimed that moving from the non-skilled to the skilled category was very difficult for refugees and was outside their control as it related to a broader legislative structure which they could not affect. They clarified that to be employed as skilled staff, applicants needed to comply with the paperwork, which required them to present an accredited diploma and apply for registration and licensing at the respective national councils for health professionals, both of which are often unavailable for refugees in Dadaab. Managers claimed that refugee health workers already contributed greatly to healthcare services, and that they do so in many ways including acting as cultural brokers within their services as they can communicate effectively with the community because they not only speak the same language but they also understand the community's cultural protocols and practices.

> "They can help us because they have the language—we do not. They can talk to the community and share their knowledge." M

Refugees are contributing to the delivery of health services in Dadaab and their need for training has been noted and addressed by the Office of the United Nations High Commissioner for Human Rights (UNHCHR), NGOs, and higher education institutions from all over the world. The following section addresses the findings relating to the current education opportunities offered in Dadaab.

(ii) Technology tools, training, and education needs

Accessing blended learning enables participants to access high-quality training, bypassing contextual constraints. Students used computers at the study sites and their smartphones to access material from the course and communicate with mentors and fellow students. They often access course material on their smartphones by using USB On-The-Go (OTG-B) adaptors for their USB sticks. WhatsApp was very popular among students and staff. Its features, voice and video features, and web versions allowed a great degree of interaction between students and mentors. The course took advantage of all available technology to facilitate training. Managers said that blended learning and the use of mobile devices and online learning tools as highly advantageous. This suggests that innovative context-sensitive health education programs and innovative information and communications technology (ICT) solutions could help to address health workforce shortages in refugee camps. The following quotation illustrates the advantages on online learning

> "We can go online and learn. We don't have a classroom, it's flexible and we can learn and continue to do our jobs and our responsibilities." 3

The large majority of this group of participants had participated in the health workforce and received on-the-job training alongside short vocational courses. Nevertheless, the participants felt that this training had little value as it did not help them to climb the career ladder within the health sector or secure a job elsewhere through choice or necessity. The possibilities for professional health education are significantly constrained in the Dadaab refugee camp. The refugee alumni interviewed were highly motivated to learn but also to gain accreditation for their learning—ideally, they would like to gain a university degree. The large majority would like to become doctors or nurses. The following quotations synthesize the participants' overall perceptions:

> "I wanted to be a doctor. I did other courses before in practical skills and nursing. But I want to learn more." 2
>
> "With the certificate, you will have opportunities. If I applied for a job, I will have more changes of getting it." 6

However, achieving the goal of becoming a doctor or a nurse is difficult when living as a refugee. Therefore, a number of post-secondary education institutions have been offering professional health education courses in Dadaab over the last five years. This study has identified a number of initiatives run by local NGOs and Kenyan and northern universities that are offering a range of professional health education and vocational health-related training to refugees in Dadaab. Such initiatives include The Windle Trust Kenya & World University Services of Canada, Kenyatta University—Campus Dadaab, the Lutheran World Federation, Borderless Higher Education for Refugees (BHER), Moi University, and North Coast Medical Training College. For the majority of these programs, it was very difficult to determine the reach of their activities, the number of students enrolled, the upcoming intake, the nature of the training, their curriculum, or the recruitment processes, due to a lack of publicly available information. However, some information about these programs was obtained through participants, particularly those in managerial positions. They also reiterated that information is hard to find and tends to be decentralized. This lack of accessibility and availability of information, coupled with infrastructural constraints to access the Internet or even to move around the camp, raises concerns about equal opportunities for refugees in receiving training and gaining opportunities for jobs and contributing to the health workforce. This lack of effective dissemination could be imposing a new layer of exclusion.

Participants' educational priorities, as pointed out above, included becoming doctors or nurses. On the other hand, the training priorities listed by managers highlighted midwives, laboratory workers, nurses, and community health workers. Education options in Dadaab are failing to meet the aspirations of young refugees. What is currently feasible to deliver in this isolated and underserved location does not match their expectations. Some of these youths could access scholarship programs, including the DAFI (Albert Einstein German Academic Refugee Initiative) scholarship program and the Bureau of Population, Refugees, and Migration program. However, access to those schemes is very limited, and removing the students from their families might come with unintended negative consequences like breaking links between the student and their community (Office of the United Nations Commissioner for Human Rights).

(iii) Governance, mobility, and views on Somalia

Mobility drives refugee lives. Refugee youths tend to be very mobile, and their future locations are often unclear, whether this is to do with facing forced repatriation, as intended by the initiative of the Kenyan government, or having to resettle in a different camp or a third country. Mobility has a strong impact and should be carefully considered in the design of capacity-building models for health workers in refugee camps.

The possibility of being repatriated was very present in the narratives of the refugee participants—sometimes as a goal and other times as the only option left to them. All participants, including managers, pointed out that if refugees have professional health education credentials even at a junior level, Somalia offers them more professional opportunities than Dadaab. These claims, which were often framed in ambiguity and complex references, were difficult to corroborate. The following quotations emphasized this:

> "My friends in Somalia told me to convert my career to medical, medical is very important in Somalia. And we are willing to come back to Somalia. As there is mass repatriation. My friends told me if you don't get medical training don't come to Somalia, for you the opportunities to get a job in Somalia are very low in other areas." 2
>
> "People are getting jobs, people from here are going, I know almost ten people who have got jobs there. If you have training here, you are ahead of people [there] (Somalia)." M

Students referred to repatriation as the most feasible option for them to develop a career as a healthcare professional. Thus, following this option was a divisive issue. Some students made reference to friends and family members who had told them that if they had a valid certificate that credited them as a junior health worker, they could most likely get a job in the health sector in Somalia and make ten times more money than they were getting as incentive staff in Dadaab. The literature on health systems has pointed out that secure livelihoods and compensation are key motivating factors for those health workers at the lower levels of the health workforce, which naturally affects recruitment and retention in low-income contexts (Tijdens, de Vries, &

Steinmetz, 2013). These findings are in line with the literature, suggesting that participants claimed that compensation is key to staff retention. Furthermore, the narratives described the health sector in Somalia as booming and suggested that refugees could benefit from it if they opted for voluntary repatriation. Refugee participants claimed that employment websites seemed to corroborate the stories of their friends. The following quotations elaborate on this point:

> "I can find information through my friends. I know there are many jobs." 10
>
> "I believe that with a certificate . . . I will leave to get a job in Somalia." FG

The findings of this research are similar to previous evidence of the movement of people between Somalia and Kenya (Mbai, 2017). The border between Somalia and Kenya is porous and people move between the two countries for different reasons that go beyond the scope of this chapter. Almost half of the refugees interviewed had recently been in Somalia and had pursued or had in the past held jobs in the health sector. All of them had come back to Dadaab. They stated that the information shared about jobs in Somalia was not fully factual and often played down the serious security concerns in the country, the barriers they would face due to tribalism, and the lack of protection for returnees. They elaborated that these issues tinted their previous experience in Somalia.

> "You might not get a job because of tribalism, even [if] you are highly qualified." FG
>
> "Tribalism is present in Somalia, and you might get a job with luck. If you get a job and another person wants your job . . . they will kill you." FG

Some of the refugees also explained that there were complex barriers to professional health education in Somalia. They mentioned that although this is technically available, not knowing the system and having to pay fees alongside the cost of living made this inaccessible for them.

> "I learned here for free because I cannot pay fees." 4
>
> "Continuing my education in Somalia will be hard. I would not be able to pay fees, here I get support. In Somalia, I not only need to pay fees, but I don't have a home there . . . I need more than only fees." 9

Furthermore, it is difficult to estimate the precise number of higher education programs on offer in Somalia. For example, the Heritage Institute for Policy Studies, an NGO based in Mogadishu, reported the existence of forty-four higher education institutions in Somalia. Later in 2016, the European Union claimed that there were now close to 1,003 higher education institutions in Somalia with over 50,000 students enrolled. However, in 2017 the *International Handbook of Universities*, published by the United Nations Educational, Scientific and Cultural Organization (UNESCO), only listed eight. Pertaining to professional health education, the Swedish Action Group for Health Research and Development in Somalia reported that in 2017 there were twenty health professional training programs and fourteen medical colleges in Somalia (Dalmar et al., 2017).

(iv) Limitations

The data collected for this research, the analysis, and the findings were treated with great caution due to the limited sample involved. This sample used in this study does not intend to be representative of all refugees in Dadaab, nor of the trends in the region. Small samples are not uncommon in research conducted in fragile contexts, as it is a well-established fact that conducting research in fragile and conflict-affected contexts is challenging due to security concerns, attitudes of distrust and restricted mobility (Raven, 2014; Martineau et al., 2017).

Conclusion

As conflict around the world continues to increase more must be done to understand the context in which refugees are living. The findings on this chapter show that available technology can allow building capacities across health workers and potentially improve service delivery in fragile context, such as refugee camps. It also shows that it is important to work toward governance structures that are more conducive to secure livelihoods and fair compensation for health workers. Enhancing the synergies between eligible young people, innovative education models, and technology to deliver professional health education and the health system could contribute to building these pathways and could contribute to strengthening health service delivery in fragile contexts such as refugee camps. Refugees are contributing to the delivery of healthcare and their contribution is valued and needed.

More research is needed in order to understand the priorities, training needs, and opportunities of formal and informal human resources for health in fragile settings. Furthermore, there is also a need to address knowledge gaps regarding the impact that fractured and fragile governance structures have on human resources constraints and service delivery. Context-sensitive technology tools can help to overpass severe constraints such as those in refugee camps and have been proven to enable the delivery of high-quality health education (Burkardt et al., 2019). This can only happen by addressing cross-cutting issues regarding the social and structural constraints faced by refugee youths. The literature analyzing how the migration of health service workers affects health systems in both high- and low-income contexts continues to grow (Jones, Bifulco, & Gabe, 2009; Kroezen, 2105; Humphries et al., 2015). There is, however, a gap in the research regarding refugee contexts and refugees as contributors to the health workforce. More research is needed to address migration and repatriation of refugees in the region through the lens of health systems research.

Acknowledgment

I would like to acknowledge invaluable support of Prof. Antoine Geissbühler and Medical students Aude Burkardt and Nicerine Krause, as well as the network for eHealth in Africa (the RAFT, Réseau en Afrique Francophone pour la Télémédecine) Geneva University Hospitals, Switzerland.

References

Burkardt, A. D., Krause, N., & Rivas Velarde, M. C. (2019). Critical success factors for the implementation and adoption of e-learning for junior health care workers in Dadaab refugee camp Kenya. *Human Resources for Health, 17*(1), 98. Retrieved from https://doi.org/10.1186/s12960-019-0435-8.

Chen, M. I., von Roenne, A., Souare, Y., von Roenne, F., Ekirapa, A., Howard, N., & Borchert, M. (2008). Reproductive health for refugees by refugees in Guinea II: Sexually transmitted infections. *Conflict and Health, 2*(1), 14.

Cropley, L. (2004). The effect of health education interventions on child malaria treatment-seeking practices among mothers in rural refugee *villages* in Belize, Central America. *Health Promotion International, 19*(4), 445–452.

Dalmar, A. A., Hussein, A. S., Walhad, S. A., Ibrahim, A. O., Abdi, A. A., Ali, M. K., … Yusuf, M. W. (2017). Rebuilding research capacity in fragile states: The case of a Somali–Swedish global health initiative: Somali–Swedish Action Group for Health Research and Development. *Global Health Action, 10*(1), 1–8.

Ehiri, J. E., Gunn, J. K., Center, K. E., Li, Y., Rouhani, M., & Ezeanolue, E. E. (2014). Training and deployment of lay refugee/internally displaced persons to provide basic health services in camps: A systematic review. *Global Health Action, 7*(1), 1–14.

George, A., Scott, K., & Govender, V. (Eds.). (2017). *Health policy and systems research reader on human resources for health*. Geneva: World Health Organization.

Humphries, N., McAleese, S., Matthews, A., & Brugha, R. (2015). "Emigration is a matter of self-preservation. The working conditions … are killing us slowly": Qualitative insights into health professional emigration from Ireland. *Human Resources for Health, 13*(1), 1–35.

Jones, A. D., Bifulco, A., & Gabe, J. (2009). Caribbean nurses migrating to the UK: A gender-focused literature review. *International Nursing Review, 56*(3), 285–290.

Kenyan Government. (2016). *Kenyan Citizen and Immigration Act No. 12 of 2011*. Nairobi, Kenya.

Kenyan Government. (2016). *Kenya: Government statement on refugees and closure of refugee camps, Department of Refugee Affairs*. Retrieved from https://minbane.wordpress.com/2016/05/06/httpwp-mep1xtjg-2ed/.

Khan, A., & DeYoung, S. (2019) Maternal health services for refugee populations: Exploration of best practices. *Global Public Health, 14*, 3, 362–374. doi:10.1080/17441692.2018.1516796

Kroezen, M., Dussault, G., Craveiro, I., Dieleman, M., Jansen, C., Buchan, J., … Sermeus, W. (2015). Recruitment and retention of health professionals across Europe: A literature review and multiple case study research. *Health Policy, 119*(12), 1517–1528.

Martineau, T., McPake, B., Theobald, S., Raven, J., Ensor, T., Fustukian, S., … Hooton, N. (2017). Leaving no one behind: Lessons on rebuilding health systems in conflict-and crisis-affected states. *BMJ Global Health, 2*(2), e000327.

Mbai, I. I., Mangeni, J. N., & Abuelaish, I. (2017). Community health workers and education in the refugee context. In *Science research and education in Africa: Proceedings of a conference on science advancement* (p. 163–188). Cambridge: Cambridge Scholars Publishing.

Mero-Jaffe, I. (2011). "Is that what I said?" Interview transcript approval by participants: An aspect of ethics in qualitative research. *International Journal of Qualitative Methods, 10*(3), 231–247.

Minden, M. (1997). Midwives for refugees. *World Health, 50*(2), 18–19.

Morris, H., & Voon, F. (2014). *Which side are you on? Discussion paper on UNHCR's policy and practice of incentive payments to refugees.* PDES PDES/2014/04/ Geneva: Policy Development and Evaluation Service, United Nations High Commissioner for Refugees. Retrieved from http://www.unhcr.org/5491577c9.html.xyz

Mutale, W., Bond, V., Mwanamwenge, M. T., Mlewa, S., Balabanova, D., Spicer, N., & Ayles, H. (2013). Systems thinking in practice: The current status of the six WHO building blocks for health system strengthening in three BHOMA intervention districts of Zambia: A baseline qualitative study. *BMC Health Services Research, 13*(1), 1–9.

Raven, J., et al. (2014). Fragile and conflict affected states: report from the Consultation on Collaboration for Applied Health Research and Delivery. *Conflict and Health, 8*(1), 15.

Sami, A., Kerber, K., Tomczyk, B., Amsalu, R., Jackson, D., Scudder, E., ... Mullany, L. (2017). "You have to take action": Changing knowledge and attitudes towards newborn care practices during crisis in South Sudan. *Reproductive Health Matters, 25*(51), 124–139. doi:10.1080/09688080.2017.1405677

Schneider, H., & Lehmann, U. (2016). From community health workers to community health systems: Time to widen the horizon? *Health Systems & Reform, 2*(2), 112–118.

Tijdens, K., de Vries, D. H., & Steinmetz, S. (2013). Health workforce remuneration: Comparing wage levels, ranking, and dispersion of 16 occupational groups in 20 countries. *Human Resources for Health, .11*, 11. doi:10.1186/1478-4491-11-11. PMID: 23448429; PMCID: PMC3787851.

Turner, C., Carrara, V., Thein, N. A. M., Win, N. C. M. M., Turner, P., Bancone, G., ... Nosten, F. (2013). Neonatal intensive care in a Karen refugee camp: A 4 year descriptive study. *PloS One, 8*(8), e72721.

United Nations (1951). *Convention Relating to the Status of Refugees*, July 28, 1951, United Nations, Treaty Series, vol. 189. Geneva: United Nations.

United Nations High Commissioner for Refugees. *Dadaab camp population statistics.* Retrieved from https://www.unhcr.org/ke/dadaab-refugee-complex#:~:text=The%20Dadaab%20refugee%20complex%20has,complex%20consists%20of%20three%20camps

United Nations High Commissioner for Refugees. (2013). *Tripartite Agreement Between the Government of the Republic of Kenya, the Government of the Federal Republic of Somalia and the United Nations High Commissioner for Refugees Governing the Voluntary Repatriation of Somali Refugees Living in Kenya, November 10, 2013.* Retrieved from http://www.refworld.org/docid/5285e0294.html.

United Nations High Commissioner for Refugees. (2014). *Seeking access to detained asylum-seekers and refugees in Nairobi, UNHCR.* Retrieved from http://www.unhcr.org/5342b35d9.html

United Nations High Commissioner for Refugees. (2017). *Camp population statistics.* Retrieved from https://www.unhcr.org/refugee-statistics/

United Nations High Commissioner for Refugees. (2017). *Dadaab, Kenya bi-weekly update.* Retrieved from https://www.unhcr.org/ke/wp-content/uploads/sites/2/2017/07/15-July-UNHCR-Dadaab-bi-weekly-Update.pdf1-15-November.pdf.

United Nations High Commissioner for Refugees. (2017). *Left behind refugee education crisis.* Retrieved from https://www.unhcr.org/left-behind/

United Nations Educational, Scientific and Cultural Organization. (2017). *World higher education database.* Retrieved from http://www.unesco.vg/INTERNATIONAL_HANDBOOK.pdf.

United Nations High Commissioner for Refugees. (2019). *Stepping up refugee education in crisis*. Retrieved from https://www.unhcr.org/steppingup/wp-content/uploads/sites/76/2019/09/Education-Report-2019-Final-web-9.pdf.

Woodward, A., Sondorp, E., Witter, S., & Martineau, T. (2016). Health systems research in fragile and conflict-affected states: A research agenda-setting exercise. *Health Research Policy and Systems*, *14*(1), 51.

World Health Organization. (2010). *Monitoring the building blocks of health systems: A handbook of indicators and their measurement strategies*. Geneva: World Health Organization.

World Humanitarian Summit Secretariat. (2015). *Restoring humanity: Synthesis of the consultation process for the World Humanitarian Summit*. New York, NY: United Nations.

14

Using Systems Thinking as a Heuristic in the Design of Interventions for Social Inclusion

"Including the excluded is a complex challenge"
(World Bank, 2013)

Tessy Huss, Euan Mackway-Jones, and Malcolm MacLachlan*

*The ideas and opinions expressed in this book/article are those of the author and do not necessarily represent the view of UNESCO.

Introduction

Social inclusion denotes an aspirational state of being where individuals or groups fully participate in all spheres of political, economic, cultural, and societal life (United Nations Department of Economic and Social Affairs, 2009; Silver 2015). Often the result of discrimination, social exclusion manifests as marginalization and deprivation. Poverty and social exclusion tend to disproportionately affect individuals who are already vulnerable and less resilient to crises (Hoogeveen, Tesliuc, Vakis, & Dercon, 2004). Social exclusion has also been recognized as a social determinant of health (O'Donnell, O'Donovan, & Elmusharaf, 2018).

The imperative of advancing social inclusion for achieving sustainable development was underscored by the international community's adoption of Agenda 2030 and Sustainable Development Goals (SDGs). The promotion of social inclusion is central to achieving Goal 3 ("Ensure healthy lives and promote well-being for all at all ages"), but also Goals 4, 8, 9, 10, and, in particular, Goal 16 ("Promote peaceful and inclusive societies for sustainable development, provide access to justice for all and build effective, accountable and inclusive institutions at all levels") (United Nations, n.d.). Through these goals, and the associated ethos of the Agenda to "leave no one behind," (see United Nations Sustainable Development Group, 2021) the importance of social inclusion as an essential enabler for driving progress toward other development objectives was recognized at the highest political level.

However, despite this popularity, significant debate still exists about how, and for what, social inclusion can be conceptually and operationally useful (du Toit, 2004). On the one hand, this can be explained by its enduring definitional ambiguity, encompassing both a process and an outcome, and being interpreted and applied differently within contrasting paradigms of political philosophy (Silver, 1994; Allman, 2013). On the other hand, it can be explained by the continuing siloed approach to

Tessy Huss, Euan Mackway-Jones, and Malcolm MacLachlan, *Using Systems Thinking as a Heuristic in the Design of Interventions for Social Inclusion* In: *Systems Thinking for Global Health.* Edited by: Fiona Larkan, Frédérique Vallières, Hasheem Mannan, and Naonori Kodate, Oxford University Press. © Oxford University Press 2023. DOI: 10.1093/oso/9780198799498.003.0014

the construction and implementation of policies on marginalization, poverty, and disadvantage, rendering the multifaceted, dynamic, and relational concept of inclusion difficult to understand or use in practice.

Indeed, it is the appreciation that many stakeholders continue to be challenged by applying the complex concept of inclusion within their own work that underpins the purpose of this chapter. Through exploring the characteristics of social inclusion, and demonstrating its inherently complex and adaptive nature, it is argued that models of "rational-technical decision-making" (Head & Alford, 2015) are insufficient to understand and operationalize inclusion in an effective manner, and instead, approaches that appreciate complexity—such as a systems thinking—are needed to render it a more useful conceptual and operational reference for tackling issues related to marginalization and development.

Systems Thinking and Complex Adaptive Systems

In recent years, systems thinking and systems approaches have been adopted across many fields and disciplines, prompted by the ever-increasing complexity of the objects and subjects of our enquiries. Systems thinking is a "discipline for seeing wholes . . . a framework for seeing interrelationships rather than things, for seeing patterns of change rather than static 'snapshots'" (Senge, 2006: 68). It provides us with a world view—a way of seeing and understanding complex realities—that is framed by the notion that the whole is more than the sum of its parts (Meadows, 2008; Davis & Stroink, 2016).

The unit of analysis within systems thinking—the singular system—has been defined as "combinations of interrelated, interdependent or interacting elements forming collective entities" (Arnold & Wade, 2015: 675). Systems always exist and are embedded within larger systems (Meadows, 2008). As pointed out by Brincat (2017), everything above the level of the most basic constitutive particles functions as a system. Systems are not immutable, unified, and static entities; rather, they are fluid, dynamic, and interrelated. While systems can be delineated by boundaries, these are permeable and they intersect or overlap with boundaries of other systems (Midgley, 2004, 2008; Brincat, 2017). Through multiple actors interacting within and across systems, and through their actions, reactions, and influences upon the system as a whole, systems grow increasingly unpredictable (de Savigny & Adam, 2009 as cited in Swanson et al., 2012).

In a world of increasing complexity, at least in part attributable to processes of globalization, and increasing interconnectedness and sophistication in technology, systems ruled by inherent dynamism are termed complex adaptive systems (CASs). The distinguishing factor between general (linear) systems and complex adaptive systems is that the latter are constantly evolving, adapting, and self-organizing; they interact with and are shaped by interactions with other systems (de Savigny & Adam, 2009, Brincat, 2017). CASs exhibit emergent properties which give rise to unexpected behaviors (Brincat, 2017). Core features of CASs include "self-organization, constant changes, feedback loops, non-linearity, . . . history dependence, unintended consequences of policy interventions", high levels of connectivity, and resistance to change (de Savigny & Adam, 2009 as cited in Swanson et al., 2012). CASs are therefore "open" systems. "Closed" systems operate rather autonomously, separate from their environment, and are intended to consistently produce the same outcomes: they are characteristic of the engineering sciences. "Open" systems, being embedded in their social environment, are much more porous, and need to be able to evolve depending on their changing inputs and outputs: this "open" evolution is a critical component of a CAS (see Antonacopoulou & Chiva, 2005; Bailie, Matthews, Brands, & Schierhout, 2013; MacLachlan & Scherer, 2018).

Recognition of the importance of systems thinking and of the value of a complex adaptive systems perspective in health is evident in the joint World Report on Health Policy and Systems Research (Alliance on Health Policy and Systems Research, 2017). The report notes the importance of the interdependence and integration of the SDGs; of balancing the health needs of individuals, communities, and populations; of supporting universal health coverage (UHC); of technological and social innovation; and of synthesizing and adapting knowledge across a wide range of contexts. While the World Report is certainly aware of the importance of reaching the most marginalized groups (via UHC), we believe that it does not adequately recognize the commonalities and opportunities between systems thinking and social inclusion.

Social Inclusion as a Complex Adaptive System

As has already been noted, the definition of social inclusion/exclusion has been complicated by the increase in its usage, the variety of issues in which it is considered, and divergence in its interpretation and application within different paradigms of political philosophy (Silver, 1994; Allman, 2013). However, certain core elements can be identified across different understandings of social exclusion/inclusion. Through delineating these commonly referenced elements and relating them to the previously identified key features of a CAS, we seek to demonstrate how social inclusion/exclusion is an exemplary case of a CAS and therefore requires and will benefit from a systems-thinking perspective.

The United Nations Educational, Scientific and Cultural Organization's *Analytical Framework for Inclusive Policy Design* (2015) was developed through synthesizing the literature on the definitional and operational boundaries of social inclusion, and identifies seven composite elements (United Nations Educational, Scientific and Cultural Organization, 2015). The first of these is multidimensionality. Social inclusion/exclusion is determined and experienced through social, cultural, political, and economic dimensions (ILO/Estivill, 2003). Exclusion, at its most basic, involves the lack or denial of resources, rights, goods, and services—thereby rendering it impossible to participate in relationships and activities available to the majority of people within any given society—across one or more of these dimensions (Levitas et al., 2007). Exclusion from one dimension is often seen to serve as a trigger or transmission channel for other forms of marginalization or disadvantage, thereby forming a self-reinforcing cycle whereby one dimension of exclusion necessarily creates or connects to another (United Nations Educational, Scientific and Cultural Organization, 2015). In this sense, social inclusion/exclusion is both *self-organizing*, since its dynamics arise from an interconnected internal structure of multiple dimensions of an individual/group's existence which evolves and adapts over time, and *governed by feedback*, since an individual or group's experience of inclusion/exclusion will adapt through feedback encountered as a result of their access to resources, rights, goods, or services in other dimensions (de Savigny & Adam, 2009: 40–41).

The second composite element identified is dynamism. Social inclusion/exclusion is best understood as both a process and an outcome: in the former sense, it refers to the developments that render an individual or group more or less included, while the latter denotes the outcome of this process (Mathieson et al., 2008; Popay et al., 2008). Silver and Miller (2003) illustrate this notion well through imagining a trajectory of inclusion/exclusion which spans from full integration to multiple exclusions. Through this imagined trajectory, it is easy to understand that the dynamics of inclusion and exclusion are highly time- and space-specific, being experienced in different ways and with different degrees of intensity in relation to specific contexts and individual/group characteristics (United Nations Educational, Scientific and Cultural Organization, 2015). Indeed, as a result of this inherent dynamism, Silver suggests that "few, if any, people ever reach the ultimate end of the imagined trajectory" of inclusion/exclusion (2007: i). Social inclusion/exclusion can therefore be understood as *constantly changing*, in that experience of it is shaped by the evolving status and position of an individual or group within a society over time. It may also be seen to be *dependent on history*, in that the inclusion/exclusion status differs over time in relation to the nature of both one's status/position and the success of interventions designed to address particular vulnerabilities (de Savigny & Adam, 2009: 40–41).

The third composite element identified is relationality. Social inclusion/exclusion is fundamentally relational since it concerns the process and outcome of an individual/group's distance from others within a society and the consequent ability of said individual/group to enjoy opportunities available to others within that society (Sen, 2000; United Nations Educational, Scientific and Cultural Organization, 2015). An individual/group's access to resources, rights, goods, or services can thereby be considered to determine their social power, the distribution of which determines one's inclusion/exclusion status. Furthermore, it has been argued by Sen (2000) that one's social inclusion/exclusion status is also determined in relation to the ability to realize one's own capabilities, both actual and potential. With these considerations in mind, social inclusion/exclusion can be considered *non-linear*, in that one's inclusion/exclusion status cannot be determined through a simple input–output calculation but is rather the sum of the complex interactions and relationships between the evolving attributes and resources of an individual/group and all other members of a society, and *tightly linked*, in that the high levels of connectivity between different individuals and groups dynamically affect the evolution of one's inclusion/exclusion status (de Savigny & Adam, 2009).

The fourth composite element identified is contextualization. As has been explained through the descriptions of the prior elements, exclusion is often understood as a lack or denial of resources, rights, goods, and services, effectively denying an individual/group participation in relationships and activities available to the majority of people in any given society (Levitas et al., 2007; United Nations Educational, Scientific and Cultural Organization, 2015). Which relationships and activities are available to most people within a society clearly varies over time and location, and is shaped by a wide range of cultural, economic, and political factors (Nussbaum & Sen, 1993; Halleröd, 1994). In this sense, social inclusion/exclusion can be considered *constantly changing*, in that the cultural, economic and political evolution of societies over time is continually (re)shaping the boundaries of what constitutes exclusion or inclusion (de Savigny & Adam, 2009).

The fifth, sixth, and seventh composite elements identified are operation at multiple levels, the presence of group and individual risks, and the intersection of risks. These have been grouped for the purpose of our exercise, owing to the linkages evident between them. Social inclusion/exclusion is determined and experienced through multiple different levels; both the risk factors that can increase vulnerability to exclusion, and the condition of inclusion/exclusion itself, can be understood to exist and be experienced at these different levels—notably, micro (such as individual and household), meso (neighborhood) and macro (national/regional) (United Nations Educational, Scientific and Cultural Organization, 2015; see also MacLachlan, 2014; MacLachlan, McVeigh, Huss, & Mannan, 2019). These processes can originate at one level, and be experienced at another, often becoming structurally rooted (Mathieson et al., 2008). In this sense, the nature and constellation of individual and group risk factors are hugely important in determining inclusion/exclusion status. Risk factors could be characteristics such as age, sexual orientation, disability status, or religious belief; or statuses, related to, for example, health, employment, or education. The intersection of these risk factors, through structures, behaviors, and the success or failures of policy interventions, can therefore be seen to determine an individual's inclusion/exclusion status, and individual risk factors alone do not necessarily lead to exclusion (Tsakloglou & Papadopoulos, 2001). Inclusion/exclusion can therefore be seen to operate as *a self-organized* system of *tightly linked* risk factors which manifest and are experienced at different levels, *feeding back* on one another to determine an individual's likelihood of inclusion/exclusion in a complex, *non-linear* manner (de Savigny & Adam, 2009).

Using Systems Thinking to Inform Interventions for Social Inclusion

Systems approaches provide us with an array of tools and innovative perspectives to grasp and untangle the complexity of social inclusion as elaborated above; it provides analysts with a coherent methodology to trace the processes of inclusion/exclusion and to identify potential opportunities for intervention within the social organization of systems. In this section we discuss operational properties of systems thinking and how they might prove useful in designing policy interventions to promote inclusion and/or reverse social exclusion. In doing so, we turn to the critical strand of systems thinking.

(i) Holistic responses

Central to the application of a systems-thinking approach is the holistic understanding of a particular system from as many perspectives as possible. Systems approaches tell us that it is important to move away from constricted perspectives and analytical models that prevent us from seeing the dynamic interactions of systems' components and subcomponents. Earlier we discussed the multi-dimensionality of social inclusion/exclusion. In systems thinking, multi-dimensionality is best captured as nested or overlapping systems. Conceptually, this helps us to realize that, for instance, economic, social, health, political, and cultural spheres interact with one another; the exclusionary processes within one (sub-) system are intimately connected with and often serve to reinforce one another. Consequently, interventions for social inclusion need to be holistic in their scope. Examples of holistic, systemic interventions are whole-of-government or joined-up policy approaches, which through collaborative efforts across problem spheres design and implement a transversal and integrated policy portfolio (United Nations Educational, Scientific and Cultural Organization, 2015). The success of joined-up approaches is largely contingent upon interministerial commitment across government, while aspiring to achieve a clear and common vision of inclusion (United Nations Department of Economic and Social Affairs, 2009; Schalock & Verdugo, 2012; Carey, McLaughlin, & Crammond, 2015). The successful promotion of social inclusion may thus hinge less on individual behavioral change and more on achieving a shift in values and norms within government (and society at large), based upon a common understanding of and strategy for achieving inclusion (Jones, 2009; World Bank, 2013; Carey, McLaughlin, & Crammond, 2015). However, paradigm shifts of this kind are unlikely to take root without transformational leadership and commitment of individuals in higher political offices (Swanson et al., 2012), civil society, or other stakeholders. Thus persuading individuals to change may well offer alternative and complementary intervention points for systems change, as individuals both construct and are constructed by the systems through which they operate (MacLachlan & McAuliffe, 2017).

(ii) Broadening boundaries of problem definition

According to Alford and Head (2015, 2017), the complexity of a problem is a function of the problem itself, the myriad of actors and institutions involved, their relationship with one another, and access to the knowledge or evidence base critical to its mitigation. The complexity of a problem becomes evident when stakeholders cannot arrive at a consensual problem definition (Alford & Head, 2017). In attempting to define a problem, stakeholders make explicit assumptions about the boundaries of a particular system. Contrary to the belief that the boundaries of systems are clearly delineated (i.e., "they are 'given' by the structure of reality"), critical systems thinkers contest this notion and argue that boundaries are socially constructed (Midgley, Munlo, & Brown, 1998: 468). They argue that when systems' boundaries are drawn, ethical values, implicit in the act of delineation, are laid bare (Midgley, 2004: 66). Similarly, Meadows (1999) contends that paradigms or value systems are the foundations of systems. Hence, those who define the boundaries of systems, ultimately ascertain and prioritize their values, knowledge and diagnosis of a problem over that of other individuals or groups. As such, they wield power over what and who is included, or excluded, from the analysis of and the solution to a problem (Midgley, Munlo, & Brown, 1998; Midgley, 2004).

Critical systems thinkers argue that complex social problems should be analyzed by those most affected by them within a given context (Ulrich 1983 as cited in Midgley, Munlo, & Brown, 1998). Similarly, they argue that marginalized individuals or groups should participate in the search for and enactment of their solutions (Midgley, Munlo, & Brown, 1998; Midgely, 2014). When policy-makers or other dominant sections of society seek to impose their definition of inclusion/exclusion, the marginalized must seek to contest it, provided they are allowed to participate in the discussions. Within critical systems thinking then, an intervention is best thought of as a "purposeful action by an agent to create change in relation to reflection upon boundaries" (Midgley, 2004: 65). Huss and MacLachlan (2016) argue that while participation in policy deliberations is a positive step toward inclusion, groups affected by exclusion should be centrally involved throughout the entire policy process (from the design, through to implementation, monitoring, and evaluation, as well as dissemination). Unless, policy *on the books* (i.e., the policy document, the strategy) is properly enacted, as intended, *on the streets*, it is unlikely to promote inclusion (Stowe & Turnbull, 2001; Huss & MacLachlan, 2016). Policy implementers (agencies, non-governmental organizations, etc.) ultimately retain power over how services are delivered and who can access them (Walker & Gilson, 2004; Brynard, 2010).

(ii) Causal modelling

The Alliance for Health Policy and Systems, based within WHO Geneva, recommends 10 steps to designing and evaluating interventions using a systems approach (de Savigny & Adam, 2009). These recommendations apply beyond the healthcare context; once convened, stakeholders ought to brainstorm "collectively" on the potential effects of interventions, in terms of their likely feedbacks (positive and negative), potential for policy resistance, and so forth. In a subsequent step, the organization recommends that stakeholders map conceptual pathways, because the visual representation of hypothetical cause and effects, embedded within actor networks, aids stakeholders with optimizing intervention design (de Savigny & Adam, 2009). Modelling tools such as knowledge synthesis, concept mapping, and social network analysis are routinely used to "map the mess" (Midgely, 2014) and in so doing try to make sense of system complexity (Willis et al., 2011 as cited in Swanson et al., 2012). Using a systems lens and its modelling tools, stakeholders are better equipped to make sense of the idiosyncrasy of a phenomenon. It is important, however, that when stakeholder convene and brainstorm that they remain cognizant of the non-linearity of the process toward full social inclusion. The journey to social inclusion is fraught with obstacles and unintended outcomes, often experienced by the excluded as adverse inclusion (Hickey & duToit, 2007; Soors, Dkhimi, & Criel, 2013; Silver, 2015). For instance, marginalized groups may be allowed to participate largely in order to authenticate the process of consultation, rather than being meaningful beneficiaries in terms of concrete outcomes (MacLachlan et al., 2014). This may in fact serve only to frustrate and further marginalize such groups. However, by explicitly considering and trying to avoid negative feedback loops, interventions can be modified in time to rectify or avoid potentially negative consequences (de Savigny & Adam, 2009).

Systems thinking provides policy-makers, practitioners, academics, politically active citizens, and service users with concepts and tools to make sense of complex adaptive systems in an effort to design and implement socially inclusive policies. We have argued that by facilitating participation and opening up discussion forums, a more inclusive, accurate, and robust definition and understanding of inclusion/exclusion can be created. While the most effective way to intervene in a system is at the "paradigm" level (Meadows, 1999), this is also the most difficult place to intervene. Yet, the potentially positive trickle-down is such that value shifts are likely to reduce policy resistance and bottlenecks significantly.

In the next section we provide two examples, from our own research, to illustrate that traditional interventions are often likely to fail because they are not grounded in a holistic understanding of social exclusion. We demonstrate that, if approached through a systems lens, interventions have the potential to be more successful. We choose to focus on homelessness and disability as they are both examples of life experiences that marginalize and may have significant consequences for health yet are often not seen systemically through a health lens.

Chronic Homelessness and Housing First

Chronic homelessness is defined by the US Department for Housing and Urban Development as the condition one experiences when having been continuously homeless for at least a year, or on four or more separate occasions in the last three years, while also experiencing a co-occurring substance abuse and/or mental or physical disability (Culhane & Metraux, 2008). Chronic homelessness is a complex problem, shaped and experienced through a range of individual and structural risks and factors which evolve over time, including traumatic events in childhood, substance misuse, poor access to welfare assistance, and possibly also the navigation of street/criminal activity to fulfil basic need (Fitzpatrick-Lewis et al., 2011). Those experiencing chronic homelessness are often characterized by their relatively poor functioning, high service usage, and especially entrenched social exclusion (Kertesz & Weiner, 2009). All these characteristics and the temporality inherent in the experience have been seen to increase the likelihood of those afflicted utilizing short-term and costly public services. Indeed, the intensive needs and associated cost of the chronically homeless are themes which have been seen to maintain both academic and political interest in the issue (Busch-Geertsema, 2011; Pleace & Bretherton, 2013).

Chronic homelessness can be considered an archetypal example of a manifestation of social exclusion operating as a CAS—its experience is determined by a self-organizing internal structure of risk factors which interact in a highly connected manner, often in feedback to one another, which evolves over time in a complex way. Policy to manage chronic homelessness has historically tended to fail to approach it as a CAS, with the most popular paradigm for addressing it viewing it one-dimensionally as a compliance/criminality issue, compelling treatment first and making access to permanent, independent social housing conditional on engagement and compliance with treatment regimes. Evidence suggests that such approaches have failed to meet service users' needs along a range of important dimensions including the provision of housing security, facilitation of consumer choice, and management of mental health and substance abuse problems (Sahlin, 2005; Tainio & Fredriksson, 2009; Johnsen & Teixeira, 2010).

However, an alternative approach has been popularized in some countries in recent years, derived from an innovative policy intervention designed through the heuristic of systems thinking. Frustrated by the stubbornness of the problem and the recidivism of the chronically homeless within traditional interventions, New York-based non-profit Pathways to Housing (PtH) designed *Housing First.* Reimagining the boundaries of the problem to understand it as a holistic health issue, they appreciated that traditional models of compliance with treatment failed to address the complex intersections of the various individual and group risk factors which lead to and sustain chronic homelessness, and that any policy intervention to address it must provide a stable basis on which service users can meaningfully engage with treatment on their own terms. They brought together interdisciplinary teams from housing support services, emergency medical centers, substance/alcohol dependency outreach and mental health treatment centers—all public services strained by their work with the (same) chronically homeless populations—and designed and tested a policy intervention (*Housing First*) which removes compliance with treatment as a condition for the provision of stable, permanent social housing. Through immediately providing permanent social housing to chronically homeless individuals, and offering assertive but non-compulsory support services from either floating or on-site multi-service practitioner teams, *Housing First* has demonstrated highly positive results for both service users and practitioners: Evaluative evidence drawn from a wide range of randomized controlled trials suggests that along the same important outcome dimensions of housing security, engagement with mental health and substance abuse treatment, ontological well-being and consumer choice, *Housing First* programs are able to provide significantly better results for service users than traditional treatment-led approaches (Tsemberis, 1999; Tsemberis, Gulcur, & Nakae, 2004). In addition, cost evaluations have shown that housing first approaches can be cost saving or cost neutral when compared with treatment led approaches (Gulcur, Stefancic, Shinn, Tsemberis, & Fischer, 2003, Kertesz & Weiner, 2009). The value added by the more holistic approach is the possibility to align factors that interplay across boundaries and to do so in a fashion that make the intervention both more coherent and more comprehensive.

The National Disability Policy in Timor-Leste

The Democratic Republic of Timor-Leste (RDTL) is one of the poorest countries in the Asia Pacific, ranking 128th out of 187 on the Human Development Index (Dos Santos & Morgan, 2016). According to the census from 2015, 38,118 people or 3.3% of this small island population live with some form of disability (Handicap International & German Federal Ministry for Economic Cooperation and Development (n.d.).). This number differs significantly from the 2010 Census, which estimated the prevalence of disability at 4.6% (Handicap International & German Federal Ministry for Economic Cooperation and Development (n.d.).). The constitution of the RDTL guarantees the non-discrimination and equality of treatment for all of its citizen, regardless of group-based characteristics or identities (Dos Santos & Morgan, 2016). However, the reality is often very different; people with disabilities in Timor-Leste continue to experience stigma and discrimination (United Nations Mission in Timor-Leste & Office of the High Commissioner for Human Rights, 2011). This is not unique to the RDTL as in most countries, disability is a ground for exclusion and discrimination (Silver, 2015). Furthermore, disability often intersects with other group-based markers of exclusion and vulnerability. As a result of this intersectionality, people with disabilities face discrimination across a variety of life domains such as health, education, employment, and so forth (Moodley & Graham, 2015). Moreover, the negative outcomes of multiple vulnerabilities are often exacerbated in lower-income contexts where access to essential goods and services is further restricted (Trani, Bakhshi, Noor, Lopez, & Mashkoor, 2010). In the Timor-Leste Strategic Development Plan (2011–2030), the government committed to improving the services available to and the living conditions for people with disabilities (Government of the Democratic Republic of Timor-Leste, 2012). In 2012, the Council of Ministers approved the *National Disability Policy for Inclusion and Promotion of the Rights of People with Disabilities*. This document is based on the core principles of the United Nations Convention on the Rights of Persons with Disabilities (UNCRPD) such as the principles of participation, coordination, responsibility, and complementarity. The policy seeks to guide a "whole of government approach to service provision," while enabling the participation of people with disabilities across all spheres of life (Ximenes & da Cunha, 2011: 74). More specifically, the policy acknowledges the importance of "multi-sectoral and multidisciplinary coordination involving the public and private entities, NGOs, governmental organizations and representatives of associations of people with disabilities" in the promotion of social inclusion (Government of the Democratic Republic of Timor-Leste, 2012). A roadmap for implementation was subsequently developed. The National Action Plan for People with Disabilities 2014–2018 (NAP) was developed under the leadership of the Ministry for Social Solidarity, with the input of ten ministries, each contributing a separate action plan to the document. The policy process was credited for having been inclusive in the sense of soliciting the input of persons with disabilities themselves (Timor-Leste National Commission for UNESCO, 2016; Ximenes and da Cunha, 2011). For instance, Ximenes and da Cunha (2011) write that during the formulation of an earlier draft of the policy, 300 people with disabilities were consulted for their input. The policy itself is a value-based document, clearly outlining the programmatic lines that were prioritized during the consultation process. The national Disability Working Group (DWG), comprising people with disabilities and their representatives, was actively involved in the development of the National Action Plan (Timor-Leste National Commission for UNESCO, 2016). At a system level, both the policy and its roadmap are indicative of horizontal alignment, that is, the documents propose, in the words of Schalock and Verdugo (2012), a logical sequencing of inputs, throughputs and outputs. Systems change, in the sense of greater inclusion for people with disabilities, however, is unlikely to happen unless the working modalities across ministries and organizations tasked with the implementation are vertically aligned to support a whole-of-government strategy (Pollitt, 2003; United Nations Department of Economic and Social Affairs, 2009; Schalock & Verdugo, 2012).

A lack of budgetary and human resources impeded the implementation of the policy (Handicap International, Kooperasaun Husi Alemaña & Asosiasaun

Defisiensia Timor-Leste, 2016). Furthermore, a 2016 mid-term review of the NAP, conducted by representatives from disability civil society organizations, found that many government officials thought that disability was solely the responsibility of the Ministry of Solidarity and as such they were unaware of their ministry's joint responsibility in progressing the disability agenda (Handicap International, Kooperasaun Husi Alemaña, & Asosiasaun Defisiensia Timor-Leste, 2016). Implementation was further delayed by the fact that, at the time of writing, the NAP had not been approved by the National Council of Ministers as an official government plan (Dyer & Tanukusum 2019; Timor-Leste National Commission for UNESCO, 2016). Ultimately, however, disability inclusion was not dealt with as a priority issue within the government (Handicap International, Kooperasaun Husi Alemaña & Asosiasaun Defisiensia Timor-Leste, 2016). To counteract many of the implementation delays, disability advocates and the Ministry for Social Solidarity were pushing for the creation of a National Disability Council, attended by powerful government officials and persons with disabilities themselves, vested with stronger powers of holding ministries accountable (Handicap International, Kooperasaun Husi Alemaña & Asosiasaun Defisiensia Timor-Leste, 2016; Timor-Leste National Commission for UNESCO, 2016). While we cannot comment on whether systems thinking was explicitly or consciously adopted in designing the policy intervention to address social exclusion for people with disabilities in Timor-Leste, in our work with the government, civil society, and UNESCO in Timor-Leste, we certainly found evidence of systems concepts. The policy process which put forward a value-based whole-of-government solution, and the action plan and indicator framework are holistic and transversal interventions aimed at creating change at the paradigm level. Despite lacking transformational leadership at the necessary levels, the creation of the National Disability Council is likely to progress the joined-up implementation of the disability agenda in Timor-Leste. Thus, in Timor-Leste a structural intervention, the National Disability Council, is being attempted as a means to link diverse systems components which left alone, act only in isolation, even though each can make a necessary, stronger, and complementary contribution to progressing inclusion when acting in unison.

Conclusion

Through elucidating how systems thinking is a relevant and useful reference to help understand and advance social inclusion, this chapter has sought to illustrate how systems thinking is related to social inclusion. Systems thinking provides a useful heuristic through which to navigate the complexity and dynamism of social inclusion/exclusion within the design and implementation of policy to promote it. It offers an approach to break down and reconceptualize solutions to the complicated problem of social exclusion where multiple different stakeholders are involved and connected. We hope that this contribution is a starting point for broader reflection on the benefits of addressing the promotion of social inclusion through a systems lens, and for eventually offering more elaborated frameworks to support the reflection of systems thinking in policy-makers' work to design and implement policies.

References

Alford, J., & Head, B. W. (2017). Wicked and less wicked problems: A typology and a contingency framework. *Policy and Society*, *36*(3), 397–413.

Alliance on Health Policy and Systems Research. (2017). *World Report on Health Policy and Systems Research*. Geneva: World Health Organization.

Allman, D. (2013). The sociology of social inclusion. *Sage Open*, *3*(1).

Antonacopoulou, E., & Chiva, R. (2005). March. Social complex evolving systems: Implications for organizational learning. In *6th International Organizational Knowledge, Learning and Capabilities Conference*, Boston, MA.

Arnold, R. D., & Wade, J. P. (2015). A definition of systems thinking: A systems approach. *Procedia Computer Science*, *44*, 669–678.

Bailie, R., Matthews, V., Brands, J., & Schierhout, G. (2013). A systems-based partnership learning model for strengthening primary healthcare. *Implementation Science*, *8*(1), 143.

Brincat, S. (Ed.). (2017). *Dialectics in world politics*. London: Routledge.

Brynard, P. A. (2010). Policy implementation and cognitive skills: The difficulty of understanding implementation. *Journal of Public Administration*, *45*(Special issue 1), 190–201.

Busch-Geertsema, V. (2011). Housing First Europe: A "social experimentation project." *European Journal of Homelessness*, *5*(2), 209–211.

Carey, G., McLaughlin, P., & Crammond, B. (2015). Implementing joined-up government: Lessons from the Australian social inclusion agenda. *Australian Journal of Public Administration*, *74*(2), 176–186.

Culhane, D. P., & Metraux, S. (2008). Rearranging the deck chairs or reallocating the lifeboats? Homelessness assistance and its alternatives. *Journal of the American Planning Association*, *74*(1), 111–121.

Davis, A. C., & Stroink, M. L. (2016). The relationship between systems thinking and the new ecological paradigm. *Systems Research and Behavioral Science*, *33*(4), 575–586.

de Savigny, D., & Adam, T. (Eds.) (2009). *Systems thinking for health systems strengthening*. Geneva: World Health Organization.

Dos Santos, J., & Morgan, E. (2016). Steps towards achieving inclusion for people with disabilities in Timor-Leste. *State, Society & Governance in Melanesia* (In Brief 2016/18). Department of Pacific Affairs, Coral Bell School of Asia Pacific Affairs, Australian National University College of Asia & the Pacific. Retrieved from: http://dpa.bellschool.anu.edu.au/experts-publications/publications/4135/steps-towards-achieving-inclusion-people-disabilities-timor

du Toit, A. (2004). "Social exclusion" discourse and chronic poverty: a South African case study. *Development and Change*, *35*(5), 987–1010.

Dyer, S., & Tanukusum, J. (2019). *Review Report: Disability Specific Partners and Program. Report prepared for the Department of Foreign Affairs and Trade Timor-Leste*. Pamodzi Consulting. Retrieved from https://www.dfat.gov.au/sites/default/files/review-report-disability-specific-partners-and-program.pdf

ILO/Estivill, J. (2003). *Concepts and strategies for combating social exclusion: an overview*. International Labour Organization. Retrieved from: http://www.ilo.org/public/english/protection/socsec/step/download/96p1.pdf

Fitzpatrick-Lewis, D., Ganann, R., Krishnaratne, S., Ciliska, D., Kouyoumdjian, F., & Hwang, S. W. (2011). Effectiveness of interventions to improve the health and housing status of homeless people: a rapid systematic review. *BMC Public Health*, *11*(1), 638. https://doi.org/10.1186/1471-2458-11-638

Government of the Democratic Republic of Timor-Leste. (2012). *The National Policy for inclusion and promotion of the rights of people with disabilities*. Government Resolution No. 14/2012.

Gulcur, L., Stefancic, A., Shinn, M., Tsemberis, S., & Fischer, S. N. (2003). Housing, hospitalization, and cost outcomes for homeless individuals with psychiatric disabilities participating in continuum of care and housing first programmes. *Journal of Community & Applied Social Psychology, 13*(2), 171–186.

Halleröd, B. (1994). *A new approach to the direct consensual measurement of poverty.* SPRC Discussion Paper No. 50. Sydney, NSW: University of New South Wales, Social Policy Research Centre.

Handicap International., & German Federal Ministry for Economic Cooperation and Development (BMZ). (n.d.). *Making it work: Good practices of implementation of UNCRPD in Timor Leste.* Dili, Timor Leste: Handicap International Indonesia & Timor Leste Programme. https://www.makingitwork-crpd.org/our-work/projects-using-miw/good-practices-implementation-uncrpd-timor-leste-2015-2017

Handicap International, Kooperasaun Husi Alemaña, & Asosiasaun Defisiensia Timor-Leste. (2016). *Looking backwards, planning forwards—Report of the mid-term review of the national action plan for people with disabilities (2014–2018).* Dili, Timor Leste: Handicap International Indonesia & Timor Leste Programme.

Head, B. W., & Alford, J. (2015). Wicked problems: Implications for public policy and management. *Administration & Society, 47*(6), 711–739.

Hickey, S., & du Toit, A. (2007). *Adverse incorporation, social exclusion and chronic poverty. CPRC Working Paper 81.* Institute for Development Policy and Management, School of Environment and Development, University of Manchester.

Hoogeveen, J., Tesliuc, E., Vakis, R., & Dercon, S. (2004). *A guide to the analysis of risk, vulnerability and vulnerable groups.* Washington, DC: World Bank. Retrieved from http://siteresources.worldbank.org/INTSRM/Publications/20316319/RVA.pdf/

Huss, T., & MacLachlan, M. (2016). *Equity and inclusion in policy processes (EquIPP): A framework to support equity & inclusion in the process of policy development, implementation and evaluation.* Dublin, Ireland: Global Health Press.

Johnsen, S., & Teixeira, L. (2010). Staircases, elevators and cycles of change: "Housing First" and other housing models for homeless people with complex support needs. London: Crisis.

Jones, H. (2009). *Equity in Development: Why it is important and how to achieve it.* London: Overseas Development Institute.

Kertesz, S. G., & Weiner, S. J. (2009). Housing the chronically homeless: High hopes, complex realities. *Journal of the American Medical Association, 301*(17), 1822–1824.

Levitas, R., Pantazis, C., Fahmy, E., Gordon, D., Lloyd, E., & Patsios, D. (2007). The multi-dimensional analysis of social exclusion. Bristol: University of Bristol.

MacLachlan, M. (2014). Macropsychology, policy & global health. *American Psychologist, 69,* 851–863.

MacLachlan, M., & McAuliffe, E. (2017). Global Health Systems: Micro, meso and macro perspectives. In I. Burić (Ed.), *20th psychology days in Zadar: Selected proceedings* (pp. 13–22). Zadar: Department of Psychology, University of Zadar.

MacLachlan, M., & Scherer, M. (2018). Systems thinking for assistive technology: A commentary on the GREAT summit. *Disability and Rehabilitation: Assistive Technology, 13*(5), 492–496.

MacLachlan, M., McVeigh, J., Huss, T., & Mannan, H. (2019). Macropsychology: Challenging and changing social structures and systems. In D. Hoggets and K. O'Doherty (Eds.), *Handbook of applied social psychology* (pp. 166–182). London: Sage.

MacLachlan, M., Mji, G., Chataika, T., Wazakili, M., Dube, A. K., Mulumba, M, … Maughan, M. (2014). Facilitating disability inclusion in poverty reduction processes: Group consensus perspectives from disability stakeholders in Uganda, Malawi, Ethiopia, and Sierra Leone. *Disability & the Global South, 1*(1), 107–127.

Mathieson, J., Popay, J., Enoch, E., Escorel, S., Hernandez, M., Johnston, H., & Rispel, L. (2008). Social exclusion meaning, measurement and experience and links to health inequalities. A review of literature. *WHO Social Exclusion Knowledge Network Background Paper, 1*, 91. Retrieved from: https://www.who.int/social_determinants/media/sekn_meaning_measurement_experience_2008.pdf.pdf

Meadows, D. (1999). *Leverage points. Places to intervene in a system*. Hartlant, VT, United States: The Sustainability Institute.

Meadows, D. (2008). *Thinking in systems: A primer*. In Diana Wright (Ed.), *Sustainability Institute*. White River Junction, Vermont: Chelsea Green Publishing.

Midgley, G. (2004). Systems thinking for the 21st century. *International Journal of Knowledge and Systems Sciences, 1*(1), 63–69.

Midgley, G. (2008). Systems thinking, complexity and the philosophy of science. *Emergence: Complexity and Organization, 10*(4), 55–73.

Midgley, G. (2014). *Systemic Intervention. Research Memorandum, No. 95*. Hull: Centre for Systems Studies, Hull University Business School.

Midgley, G., Munlo, I., & Brown, M. (1998). The theory and practice of boundary critique: developing housing services for older people. *Journal of the Operational Research Society, 49*(5), 467–478.

Moodley, J., & Graham, L. (2015). The importance of intersectionality in disability and gender studies. *Agenda, 29*(2), 24–33.

Nussbaum, M., & Sen, A. (Eds.). (1993). *The quality of life*. Oxford: Oxford University Press.

O'Donnell, P., O'Donovan, D., & Elmusharaf, K. (2018). Measuring social exclusion in healthcare settings: a scoping review. *International Journal for Equity in Health, 17*(1), 15.

Pleace, N., & Bretherton, J. (2013). The case for Housing First in the European Union: A critical evaluation of concerns about effectiveness. *European Journal of Homelessness, 7*(2), 21–41.

Pollitt, C. (2003). Joined-up government: A survey. *Political Studies Review, 1*(1), 34–49.

Popay, J., Escorel, S., Hernández, M., Johnston, H., Mathieson, J., & Rispel, L. (2008). Understanding and tackling social exclusion. Final report to the WHO Commission on Social Determinants of Health, from the Social Exclusion Knowledge Network. Geneva: World Health Organization.

Sahlin, I. (2005). The staircase of transition: Survival through failure. *Innovation: The European Journal of Social Science Research, 18*(2), 115–136.

Schalock, R. L., & Verdugo, M. A. (2012). A conceptual and measurement framework to guide policy development and systems change. *Journal of Policy and Practice in Intellectual Disabilities, 9*(1), 63–72.

Sen, A. (2000). *Social exclusion: Concept, application, and scrutiny*. Manila, Philippines: Asian Development Bank.

Senge, P. (2006). *The Fifth Discipline: The Art and Practice of the Learning Organization*. New York, NY: Currency.

Silver, H. (1994). Social exclusion and social solidarity: Three paradigms. *International Labor Review, 133*, 531–578.

Silver, H. (2007). The process of social exclusion: The dynamics of an evolving concept. Chronic Poverty Research Center Working Paper No. 95. Retrieved from https://ssrn.com/abstract=1629282 and http://dx.doi.org/10.2139/ssrn.1629282.

Silver, H. (2015). *The contexts of social inclusion. DESA Working Paper No. 144*. New York, United States: Department of Economic & Social Affairs.

Silver, H., & Miller, S. M. (2003). Social exclusion. *Indicators, 2*(2), 5–21.

Soors, W., Dkhimi, F., & Criel, B. (2013). Lack of access to healthcare for African indigents: A social exclusion perspective. *International Journal for Equity in Health, 12*, 91.

Stowe, M. J., & Turnbull, H. R. (2001). Tools for analyzing policy "on the books" and policy "on the streets". *Journal of Disability Policy Studies, 12*, 206–216.

Swanson, R. C., Cattaneo, A., Bradley, E., Chunharas, S., Atun, R., Abbas, K. M., … Best, A. (2012). Rethinking health systems strengthening: Key systems thinking tools and strategies for transformational change. *Health Policy and Planning, 27*(suppl 4), iv54–iv61.

Tainio, H., & Fredriksson, P. (2009). The Finnish homelessness strategy: From a "staircase" model to a "housing first" approach to tackling long-term homelessness. *European Journal of Homelessness, 3*, 181–199.

Timor-Leste National Commission for UNESCO. (2016). *Promoting Social Inclusion in Timor-Leste: Analysis of the National Disability Policy Framework in Timor-Leste*. Retrieved from http://www.unesco.or.id/download/Report_Social_Inclusion_PwD_TimorLeste.pdf

Trani, J. F., Bakhshi, P., Noor, A. A., Lopez, D., & Mashkoor, A. (2010). Poverty, vulnerability, and provision of healthcare in Afghanistan. *Social Science and Medicine, 70*(11), 1745–1755.

Tsakloglou, P., & Papadopoulos, F. (2001). *Identifying population groups at high risk of social exclusion: Evidence from the ECHP. IZA Discussion Paper No. 392.* Retrieved from https://ssrn.com/abstract=290600

Tsemberis, S. (1999). From streets to homes: An innovative approach to supported housing for homeless adults with psychiatric disabilities. *Journal of Community Psychology, 27*(2), 225–241.

Tsemberis, S., Gulcur, L., & Nakae, M. (2004). Housing first, consumer choice, and harm reduction for homeless individuals with a dual diagnosis. *American Journal of Public Health, 94*(4), 651–656.

United Nations. (n.d.). *The 17 Goals.* Retrieved from https://sdgs.un.org/goals

United Nations Department of Economic and Social Affairs. (2009). *Draft report. Creating an inclusive society: Practical strategies to promote social integration.* Retrieved from https://www.un.org/esa/socdev/egms/docs/2009/Ghana/inclusive-society.pdf

United Nations Educational, Scientific and Cultural Organization. (2015). *UNESCO analytical framework for inclusive policy design: Of why, what and how.* Paris: UNESCO.

United Nations Mission in Timor-Leste (UNMIT) & Office of the High Commissioner for Human Rights. (2011). *Report on the rights of persons with Disabilities in Timor-Leste.* Retrieved from http://www.ohchr.org/Documents/Countries/TP/UNHR_Report2011_en.pdf

United Nations Sustainable Development Group. (2021). Leave No One Behind. Retrieved from https://unsdg.un.org/2030-agenda/universal-values/leave-no-one-behind

Walker, L., & Gilson, L. (2004). "We are bitter but we are satisfied": Nurses as street-level bureaucrats in South Africa. *Social Science and Medicine, 59*(6), 1251–1261.

Willis, C. D., Mitton, C., Gordon, J., & Best, A. (2011). System tools for system change. *BMJ Quality & Safety, 21*, 250–62.

World Bank. (2013). *Inclusion Matters: The Foundation for Shared Prosperity. New Frontiers of Social Policy* (advance edition). Washington, DC: World Bank.

Ximenes, T., & da Cunha, D. (2011). Developing a national disability policy: The Timor-Leste experience. Implementing disability-inclusive development in the Pacific and Asia: Aspects of human resource development. *Development Bulletin, 74*, 72–74.

15

Using a Systems Approach to Understand Quality Improvement in a Nursing Home in Japan

Robotics-aided Care and Organizational Culture

Naonori Kodate, Kazuko Obayashi, Hasheem Mannan, and Shigeru Masuyama

Introduction

The global population aged sixty years and above reached 962 million in 2017, more than twice the population reported in 1980. By 2050, this figure is projected to reach more than 2 billion. In 2017, the United Nations Department of Economic and Social Affairs published the 2030 Agenda for Sustainable Development, recognizing the significance of a life-course approach to aging and calling for the protection and promotion of the rights of older people in its implementation of the Agenda. Similarly, the World Health Organization (WHO) published a 2015 report outlining a framework for action to foster healthy aging based on the new concept of *functional ability*, or "the health-related attributes that enable people to be and to do what they have reason to value" (World Health Organization, 2015). With this new concept, the environment in which an older person lives plays an essential role in enabling her or his functional ability. Emerging technologies are expected to enhance the environment, which will lead to healthy aging and *aging in place*, or "the ability to live in one's own home and community safely, independently and comfortably, regardless of age, income or level of capacity" (The United States Centers for Disease Control and Prevention, n.d.).

Population aging is considered to be a key issue in global health, with people of older age now categorized as a vulnerable group (e.g., EquiFrame, see Chapter 26). Therefore, understanding, protecting, and improving the environment for healthy aging requires the consideration of multiple factors that constitute a health system including housing, economy, attitudes and values, health and social care services, and human relationships. More recently, the COVID-19 pandemic has affected the lives of older people particularly harshly, reinforcing the view that building capacity in health systems by utilizing technologies should be a priority.

Long influenced by Confucianism, East Asia can be regarded as family-oriented and socially conservative, with strong family values including filial piety (e.g., the relationship between parents and the child), gender inequality, and social hierarchy

Naonori Kodate, Kazuko Obayashi, Hasheem Mannan, and Shigeru Masuyama, *Using a Systems Approach to Understand Quality Improvement in a Nursing Home in Japan* In: *Systems Thinking for Global Health*. Edited by: Fiona Larkan, Frédérique Vallières, Hasheem Mannan, and Naonori Kodate, Oxford University Press. © Oxford University Press 2023.
DOI: 10.1093/oso/9780198799498.003.0015

(i.e., human relationships: father–son, husband–wife, and elder–younger friend, etc.) (Ochiai, 2009). Recent changes, including rapid economic growth and political democratization, combined with dramatic demographic change (e.g., ultra-low fertility rate) have seen social policy emerge as a key factor to help ensure economic and political stability as well as governmental legitimacy in East Asia. At the same time, changing traditional family structures, living arrangements, and increased levels of female labor market participation have created gaps in long-term care provision. So, while prevailing social norms and customs still pose a challenge to the government's investment in publicly funded long-term care (Holliday, 2000; Lee & Ku, 2007), long-term care policies have been developed, proposed, and implemented in many East Asian economies. Japan, as a global harbinger of this phenomenon with a rapidly aging population, introduced publicly funded long-term care insurance (LTCI) in 2000 (Kodate & Timonen, 2017).

While longevity and a healthy life expectancy are cause for celebration, an increasing demand for care and a shortage of care workers have given rise to a crisis of care in Japan. As the proportion of older people (aged sixty-five years old and over) grows at a rapid pace (29.1% as of 2021), the size of the older population is overwhelming in comparison to other countries. The government estimates that by 2025, there will be a shortfall of 380,000 nurses and care workers (Ministry of Health, Labour and Welfare, 2016; Cabinet Office, Government of Japan, 2018). Consequently, the Japanese government has also begun to relax its strict immigration restrictions, introducing a new visa scheme for foreign workers with designated skills in April 2019. While this move was welcomed by the business community, including the care sector, it also faced criticisms from media and policy analysts for various reasons. A nationwide opinion poll conducted by *Yomiuri Shimbun* newspaper in May 2019 ($N = 2{,}103$, the response rate of 70%), for example, suggested that while 57% were in favor of the government policy, 59% said they were reluctant to have a migrant carer take care of them (*Yomiuri Shimbun*, 2019). The implications of this new immigration policy as a way to address the shortage of care workers are therefore unlikely to be immediate.

Studies worldwide have shown support for promising technological solutions that could potentially support "aging in place" by creating an ambient assisted-living system with in-home monitoring (Pilotto, D'Onofrio, Benelli, et al., 2011; Takayanagi, Kirita, & Shibata, 2014; Moyle, Jones, Murfield, et al., 2017). Correspondingly, robotics-aided care is seen as not only promising but as an almost inevitable innovation to tackle the aforementioned caring crisis. In March 2016, a robot-assisted walker was added, for the first time, to the list of reimbursable items under the LTCI scheme. The list of items was expanded in 2017. In April 2018, the Ministry of Health, Labour and Welfare established the Office for Nursing Care Robot Development and Promotion and appointed special staff to lead it (Ministry of Economy, Trade and Industry, 2017). There is now a strong impetus for bringing this innovation to the next level of policy implementation. Having produced a string of robots, ranging from industrial types to humanoid and companion types, Japan is leading in this effort (Cabinet Office of Japan, 2014). Table 15.1 shows three different types of care robots.

Table 15.1 Three types of care robots

Type	Examples	
Physical support type	Power suits, a modular robot arm (e.g., RIBA) and robots that assist with bathing, dining, excretion, and sleep (e.g., Nemuri-scan) and transferring (e.g., Toyota Porte)	
Independence support type	Powered exoskeletons (e.g., HAL, WPAL), and mobile arm/hand support (e.g., MARo, RAPUD)	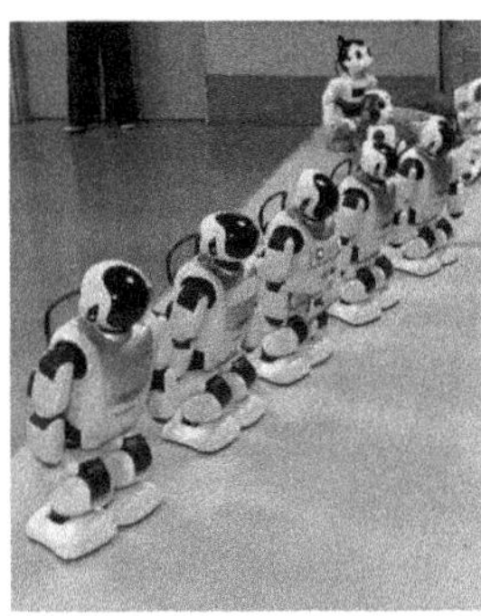
Communication, comfort and safety monitoring type	Safety monitoring (e.g., WAKAMARU), giving guidance to people with dementia (e.g., Sota), and companionship (e.g., Aibo, Paro, Qoobo).	

Reproduced with permission from National Institute of Advanced Industrial Science and Technology (AIST), Japan, 2017.

Setting

In Japan, there are three types of care facilities. Of these, the Social Welfare Corporation (SWC) operates two different types: special nursing homes for older people (known as Tokuyō), and geriatric health services facilities (known as Rōken). The difference between the two lies in the level of care required, with greater levels of care typically needed within Tokuyō. People living in Tokuyō tend to stay for the rest of their life, whereas Rōken serve more as a "step-down" facility, preparing residents for independent living at home. Taken together, the SWC-operated facilities observed in this study comprise 100 beds and approximately 100 staff members, including doctors, care professionals, care managers, nurses, nutritionists, and counselors who handle admission procedures and contract work.

(i) Introduction of robotics-aided care—pilot testing

In 2016, the Japan Agency for Medical Research and Development (AMED), with support from the Ministry of Economy, Trade, and Industry, funded pilot studies to assess the effectiveness of robots with communication and social support functions for older people (Japan Agency for Medical Research and Development, 2016). SWC became one of the test sites, where robotics came to be seen as a potential organizational strengthening mechanism. Importantly, robotic-aided care in the SWC was introduced and tested to complement and improve standards of care, instead of *replacing* personal care. Ultimately, a total of sixty-seven people aged sixty-five years and older (sixty females and seven males; aged 86.1 +/– 19.9 years) participated in the pilot between September 2016 and August 2017, which was designed as a twenty-four-week-long, pre-post, quasi-experimental study involving five nursing homes. Three types of socially assistive robots (SARs) were brought into the SWC and used as a robot intervention group. The three types of SARs (e.g., A.I. Sense (AIS), Palro, and Sota) share some common features, such as cloud computing and a programmed alert system, but differ in their degree of interactivity. All three types of robot speak and encourage residents to do certain tasks. They also monitor the person with a bedside infrared camera, which sends alerts to the person as well as the central nursing station in case of emergencies such as falls (see Figure 15.1).

As a first step, a nursing care program was devised for each participant. A set of goals in the areas of participation and activities was also identified by a care team using the World Health Organization's (WHO) International Classification of Functioning, Disability and Health (ICF) framework, in consultation with each participant (World Health Organization, 2002). Developed by the WHO, and widely used in the curriculum of social care professionals in Japan, the ICF is regarded as the most encompassing taxonomic model for looking at one's functioning and disability from a universal accessibility perspective (World Health Organization, 2002). The ICF therefore acted as the standardized tool to collect and measure data for this pilot study and included indicators across the domains of (i) communication, (ii) movement, (iii) self-care, (iv) domestic life, (v) interpersonal activities, (vi) performing tasks in a major life area, and (vii) tasks in social and civic life.

The results of the pilot study have been reported elsewhere (Obayashi, Kodate, & Masuyama, 2018), and clearly demonstrated improved scores for "communication," "self-care," and "tasks in social and civic life" among the residents after the introduction of communication and monitoring robots. Furthermore, results suggest no disruption to the care delivery process when these new technologies were introduced, and no care professional expressed discomfort or concern in relation to the shift toward a robotics-aided care system.

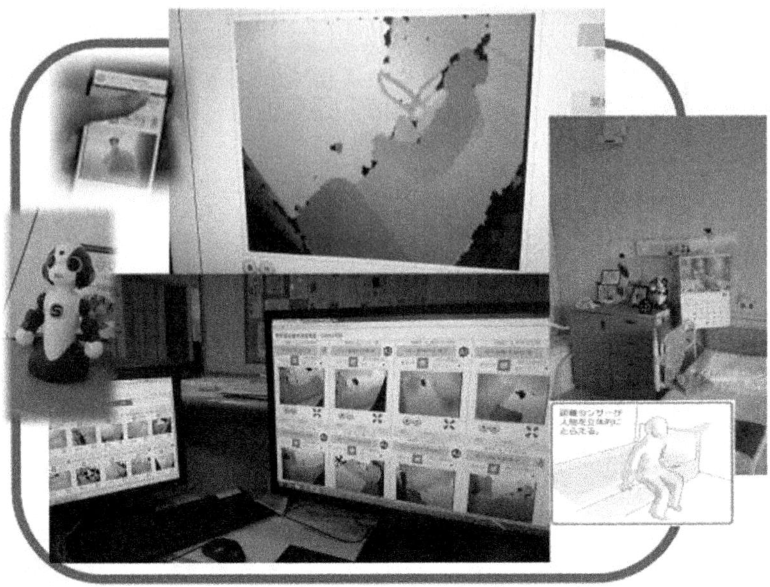

Figure 15.1 Communication robot alerting system

Reproduced with permission from Obayashi K, Kodate N, Masuyama S. Can connected technologies improve sleep quality and safety of older adults and care-givers? An evaluation study of sleep monitors and communicative robots at a residential care home in Japan. Technology in Society 62 (2020) 101318. https://doi.org/10.1016/j.techsoc.2020.101318.

Despite the strong policy drive and early evidence of success, however, there is still a strong belief that care should be delivered by human beings rather than by robots (Suwa et al., 2020). Previous studies highlight the difficulty of successfully implementing assistive technologies in care settings (Lauriks et al., 2011; Wigfield, Wright, Burtney, & Buddery, 2013). This view, however, must be balanced with the challenge of the under-resourced social care sector, recognizing the benefits that can be brought by assistive technologies, including robots, for improving the quality of the workplace for caregivers. The question should therefore not be *whether* but *how* can these technologies be best implemented and integrated to ensure person-centered care delivery. Specifically, the application of assistive technologies requires careful consideration of users' needs, human rights, and workforce development implications (Bennett et al., 2017). So, while results of the pilot phase were interpreted as a success, the identification of facilitating and inhibiting factors (i.e., enablers and obstacles) for successful implementation remain unclear. Against this background, we therefore explore care professionals' experiences with and perceptions of these assistive technologies.

Successful implementation requires multi-level thinking (from user experience and organizational processes to policy and industry context) (Greenhalgh, Shaw, Wherton, et al., 2016) and the understanding that technology-supported work is cooperative and embedded in organizational processes (Greenhalgh et al., 2019). Although the inertia of established routines can be a hindrance to achieving the goal of smooth implementation, certain types of organizational routines can serve as enablers in the process of adapting "disruptive" technologies within care settings. Systems thinking therefore provides a useful tool through which to understand such enablers and obstacles as it allows a care delivery unit to be analyzed as work system, processes, and outcomes (Carayon et al., 2006).

(ii) Systems approach

While the effectiveness of assistive technologies and their positive impact on safety have been reported, the *mechanism* through which technology-driven systems improve care and residents' quality of life remains unclear. Moreover, little is known as to how to ensure that person-centered care is maintained when assistive technologies are introduced, as they undoubtedly affect one's work systems, processes, and outcomes. This chapter therefore uses a framework, known as the Concepts for Applying Resilience Engineering (CARE) model, which builds upon systems thinking (Figure 15.2) to measure and analyze the care system's resilience for delivering high-quality and safe care. The CARE model seeks to capture the alignment between "work as imagined" (WAI) and "work as done" (WAD). According to this model, a successful outcome is reliant on team members' ability to make adaptations and adjustments to fill the gap between WAI and WAD. This model can therefore be applied to explore the interconnection between external and internal components (e.g., technology, leadership, tools, organizational culture) in the context of the introduction of new "disruptive" technologies.

We argue that by examining the context in which use of technology was deemed successful, and how care professionals felt about the technologies in relation to effectiveness and their workplace, we can improve our understanding of the key mechanisms that are necessary for an organization (i.e., a system) to implement such devices successfully (Wiig & Fahlbruch (Eds.), 2019).

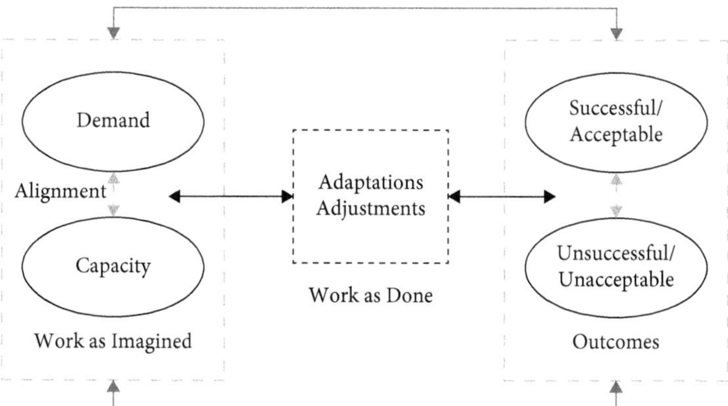

Figure 15.2 Concepts for Applying Resilience Engineering (CARE) model

Reproduced with permission from Anderson, J. E., et al. (2016). Implementing resilience engineering for healthcare quality improvement using the CARE model: A feasibility study protocol. *Pilot and Feasibility Studies*, *2*, 1–9.

In support of this argument, we analyzed key documents and sixteen semi-structured interviews with care professionals conducted in July 2018, after the aforementioned introduction of robotics within the SWC in Tokyo.

Applying Systems Thinking for the Successful Implementation of Assistive Technologies in Care Settings

(iii) Interview results

Interviews asked about participant's perceptions of care, patient experience, teamwork, leadership, and perceived usefulness of the SARs (communication robots and monitoring sensors). The results are summarized in Tables 15.2 and 15.3.

First, issues around the difficulty of adjusting the SARs were raised. Their limited two-way communication, though anticipated, was particularly emphasized. However, one person responded very positively, stating that he felt the great impact of the robot on humans. In addition, other care professionals recalled positive elements such as residents' interest in the existence of the robot itself (irrespective of their functions

Table 15.2 Views about the communication robots

	Themes / roles of robots	Illustrative quotes
Positive	Having something in common to talk about	"Having robots around, they became the talking point between us and the residents, which was good."
	Acting as an alarm clock that speaks at a regular time	"The robots alert residents about something . . . for example, 'come out to have snacks together.'"
	Buying time before care staff rush to their room	"When a resident who could not press a nurse call button tried to go to toilet herself, the robot said, 'is there anything wrong?' . . . so it buys time."
Negative	Frightening appearance	"There were residents who refused to use it and switched it off. The robots' eyes flash, and they flash at night."
	Very limited verbal / communication capacity	"When the residents want the robots to listen to them, they did not hear the robot's reply, so they asked, 'what is it saying?' We tried to relay the message and said, 'the robot says wait a little', but the residents lost interest and did not strike up any conversation."
	Waking up residents at night	"Some residents have very good hearing, and responded and woke up to the robot's voice."

Source: data from Obayashi, K., Kodate, N., & Masuyama, S. (2018). Enhancing older people's activity and parwith socially assistive robots: A multicentre quasi- experimental study using the ICF framework. *Advanced Robotics*, 32, 22. Retrieved from https://doi.org/10.1080/01691864.2018.1528176.

Table 15.3 Views about the monitoring sensors

	Themes / roles of sensors	Illustrative quotes
Positive	Learning about safety-related incidents	"Thanks to the introduction of the sensors, we could understand how the resident got up and stood up and why she fell." "Because we can verify and investigate incidents later."
	Providing peace of mind and preventing falls	"We actually prevented some accidents from happening."
	Providing an effective tool during night shifts, reducing stress at work	"There are only two people on the night shift, and sometimes there is one person . . . Then, if someone goes to the toilet frequently, and someone else gets up . . . we could look at the sensors, and say 'now, ah, someone's in the toilet for a long time, let's go and take a look' etc.'"
Negative	Technical limitations (1)—multiple calls	"However, the difficult challenge was that there were times when you can't see all of them, as several calls come in all at once."
	Technical limitations (2)—screen time is too short	"In a few dozen seconds, the alert will disappear . . . I wish I could see it (the screen) for a little longer. And if there was an accident, it would cut off on the way."

Source: data from Obayashi, K., Kodate, N., & Masuyama, S. (2018). Enhancing older people's activity and parwith socially assistive robots: A multicentre quasi- experimental study using the ICF framework. *Advanced Robotics*, 32, 22. Retrieved from https://doi.org/10.1080/01691864.2018.1528176.

and capabilities) and their sense of ownership, as well as the interactions between caregivers and the residents. With regard to the monitoring sensor, the overall response was very positive, and care professionals provided some details about how they worked.

One of the reasons for the largely positive responses to monitoring robots is that they had a direct effect on the caregivers' stress level and workload, whereas the communication robots had only an indirect relationship with care professionals. It was considered that the relative utility of the monitoring sensor was higher. However, it is important to stress that the interview data revealed care professionals' observation of both direct and less direct (subtle) interactions between older people and robots. They also underlined the role played by assistive technologies in filling the gap between WAI and WAD, while referring to the required adjustments. Care professionals also displayed a clear understanding of the distinction between their work and outcomes of their care and found pros and cons of robotics-aided care accordingly. This was supported by the consensus among care professionals on perceptions of care (person-centered care, based on the capability approach) and the importance of communication channels and tools that are shared between care professionals for delivering high-quality care.

Unearthing Enabling Factors for Successful Implementation of Assistive Technologies

In addition to the key enabling factors of strong awareness of tangible benefits of technologies and positive perceptions of care and workplace, a number of facilitating conditions were also found to be present in the SWC *prior* to the introduction of the robotics-aided care system.

First, the SWC had several well-trained care professionals, including leaders, who shared an understanding of the importance of "person-centered care" and the "capability approach." Secondly, there was a tacit understanding between managers and care professionals that the introduction and testing of robots was not aimed at possible substitution of human carers, but rather as a way to complement their existing roles. The embedded culture of person-centered care was therefore understood as a broader concept which includes support for staff, ensuring a good work environment.

Third, a number of initiatives had been undertaken by the current SWC Director to improve the work environment within the SWC. Underpinned by Maslow's hierarchy of needs (Maslow, 1954), the SWC Director's goal was not just to create a workplace to meet basic and psychological needs of frontline care professionals, but also to produce an environment where a sense of community, respect, recognition and self-actualization can be achieved. In this sense, reduction of workloads was seen as insufficient and instead, a sense of purpose at work/intangible rewards ("*yarigai*," in Japanese) needed to be instilled within the organization.

The *Kiduichatta* Sheet

One of the ways in which the SWC has tried to achieve yarigai is through the use of a unique reporting form called "Something I noticed today" (the *Kiduichatta* sheet). "Kiduichatta" literally means "(one) happened to notice" and implies a sense of happy surprises. Introduced in the SWC in 2009, this complementary reporting form to the existing incident reporting system was introduced to (i) improve the observation skills of care professionals; (ii) provide person-centered care by improving the quality of life among residents (those with dementia in particular); and (iii) activate the capability approach by encouraging residents (those with dementia in particular) to participate in social activities and the local community. This form is thus used to reflect on what care professionals notice in an individual resident's care plan, placing a greater emphasis on what an older person *can do* rather than what one cannot do, or on adverse events (Obayashi, 2014), while also translating professionals' abilities into care in a visible manner. This reporting process of observing a slight behavioral change and sharing it verbally among the team heightened awareness of the care that participants collectively provide (through the work system) and produced positive outcomes for care recipients.

Proactive attitudes toward involvement in research activities (including the study of robotics and disruptive technologies) were also reportedly used to achieve yarigai within the SWC. The form was also used to share information and facilitate communications among care professionals. The range of activities that were uncovered to have

Table 15.4 Organizational mechanisms for improving care and society by supporting professionals, service users, and the community

	Enhancement of organizational culture		**Contributions to community and society**
Purposes	Continuous professional development	Improvement in workplace environment	Community participation Dissemination of information
Examples of tools and forums	Regular training and seminars; Reporting form ("*Kiduichatta*" sheet); Research skills; Conference presentations	Appropriate proportion and division of labor. Appraisal; Support for career progression; Efforts to welcome migrant care workers; Introduction of technologies (e.g., robots)	Community radio program (seven years) Free seminars on care Employment support Local festivals (eighteen years) Disaster-prevention drills

taken place in the SWC to strengthen the organizational culture is summarized in Table 15.4.

Discussion and Conclusion

Care facilities are a complex system, with many constituent parts, involving multifaceted interactions, which change over time. A nursing home such as SWC displays the very nature of a complex system, within which certain properties have to be proactively maintained over time to instil a sense of belonging and ownership. The above results highlight the significance of the "temporal" dimension in which a positive culture is nurtured by dedicated staff with long-term planning and a series of initiatives that create a clear sense of work system as a well-coordinated whole.

Good governance, dignity, respect, and a strong sense of teamwork are all key enablers for the successful implementation and sustainable maintenance of assistive technologies in a residential care home setting. The SWC created an environment to nurture a sense of community, respect, recognition, and self-actualization. Although it requires further research to fully understand the mechanism(s) through which the technology-driven system improves care and residents' quality of life needs, this study, based on the CARE framework, found that care professionals' strong sense of belonging and community functioned as a valve to close the gaps between WAI and WAD. As the interview data demonstrate, the robots and other ATs were not seen as externally imposed gadgets but as potentially useful tools for quality improvement of their care delivery. This perceived usefulness of assistive technologies was filtered through their strong sense of person-centered care.

The inhibitors for the successful implementation, on the other hand, include technical glitches, insufficient infrastructure, lack of time for staff training and work coordination. With regard to communication robots, user-centered design is still under-utilized in Japan. Older adults' needs and preferences, particularly those with cognitive impairments, should be reflected in the design (appearance) and functions (tone of voice, pace of speech) of assistive technology.

With the advancement of research, the COVID-19 pandemic, and rising expectations for high-quality and safer care, complex care systems are now under stricter scrutiny in many countries. In England, the third-party regulator of all health and social care services, called the Care Quality Commission, has thirteen fundamental standards for care provision. These include person-centered care; dignity and respect; consent; safety; safeguarding from abuse; food and drink; premises and equipment; complaints; good governance; staffing; fit and proper staff; duty of candor; and display of ratings (Care Quality Commission, United Kingdom, n.d.). According to the 2017/18 Annual Review of complaints submitted to the Local Government and Social Care Ombudsman, the Chairperson states that "the issues we see are often not mistakes occurring in one-off circumstances, but systemic issues where a policy or procedure is being regularly incorrectly applied" (Local Government and Social Care Ombudsman, 2018). Care homes' handling of care and data were also put under the spotlight during the pandemic, given the high proportion of deaths occurred in residential care homes across Europe and the United States (Declercq, de Stampa, Geffen, et al., 2020).

In the coming post-COVID-19 era of global aging, there will be higher expectations and an increasing demand for care, while the shortage of care professionals will continue to be a key matter of public policy. Despite chronic underfunding and under-investment, many "culture change" initiatives have been adopted in the last three decades, including outside Japan (Grabowski et al., 2014). However, a systems approach and thinking does not appear to have penetrated the sector. Care recipients and caregivers (both professionals and family/relatives) need innovation that adapts to their individual needs, as well as their work environment to live up to their expectations. The "disruptive" technologies such as robots and monitoring devices can address some of this need, and potentially make the care sector more attractive to care workers, while also upholding the concept of "person-centered care." However, the effectiveness and potential issues of robotics solutions in caring for older people will depend on how implementation processes are designed and managed to maximize benefits, all of which need to be examined from the perspective of systems and individuals (users, professionals, and policy-makers).

Acknowledgements

We would like to thank the funding bodies, all the participants and staff members who provided help. This study was in part supported by the Tokyo Metropolitan Government's Model Project 'Utilization of Robotics-Aided Nursing Care and Social Welfare Equipment' (H29-Fukuhoko330) and the Toyota Foundation-funded project 'Harmonisation towards the establishment of Person-centred, Robotics-aided Care System (HARP: RoCS)' (D18-ST-0005).

References

Anderson, J. E., Ross, A., Back, J., Duncan, M., Snell, P., Walsh, K., & Jaye, P. (2016). Implementing resilience engineering for healthcare quality improvement using the CARE model: A feasibility study protocol. *Pilot and Feasibility Studies, 2*, 1–9.

Bennett, B., McDonald, F., Beattie, E., Carney, T., Freckelton, I., White, B., & Willmott, L. (2017). Assistive technologies for people with dementia: Ethical considerations. *Bulletin of the World Health Organization, 95*, 749–755. doi:http://dx.doi.org/10.2471/BLT.16.187484

Cabinet Office of Japan. (2014). FY2014 Report on Priority Policy Measures etc. for Industrial Competitiveness Enhancement, 2014. Retrieved from https://www.kantei.go.jp/jp/singi/keizaisaisei/pdf/houkoku_honbun_150210en.pdf.

Cabinet Office, Government of Japan. *White paper on ageing society* (Heisei 30). 2018 (Japanese). Retrieved from http://www8.cao.go.jp/kourei/whitepaper/w-2018/zenbun/pdf/1s1s_01.pdf.

Carayon, P., Hundt, A. S., Karsh, B., Gurses, A. P., Alvarado, C., Smith, M., & Brennan, P. F. (2006). Work system design for patient safety: The SEIPS model. *BMJ Quality Safety, 15*(suppl 1), i50–ii8. doi:10.1136/qshc.2005.015842

Care Quality Commission, United Kingdom. (n.d.). The fundamental standards. https://www.cqc.org.uk/what-we-do/how-we-do-our-job/fundamental-standards.

Declercq, A., de Stampa, M., Geffen, L. Heckman, G., Hirdes, J., Finne-Soveri, H., Lum, T., Millar, N., et al. (2020). *Why, in almost all countries, was residential care for older people so badly affected by COVID-19? OSE Working Paper Series, Opinion Paper No. 23.* Brussels: European Social Observatory.

Grabowski, D. C., O'Malley, A. J., Afendulis, C. C., Caudry, D. J., Elliot, A., & Zimmerman, S. (2014). Culture change and nursing home quality of care. *The Gerontologist, 54*(Suppl 1), S35–S45.

Greenhalgh, T., Shaw, S., Wherton J., Hughes, G., Lynch, J., A'Court, C., Hinder, S., Fahy, N., et al. (2016). SCALS: A fourth-generation study of assisted living technologies in their organisational, social, political and policy context. *BMJ Open, 6*, 1–13. doi:10.1136/bmjopen-2015-010208

Greenhalgh, T., Wherton, J., Shaw, S., Papoutsi, C., Vijayaraghavan, S., Stones, R. (2019). Infrastructure revisited: An ethnographic case study of how health information infrastructure shapes and constrains technological innovation. *Journal of Medicine and Internet Research, 21*(12), e16093. doi:10.2196/16093

Holliday, I. (2000). Productivist welfare capitalism: Social policy in East Asia. *Political Studies, 48*, 706–723.

Hollnagel, E., Pariès, J., Woods, D. D., & Wreathall, J. (Eds.). (2011). *Resilience engineering in practice. A guidebook (Resilience Engineering Perspectives Volume 3).* Farnham: Ashgate.

Japan Agency for Medical Research and Development (2016). Press Release "The list of robots announced for the use of large-scale experimental study" (May 18, 2016). Retrieved from https://www.amed.go.jp/news/release_20160518.html.

Kodate, N., & Timonen, V. (2017). Bringing the family in through the back door: The stealthy expansion of family care in Asian and European long-term care policy. *Journal of Cross-Cultural Gerontology, 32*(3), 291–301.

Lauriks, S., Reinersmann, A., Van der Roest, H. G., Meiland, F. J., Davies, R. J., Moelaert, F., . . . Droes, R. M. (2011). Review of ICT-based services for identified unmet needs in people with dementia. In M. D. Mulvenna & C. D. Nugent (Eds.), *Supporting People with Dementia using Pervasive Health Technologies* (pp. 37–62). London: Springer.

Lee, Y.-J., & Ku, Y. (2007). East Asian welfare regimes: Testing the hypothesis of the Developmental Welfare State. *Social Policy and Administration, 41*, 2, 197–202.

Local Government and Social Care Ombudsman. (2018). *Review of adult social care complaints 2017–2018.* Retrieved from https://www.lgo.org.uk/information-centre/news/2018/nov/social-care-pressures-reflected-in-ombudsman-s-annual-review-of-complaints.

Maslow, A. H. (1954). *Motivation and personality.* New York, NY: Harper & Row Publishers.

Ministry of Economy, Trade and Industry. (2017). *Priority areas for the utilization of robotics technology in long-term care, 2017.* Retrieved from http://www.meti.go.jp/press/2017/10/20171012001/20171012001.html.

Ministry of Health, Labour and Welfare. (2016). *White paper on long-term care personnel and labour.* Tokyo: Ministry of Health, Labour and Welfare.

Moyle, W., Jones, C. J., Murfield, J. E., Thalib, L., Beattie, E. R. A., Shum, D. K. H., O'Dwyer, S. T., Mervin, M. C., et al. (2017). Use of a robotic seal as a therapeutic tool to improve dementia symptoms: A cluster-randomized controlled trial. *Journal of the American Medical Directors Association, 18*, 9, 766–773.

National Institute of Advanced Industrial Science and Technology (AIST), Japan. (2017). *Large-scale empirical studies on utilization of communication robots in the field of nursing care.* Retrieved from http://robotcare.jp/wp-content/uploads/2017/07/communi_robo_veri_test_report.pdf.

Obayashi. K. (2014). Increased "awareness" of care staff reduces adverse events: A research note (*in Japanese*). *The 15th Japanese Society for Dementia Care Annual Conference.* Tokyo, Japan. 29 May 2014.

Obayashi, K., Kodate, N., & Masuyama, S. (2018). Enhancing older people's activity and participation with socially assistive robots: A multicentre quasi-experimental study using the ICF framework. *Advanced Robotics, 32*, 22. Retrieved from https://doi.org/10.1080/01691864.2018.1528176.

Obayashi, K., Kodate, N., & Masuyama, S. (2020). Can connected technologies improve sleep quality and safety of older adults and care-givers? An evaluation study of sleep monitors and communicative robots at a residential care home in Japan. *Technology in Society, 62*, 101318. Retrieved from https://doi.org/10.1016/j.techsoc.2020.101318.

Ochiai, E. (2009). Care diamonds and welfare regimes in East and South-East Asian societies: Bridging family and welfare sociology. *International Journal of Japanese Sociology, 18*(1), 60–78. Retrieved from https://doi.org/10.1111/j.1475-6781.2009.01117.x.

Pilotto, A., D'Onofrio, G., Benelli, E., Zanesco, A., Cabello, A., Margelí, M. C., Wanche-Politis, S., Seferis, K., et al. (2011). Information and communication technology systems to improve quality of life and safety of Alzheimer's disease patients: A multicenter international survey. *Journal of Alzheimers Disorders, 23*, 131–141.

Suwa, S., Tsujimura, M., Kodate, N., Donnelly, S., Kitinoja, H., Hallila, J., … Yu, W. (2020). Exploring perceptions toward home-care robots for older people in Finland, Ireland, and Japan: A comparative questionnaire study. *Archives of Gerontology and Geriatrics, 19*, 1–15. https://doi.org/10.1016/j.archger.2020.104178.

Takayanagi, K., Kirita, T., & Shibata, T. (2014). Comparison of verbal and emotional responses of elderly people with mild/moderate dementia and those with severe dementia in responses to seal robot, PARO. *Frontiers in Aging Neuroscience, 6*, 257. doi:10.3389/fnagi.2014.00257

The United States Centers for Disease Control and Prevention. Healthy Places Terminology. Retrieved from https://www.cdc.gov/healthyplaces/terminology.htm.

Wigfield, A., Wright, K., Burtney, E., & Buddery, D. (2013). Assisted living technology in social care: Workforce development implications. *Journal of Assistive Technologies, 7*, 4, 204–218. Retrieved from https://doi.org/10.1108/JAT-01-2013-0001.

Wiig, S., & Fahlbruch, B. (Eds.). (2019). *Exploring resilience: A scientific journey from practice to theory*. Cham, Switzerland: Springer. Retrieved from https://doi.org/10.1007/978-3-030-03189-3_9.

World Health Organization. (2002). *Towards a common language for functioning, disability and health ICF, WHO/EIP/GPE/CAS/01.3*. Retrieved from http://www.who.int/classifications/icf/training/icfbeginnersguide.pdf.

World Health Organization. (2015). *World report on ageing and health*. Geneva: World Health Organization.

Yomiuri Shimbun, 57 percent in favour of more foreign workers: Yomiuri Shimbun opinion poll results. May 5, 2019.

16

Capability Approach to Aid Systems-Thinking in Addressing Right to Health of Persons with Disabilities

Thilo Kroll and Hasheem Mannan

The Evolution of Systems Thinking and the Capability Approach in Disability and Health Research

In this chapter, we place systems thinking and capabilities into the context of how disability has been historically understood and we examine a concrete policy evaluation drawing on the capabilities approach.

(i) Reconciling disability and health: a contested and complex relationship

Over the centuries the conceptualization of disability has undergone profound changes, and even in the twenty-first century we are far from a uniform, global understanding of what constitutes a disability due to sociocultural and historical differences. The view of disability as a "personal fault," "a sin," "a curse," or "punishment" resulted in many people with disabilities being ostracized and marginalized by those who considered themselves as able-bodied (Stiker, 2019). In the nineteenth and twentieth centuries, with advances in the medical sciences, disability was largely regarded as an "individual aberration" that need to be corrected. When correction was not "possible," society had to be protected from those who did not conform. People with disabilities were largely seen as inferior, defective, or lacking in fundamental capacity to contribute productively to society. Charities supporting those who did not "fit in" with society and who required help and assistance in life sprung up in most Western societies at the turn of the nineteenth century, initially supporting those who became disabled as a result of war or in factories in the wake of industrialization (Turner & Blackie, n.d.). Interestingly, the principal links were drawn between the human capacity to work and be productive to society. Disability was equated with being unproductive, and the charitable response was to support people with disabilities through donations and taxes, but society as a whole did not see any productive benefit. The thought of focusing on individuals' capabilities, their potential for development and re-habilitation or the design of barrier-free environments that would be conducive for social and labor force participation was alien at this time. A whole-system understanding

Thilo Kroll and Hasheem Mannan, *Capability Approach to Aid Systems-Thinking in Addressing Right to Health of Persons with Disabilities* In: *Systems Thinking for Global Health.* Edited by: Fiona Larkan, Frédérique Vallières, Hasheem Mannan, and Naonori Kodate, Oxford University Press. © Oxford University Press 2023. DOI: 10.1093/oso/9780198799498.003.0016

was non-existent. Along with two globally fought wars (Word Wars I and II), medical technology focused on improving prosthetics and assistive devices for those who lost limbs, eyesight, or suffered shock trauma (McGuire, 2019). The field of medical rehabilitation developed with the aim to restore lost physical function to a maximum level. Physiotherapy became established as an important discipline allied to medicine. The focus very much remained on fixing individuals to enable them to reintegrate into normative ableist societies.

In the latter half of the twentieth century, human and civil rights movements gained momentum. In 1948, the United Nations General Assembly adopted the Universal Declaration on Human Rights (UDHR) and, while not specifically mentioning disability, this document emphasized that all human beings have the unalienable "rights and freedoms set forth in this Declaration, without distinction of any kind, such as race, color, sex, language, religion, political or other opinion, national or social origin, property, birth or other status" (Article 2) (United Nations, 1948). The UDHR was the first powerful tool for civil rights advocates who fought for equal societal recognition and participation for people irrespective of gender and race. And in the 1960s, people with disabilities began to advocate strongly for their civil rights. In the United States, Edward Roberts fought for his way into the University of California at Berkley. He challenged the "medicalization" and "individualization" of disability and shifted the focus from the person to the societal institutions, ableist social attitudes, patronizing behaviors, and barriers of the built environment. Ed Roberts is largely viewed as the father of the independent living movement (DeJong, 1979) that expanded rapidly in the United States and throughout the world in the 1970s. In the United Kingdom, the Union of Physically Impaired Against Segregation (UPIAS) was formed by disability activists to fight against segregated facilities for people with disabilities and to ensure that people with disabilities have the same opportunities as others to participate fully in society (The Union of the Physically Impaired, 1975.). It wanted to give people with disabilities the control back over their own lives. The so-called social model of disability regarded society as disabling and that disability was the product of societal forces that exclude people with impairments from participation. Much legislative, political, and arguably social progress has been made in many countries half a century later. In the United States, the American with Disabilities Act (ADA) was a landmark piece of legislation in 1990 that was passed to ensure that civil rights of people with disabilities in public life are protected as they are for other people irrespective of gender or race (The Union of the Physically Impaired, n.d.). Since its signing, access to public services, the built environment has greatly improved in the United States. While the proportion of people with disabilities in education and employment grew, disparities are still considerable in terms of equitable opportunities in relation to employment, income, transportation, health and healthcare, and housing. The ADA served as a template for legislation in many other countries. Globally, it was superseded by the UN Convention on the Rights of Persons with Disabilities (CRPD) in 2006 (World Health Organization, 2001; United Nations, 2006) The UN CRPD affirmed equality of opportunities for persons with disabilities, and currently 181 state parties have ratified it as of March 2020. The importance of equity and human rights permeates the articles of the CRPD (Mannan, MacLachlan, & McVeigh, 2012; Shogren & Turnbull, 2014), and these concepts have been incorporated into disability and international development policies (Andersen & Mannan, 2012). People with disabilities are entitled under human rights legislation to receive the same level and quality of affordable healthcare as people without disabilities, according to Article 25 of the UN CRPD.

The continued relevance of the social model is interpreted differently by disability scholars. Some emphasize it is as relevant as ever in the wake of neoliberal policies that continue to threaten the position of and opportunities for people with disabilities in society (Oliver, 2013), others see the need to strengthen the human rights element (Berghs, Atkin, Hatton, & Thomas, 2019) and emphasize the need to reform the social model (Gabel & Peters, 2004), and yet others see it as a slightly outdated ideology that fails to address key issues of importance for people with disabilities (Shakespeare & Watson, 2001; Beaudry, 2016).

The discussion of health in relation to disability has been considered with extreme suspicion by disability scholars and activists (Hayes & Hannold, 2007). Many outrightly refused to go near health as they feared it would again equate disability with an individual, biomedically framed condition that requires cure or treatment. The concept of health has evolved over time, as has the understanding of disability; even the World Health Organization (WHO) has provided further clarification. Health per se is no longer seen as a "state of complete physical, mental, and social well-being" (WHO Constitution, 1948) but as "a positive concept emphasizing social and personal resources, as well as physical capacities" (World Health Organization, 1986). Health is a resource that enables societal participation. In 2009, authors of an article in *The Lancet* characterized "health" as "the ability of a body to adapt to new threats and infirmities."(Chatterji, Byles, Cutler, Seeman, & Verdes, 2015). Interestingly, the latest understanding has moved health into a dynamic systems framework and emphasized the fact that health varies from person to person. What this characterization has lost is the agency through health for social well-being and participation that was implicit in the 1986 WHO clarification. Moreover, there remains an emphasis on the biological and physiological aspects of health and does not fully appreciate the dynamic biopsychosocial interactions that determine objective and subjective states of health and well-being at any given time.

National statistics, where available, have repeatedly documented that people with disabilities overall have worse health outcomes, increased mortality, and more difficulties in accessing needed healthcare services (Krahn, Walker, & Correa-De-Araujo, 2015). Health along with opportunities for education, employment, housing, voting and participation in leisure activities cannot be ignored. Census data, health surveys and other instruments have documented health and health care outcomes for people with disabilities since the 1990s in the United States. Disability questions are included in many national survey instruments globally now. The Global Burden of Disease Survey and the Word Report on Disability highlighted health disparities for people with disabilities (World Health Organization, 2011) and strategic initiatives such as Healthy People in the United States and the WHO *Global Disability Action Plan 2014–2021* (World Health Organization, 2018) monitor and confront health inequalities and service disparities. While disability and health are increasingly seen as distinct constructs, the academic discussion of how to understand, conceptualize, and measure the former continues. Pragmatically, work at the intersection of disability and health has continued.

(ii) Reimagining disability and health: disability as a relational construct

A major milestone in promoting a relational or transactional understanding of disability is the International Classification of Functioning, Disability and Health (World Health Organization, 2001) The ICF was endorsed by 191 WHO member states in the Fifty-fourth World Health Assembly on 22 May 2001 (Resolution WHA 54.21). This new system of classification represented a radical shift in conceptualizing disability along a continuum of activity limitation, and it recognized that because everyone experiences some degree of activity limitation during their life span, disability is a universal experience and not just one that happens to a minority of the population. Persons with disabilities are not a homogenous group, and the experience of disability is unique to each individual and is influenced by a range of context-specific social and economic factors.

Over the past three decades "activity limitation" has emerged as a global population-level challenge and as a result, "disability" has gathered wider attention (Loeb, Eide, & Mont, 2008; Palmer et al., 2011; Trani, Bakhshi, Bellanca, Biggeri, & Marchetta, 2011; Trani & Loeb, 2012; Eide, Amin, MacLachlan, Mannan, & Schneider, 2013; Lamichane, 2013; Eide et al., 2015). Yet, to date there is little understanding or empirical evidence in relation to what contextual factors would enable or prevent access to healthcare, education, and employment for persons with disabilities. We simply do not know what works for whom and under what circumstances. The link between disability and access to public services is also influenced by personal factors (coping skills, extent of activity limitation, type of impairment, experience of secondary health problems, gender, age, and ethnicity), community factors (cultural understandings of disability, extent of family support, and opportunities for inclusion), and environmental factors (physical and information access). For example, transport to healthcare facilities may be inaccessible to persons with disabilities, and the educational opportunities and social welfare support available to such individuals may not be appropriate or adequate to enable them to utilize the health and rehabilitation services they need. Equitable access to healthcare, education, and employment for persons with disabilities requires consideration of the interplay between disability, personal, community, and environmental factors (Palmer et al., 2011; Mannan et al., 2012; Lamichane, 2013).

Currently, the ICF is being implemented in a range of high-income countries to inform policy, research, education, and clinical practice. For example, in the United States, the American Speech-Language-Hearing Association (ASHA) has used the ICF as the organizing framework for its person-centered focus on functioning (American Speech-Language-Hearing Association, 2015). In Sweden, the ICF has been demonstrated to be useful in the electronic health record for social service management processing among the elderly population (Almborg & Welmer, 2012). Furthermore, ICF terminology has been incorporated into Japan's comprehensive rehabilitation planning form, a required document for billing of rehabilitation services (Threats, 2015). Koutsogeorgou et al. (2014) have suggested that the ICF could offer an informational platform for conceptualizing and potentially measuring the causal linkages between disability and the networks of supports to which people have access.

The relationship between disability and public health has always been complicated. If medicine has been accused of seeking to cure social diversity, the role of population and public health in the context of disability has been even more complex. The focus of public health is the prevention of illness and the promotion of health in populations. The normative view of disability as something that must be prevented rather than being an expression of human diversity still prevails in many societies. Disability scholars and activists have been vocal in their opposition to eugenic and prenatal policies, laws, and behavior that are in breach of fundamental human rights (Parens & Asch, 1999; Giric, 2016; Steinbach, Allyse, Michie, Liu, & Cho, 2016).

Over the past three decades a new perspective in relation to disability emerged in public and population health, primarily in North America. The focus has shifted from the primary prevention of impairment to a focus on the social determinants of health, specifically inequities in health outcomes for people with disabilities and access barriers to equitable healthcare (Lollar & Andresen, 2011; Krahn et al., 2015; Frier, Barnett, Devine, & Barker, 2016;). The traditional medical view of disability has been gradually replaced by a social justice and human rights focus. The first textbooks reflecting public health perspectives on disability were published in 2009 and 2011 (Drum, Krahn, & Bersani, 2009; Lollar & Andresen, 2011). This renewed understanding of disability has also transformed the discipline of public and population health to an extent. Arguably, the field has become more interdisciplinary. In the United Kingdom, scholars like Hanlon and his colleagues in the "After Now Project" have argued that a new phase in public health is needed that combines the objective socio-environmental factors and subjective and interpersonal experiences in our understanding of health and wellbeing in populations (Hanlon, Carlisle, Hannah, Lyon, & Reilly, 2012). Personal values, cultural meanings, and cultural assets are equally relevant to our understanding of what creates population health as are biological and environmental factors. Individual and collective capabilities as assets need to be made visible (Blickem et al., 2018).

The *World report on disability* noted that 1 billion people experience some form of disability, and disability prevalence is even higher in developing countries (World Health Organization, 2011). The report also highlighted that one-fifth of the estimated global population, or between 110 million and 190 million people, experience significant disabilities. However, the exact number of people with disabilities is unknown because counting and measurement depend on the conceptual definition of disability, its operationalization in national surveys and censuses, the resources deployed to collect national and regional data, and the quality of the resulting data. National prevalence estimates from census or survey data in relation to disability vary between countries as well as within them (Altman & Gulley, 2009). The reasons are manifold. Conceptually, there are substantial variations of how disability is characterized in these instruments. Many surveys do not measure disability but contain lists of functional activity limitations and medical descriptions of medical conditions associated with disability. Rarely, these instruments contain measures of social and built-environment factors or of assistive technologies that mitigate impairments. Thus, population data estimates still rely very much on a static model of disability as a person characteristic. One of the principal challenges for national surveys is feasibility and practicality of administration so that samples remain representative and current. Reflecting the dynamic production of disability as a result of person and environment factors would require substantial economic resources. Despite efforts from the UN and some progress to reach agreement on key national metrics, international disability data continue to vary substantially.

Irrespective of specific enumeration challenges, people with disabilities as a group find themselves consistently at the lower end of national household income scales and are more likely to live in poverty than others (Mitra, Posarac, & Vick, 2013). In many countries, including the United States, employees with disabilities earn less than people with no disabilities, are more likely to be employed below their level of education, less likely to receive promotions, and are less likely to retain their job. Despite legislative advances, for many health insurance and healthcare services remain unaffordable or they remain excluded from insurance coverage (Silvers & Francis, 2013).

Global Challenges for Disability and Health

Nowhere are systems challenges in relation to health and disability more evident than in the field of global health. Ten years after the World Bank and WHO released the *World report on disability* and the launch of Agenda 2030 and arguably after some progress being made, many health inequities related to people with disabilities still prevail around the globe. In many countries, we see complex interrelationships between the risk for being born with a congenital disability (e.g., due to insufficient prenatal diagnostics and maternal health provision), the development of traumatic impairments and disability as a result of violence or unsafe infrastructure and environments, the failure to identify and adequately support individuals with intellectual disabilities on the one side, and the limited opportunities for people with disabilities to participate in society on the other. Public attitudes, barriers in the built or communication environment, lack of accommodation and assistance in education or employment all still marginalize people with disabilities in most countries around the world, primarily in resource-poor settings. Some global system phenomena have made health and social inequities more visible and prescient, as the following examples illustrate.

Global population aging. In many high- and middle-income countries, medical progress has led to greater longevity, while fertility rates have declined in many of these settings (Chatterji et al., 2015). As populations age, many healthcare systems are struggling to keep up with providing appropriate care for people who are sixty-five-years old or older and who are increasingly likely to have to manage more than one long-term condition (Lafortune & Balestat, 2007). Many of these conditions are associated with complex impairments (Mitra & Sambamoorthi, 2014). Multi-morbidity treatment and poly-pharmacy guidelines are slow to emerge, integrated care and support pathways are missing, and the infrastructure to assist people in their homes or adequately staffed and prepared care facilities are non-existent, especially in rural areas. Many people with congenital disabilities now live into late adulthood. However, they lack access to adequate independent living facilities, personal assistance services, and affordable assistive technologies. Failure to meet these requirements places them at risk for health-related complications and excludes them from societal participation.

Primary preventative healthcare and health promotion. People with disabilities continue to face many barriers to accessing healthcare services, including preventative diagnostics and services, such as breast health information and mammography screenings and prostate checks (Wei, Findley, & Sambamoorthi, 2006; Roll, 2018). Health risk behavior counselling (in relation to smoking, alcohol consumption, diet, and sexually transmitted diseases) is not routinely provided to many people with disabilities (Marks & Heller, 2003; Kroll, Jones, Kehn, & Neri, 2006; Kehn, Ho, & Kroll, 2013;) and there is extensive evidence that considerable physical, social, and economic barriers to the receipt of basic and routine primary care services exist for people with disabilities (Kroll et al., 2006). Health education and promotion initiatives (e.g., smoking cessation, dietary advice, physical activity promotion) that are frequently aimed at the general population often ignore accessibility and usability of recommendations and interventions by people with physical, cognitive, or sensory disabilities. For example, evidence-based exercise programs for people with intellectual disabilities are rare, diabetes self-management programs for people with visual impairments are difficult to find, and the equivalent of walking or running initiatives (e.g., Park Run programs) for wheelchair users are the exception. Health and disability remain disconnected concepts unless health consequences are the immediate result of a physical condition (e.g., bladder infections among people with spinal injuries). Unsurprisingly, health outcome disparities between the general population and people with disabilities remain strikingly large. US data have shown that rates for smoking and alcohol consumption, overweight and obesity, diabetes, cardiovascular disease, exposure to violence, and preventable mortality are substantially higher for people with disabilities than those without (Krahn et al., 2015). It is reasonable to assume that what holds true in the United States, one of the world's most highly developed countries, can also be found globally, especially in resource-poor settings.

Climate and environmental change. Climate change has become manifest in the form of flooding, storms, and droughts, and it has threatened lives, ways of living, and livelihoods around the globe. Hurricane Katrina in 2005 was the one of the first major events that triggered awareness of how severe weather events impact and jeopardizes the lives of people with disabilities (Administration for Community Living, 2005.). There was acute realization that emergency preparedness plans in the United States had to be revised specifically to include guidance on response to the needs of vulnerable populations including people with disabilities. We are yet to appreciate fully the systemic impact of environmental hazards and weather events on the health and well-being of people with disabilities around the globe, especially in low-resource settings where little is known about disability in the first place. To date, many countries still lack detailed and comprehensive plans for people with disabilities. This is particularly disconcerting as other global threats appear to be on the rise (e.g., international terrorism, the emergence of new viral diseases such as COVID-19). Emergency preparedness stretches beyond evacuation and immediate support. It requires assistance, clear and tailored communication, and flexibility in providing support before, during, and after national and global emergencies. The concept and existence of disability illustrate the need for systems thinking to connect health with assistance, housing, technology, transportation, and many other areas.

Violence and conflict. Violence as a result of war, interpersonal conflict, or domestic abuse affects people with disabilities disproportionally (Jones et al., 2012; Mikton &

Shakespeare, 2014). Gun violence is on the rise globally. Media attention is mostly directed at those who die as a consequence of violent acts but rarely focuses on survivors who have to adapt to a life with a disability (Buchanan, 2014). While disabling physical and emotional trauma is the direct consequence of violence and combat, people with existing disabilities are at risk of financial, physical, and emotional abuse and hate crimes. Violence negatively impacts the thinner margin of health among people with disabilities (DeJong, Palsbo, Beatty, Jones, Kroll, & Neri, 2002). Studies have highlighted that women with disabilities are particularly vulnerable to violent abuse (Astbury & Walji, 2014; Ballan et al., 2014).

Communication and information technologies. Contemporary information and communication technology, the Internet, smart phones, and tablets have equipped populations, including people with disabilities, with unprecedented access to information and opportunities to connect and interact with each other (Schroeder, 2010; Barlott et al., 2020). While not everyone benefits from these technologies, the Internet has enabled the spread of information in volumes and at speeds that no previous generation has enjoyed. Social media have created opportunities for network formation, be it for support or advocacy. The Internet, which was in its infancy just twenty-five years ago has radically reformed the way people live, communicate, and share information. For people with disabilities, it has created new assisted technologies with the potential of supporting independent living in unprecedented ways. Smart homes and digital monitoring devices, new mobility technologies, assisted and augmented communication tools have all emerged in rapid succession. The Beijing and London Paralympics Games, both broadcast to a large global audience, offered a different portrait of people with disabilities, one of success and capability. While a new wave of citizen activism has swept around the world to challenge autocratic regimes, neoliberal attitudes to economic development, and inaction on climate change, people with disability have not yet fully capitalized on this momentum to strengthen their demands for inclusion and social justice.

As these challenges unfold, we are tempted to view them in isolation and without interconnection. However, we know that the impact of climate change will affect the lives of people with disabilities even more profoundly. Weather hazards, droughts, and power failures generate new vulnerabilities. Pandemics such as the COVID-19 virus hit those who live in precarious conditions or have a "thinner margin of health" particularly hard. Challenging decisions among healthcare staff about who will have priority in case of a ventilator shortage is most likely to disfavor those with complex conditions. As the global economy is moving toward recession, people with disabilities find themselves competing with other parts of society for social and financial support. Violence against people who are receiving assistance or care us rising in times of crisis beyond already comparatively higher levels and compared to the levels experienced by the general public.

Connecting the Dots: Human Rights, Systems Thinking and the Capability Approach

At the end of the first two decades of the new Millennium, there is growing awareness that traditional, siloed approaches to health and disability are not fit for purpose in a new, interconnected, globalized world. The Sustainable Development Goals (SDGs)—contrary to the Millennium Development Goals (MDGs)—have clearly stipulated action to reduce disparities for people with disabilities across all seventeen goals. The *Disability and development report* (United Nations, 2019) released in 2018 illustrated the relative greater disadvantage of people with disabilities compared to the general public in all areas, including access to needed healthcare service. As our understanding of disability has evolved from viewing it as a medical deficiency toward seeing it as the time- and context-bound product of dynamic interactions between person and environment factors, the right to health can only be fulfilled if it acknowledges the multilayered social dimensions associated with it. Individual characteristics such as gender, age, disability, ethnicity, social circumstances relating to family size, household composition, and living conditions, cultural context, and macro-economic context (i.e., living in resource-poor or affluent environments) can only explain parts of the puzzle of why some individuals with disabilities flourish and others do not. Whole systems thinking and awareness are needed to delineate the complex balancing and reinforcing of relationships between health, socio-environmental, and individual-level factors. The health disparities experienced by people with disabilities point to a complex picture of interrelated challenges. Siloed approaches that only seek to address one particular aspect, such as healthcare provision or economic support, are likely to be ineffective. Systems thinking to fulfil the health rights of people with disabilities requires a multilayered approach that considers individual, social, environmental, and political factors. Trochim et al. refer to systems thinking as a "general conceptual orientation concerned with the interrelationships to a functioning whole, often understood within the context of an even greater whole" (Trochim, Cabrera, Milstein, Gallagher, & Leishow, 2006: 541). They developed a concept map of practical challenges that need to be addressed to encourage and support effective systems thinking in public health work. One of the concepts relates to "use systems measures and models" and the practical challenge within the concept was "to develop new evaluation approaches that will demonstrate the value of systems approaches" (Trochim et al., 2006: 543).

Public policies have the potential to shape individual capabilities through creating opportunities for agency. They can expressively promote a respect for individual's freedom to make choices. Individual capabilities are the set of all potential functions from which a person can freely chose, and they are influenced by circumstances, efforts, and public policies. The capability approach enables us to consider disability "as inherently relational and multidimensional, as one aspect of human diversity that has to be considered when evaluating the reciprocal positions of individuals and the distribution of benefits and burdens in social arrangements" (Terzi, 2005: 215). Scholarship has also extended the capability approach to incorporate collective capabilities, in order to understand choices made with (and by) families and communities (Trani, Bakhshi, Noor, & Mashkour, 2009; Trani et al., 2011). Over the last decade, the capability approach has been used in multiple disciplines to study various disabilities issues related to health, educational, and economic well-being, mainly by non-disabled scholars. It has also been used to analyze intentions of disability policy and to conceptualize disability as capacity deprivation. If health policies are to have a positive impact on the lives of disabled people, these policies need to enhance their capabilities. However, there is limited scholarship regarding the contexts in which the capability approach works and why.

Sherlock and Barrientos (2002) have argued that Nussbaum's capability approach can be considered a useful tool for understanding the condition of older people in developing countries. Baylies reviewed human rights discourses related to disability and argued that the capability approach may provide a better framework "for identifying the responsibilities of governments and external agencies in genuinely equalizing opportunities" (Baylies, 2002: 725). Terzi has argued that the capability approach is "an ethical, normative framework based upon justice and equality" (Terzi, 2005: 197), which provides an essential view for reconceptualizing disability and special needs. In particular, Terzi believes that the capability approach is an appropriate framework for "assessing the relevance of impairment and disability in designing just and inclusive institutional and social arrangements" (Terzi, 2006: 203). She believes that the capability perspective on disability provides appropriate directions for inclusive educational policies to respect human diversity and to consider the special needs of children with disabilities. Terzi (2007) has also developed a conceptual framework based on the capability approach for a just distribution of opportunities and effective access to educational functioning for children with disabilities.

Sen has noted that the concepts of human rights and capabilities "go well with each other, so long as we do not try to subsume either concept entirely within the territory of the other" (Sen, 2005: 151). He goes on to indicate that many human rights can be seen as rights to particular capabilities. The current program of research will empirically validate the extent to which human rights are illustrated as rights to particular capabilities. Both human rights scholarship and the capability approach focus on the dignity and liberty of the individual (Vizard, Fakuda-Parr, & Elson, 2011). As an approach to public policy, the capability approach brings to the fore opportunities, while human rights highlights core concepts such as liberty, dignity, participation, non-discrimination, autonomy, accountability, protection from harm, entitlements, and accountability (Vizard et al., 2011). Burchardt and Vizard (2011), in discussing a capability-based measurement framework that evaluates the equality and human rights positions of individuals and groups, contend that one needs to consider three aspects of the positions of individuals and groups. These include functioning (what people are actually doing and being); treatment (how are they being treated, including the core concepts of non-discrimination, dignity, and respect); and autonomy (participation and decision-making) (Burchardt & Vizard, 2011). These fall within ten domains of substantive freedoms and opportunities including health, education, employment, and family and community life, among others, and they identify several disaggregation characteristics, including gender, disability, sexual orientation, age, and religion, among others (Burchardt & Vizard, 2011). They note that the list of capabilities can emerge from "bottom-up" processes that engage individuals and groups concerned and caution that these "might conflict with standards and principles that are recognized and embedded in international human rights law" (Burchardt & Vizard, 2011: 92). They have also demonstrated how information about functioning and social participation metrics in relation to the WHO ICF can be found in administrative and social survey data. Finally, they argue that evaluating the equality and human rights position of individuals and groups using the capability approach, while informationally demanding, is feasible.

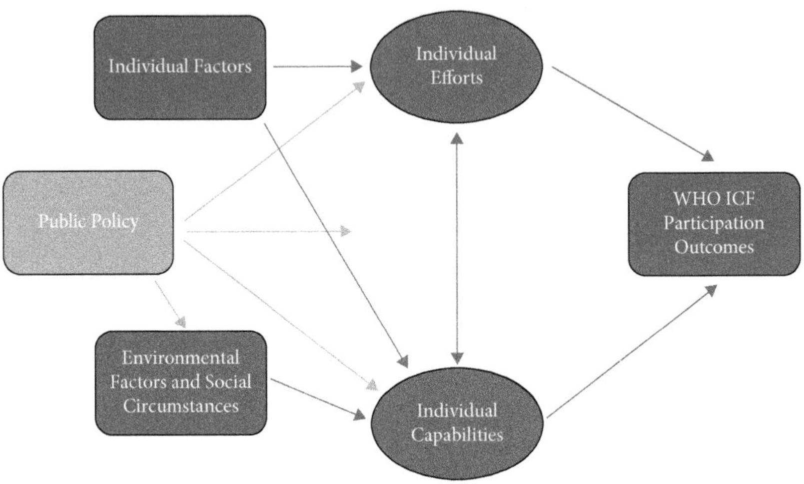

Figure 16.1 Public Policies Effect on Living Conditions

Opportunities for equal and equitable social inclusion and participation for people with disabilities arise best in an ecosystem that maximizes human capabilities. Thus, health policies may not explicitly and directly shape circumstances such as disability, gender, household composition, or living conditions, but they do shape the extent to which these circumstances affect individual's capabilities to consider themselves as free and equal agents who have a fair and equitable chance of a good life in society. Figure 16.1 illustrates how public policies can exert a direct effect on living circumstances (i.e., in making public infrastructure and systems more accessible and ensuring equal employment opportunities, access to education, and fair insurance policies) but also how policies can promote social participation and inclusion through the creation of choice and opportunity. The illustration combines components of the WHO ICF and the capabilities approach.

Conclusion

The conceptualization of health as a human right for people with disabilities has been fraught with historical and political obstacles. The UN CRPD has created a political instrument to guide national legislation and practice. Over the past fifty years, disabilityhas been established as a relational and dynamic phenomenon which policy-makers and practitioners still find hard to grasp. The time- and context-bound nature of disability and its systemic quality create major challenges for national and international data capture. Classifications such as the WHO ICF reflect the dynamic interplay of person and environment factors in producing or preventing disability. The shift from deficit to difference and diversity, from dysfunction to capability and human assets still presents major challenges for policy decision-makers. Public policy has the potential to influence the dynamic interplay between person and environment that generates or abates disability in numerous ways. It can directly remove barriers of the physical infrastructure and strive to educate the public about human diversity. But perhaps, even more importantly, it can strengthen the personal agency of people with disabilities by creating both the necessary environment as well as the opportunities to become dignified and equitable partners in society.

References

Administration for Community Living. (2005.) *No one left behind: Including older adults and people with disabilities in emergency.* Retrieved from https://acl.gov/news-and-events/acl-blog/no-one-left-behind-including-older-adults-and-people-disabilities.

Almborg, A. H., & Welmer, A.-K. (2012). Use of the International Classification of Functioning, Disability and Health (ICF) in social services for elderly in Sweden. *Disability and Rehabilitation, 34*(11), 959–964.

Altman, B. M., & Gulley, S. P. (2009). Convergence and divergence: Differences in disability prevalence estimates in the United States and Canada based on four health survey instruments. *Social Science and Medicine, 69*(4), 543–552. Retrieved from https://doi.org/10.1016/j.socscimed.2009.06.017.

Andersen, A., & Mannan, H. (2012). Assessing the quality of European policies on disability and development cooperation: A discussion of core concepts of human rights and coherence. *Behinderung und Internationale Entwicklung/Disability and International Development, 23*(1), 16–24.

Astbury, J., & Walji, F. (2014). The prevalence and psychological costs of household violence by family members against women with disabilities in Cambodia. *Journal of Interpersonal Violence, 29*(17), 3127–3149. Retrieved from https://doi.org/10.1177/0886260514534528.

Ballan, M. S., Freyer, M. B., Marti, C. N., Perkel, J., Webb, K. A., & Romanelli, M. (2014). Looking beyond prevalence: A demographic profile of survivors of intimate partner violence with disabilities. *Journal of Interpersonal Violence, 29*(17), 3167–3179. Retrieved from https://doi.org/10.1177/0886260514534776.

Barlott, T., Aplin, T., Catchpole, E., Kranz, R., Le Goullon, D., Toivanen, A., & Hutchens, S. (2020). Connectedness and ICT: Opening the door to possibilities for people with intellectual disabilities. *Journal of Intellectual Disabilities, 24*(4), 503–521. Retrieved from https://doi.org/10.1177/1744629519831566.

Baylies, C. (2002). Disability and the notion of human development: Questions of rights and capabilities. *Disability & Society, 17*(7), 725–739.

Beaudry, J.-S. (2016). Beyond (Models of) Disability? *The Journal of Medicine and Philosophy, 41*(2), 210–228. Retrieved from https://doi.org/10.1093/JMP/JHV063.

Berghs, M., Atkin, K., Hatton, C., & Thomas, C. (2019). Do disabled people need a stronger social model: A social model of human rights? *Disability and Society, 34*(7–8), 1034–1039. Retrieved from https://doi.org/10.1080/09687599.2019.1619239.

Blickem, C., Dawson, S., Kirk, S., Vassilev, I., Mathieson, A., Harrison, R., ... Lamb, J. (2018). What is asset-based community development and how might it improve the health of people with long-term conditions? A realist synthesis. *SAGE Open, 8*(3), ISSN 2158-2440. Retrieved from https://doi.org/10.1177/2158244018787223.

Buchanan, C. (2014). *Gun violence, disability and recovery.* Bloomington, United States of America: XLibris.

Burchardt, T., & Vizard, P. (2011). Operationalizing the capability approach as a basis for equality and human rights monitoring in twenty-first-century Britain. *Journal of Human Development and Capabilities, 12*(1), 91–119.

Chatterji, S., Byles, J., Cutler, D., Seeman, T., & Verdes, E. (2015). Health, functioning, and disability in older adults—Present status and future implications. *The Lancet, 385*(9967), 563–575. Retrieved from https://doi.org/10.1016/S0140-6736(14)61462-8.

DeJong, G. (1979). Independent living: From social movement to analytic paradigm. *Archives of Physical Medicine and Rehabilitation, 60*(10), 435–446.

DeJong, G., Palsbo, S. E., Beatty, P. W., Jones, G. C., Kroll, T., & Neri, M. T. (2002). The organization and financing of health services for persons with disabilities. *Milbank Quarterly, 80*(2), 261–301. doi:10.1111/1468-0009.t01-1-00004. PMID: 12101873; PMCID: PMC2690107.

Drum, C. E., Krahn, G. L., & Bersani, H. Jr. (2009). *Disability and public health*. Washington, DC: American Public Health Association.

Eide, A. H., Amin, M., MacLachlan, M., Mannan, H., & Schneider, M. (2013). Addressing equitable health of vulnerable groups in international health documents. *ALTER: European Journal of Disability Research, 7*(3), 153–162.

Eide, A. H., Mannan, H., Khogali, M., Van Rooy, G., Swartz, L., & Munthali, A. (2015). Perceived barriers for accessing health services among individuals with disability in four African Countries. *PLoS One, 10*(5).

Frier, A., Barnett, F., Devine, S., & Barker, R. (2016). Understanding disability and the "social determinants of health": How does disability affect peoples' social determinants of health? *Disability and Rehabilitation, 40*(5), 538–547.

Gabel, S., & Peters, S. (2004). Presage of a paradigm shift? Beyond the social model of disability toward resistance theories of disability. *Disability and Society, 19*(6), 585–600. Retrieved from https://doi.org/10.1080/0968759042000252515.

Giric, S. (2016). Strange bedfellows: Anti-abortion and disability rights advocacy. *Journal of Law and the Biosciences, 3*(3), 736–742. Retrieved from https://doi.org/10.1093/JLB/LSW056.

Hanlon, P., Carlisle, S., Hannah, M., Lyon, A., & Reilly, D. (2012). A perspective on the future public health: An integrative and ecological framework. *Perspectives in Public Health, 132*(6), 313–319. Retrieved from https://doi.org/10.1177/1757913912440781.

Hayes, J., & Hannold, E. M. (2007). The road to empowerment: A historical perspective on the medicalization of disability. *Journal of Health and Human Services Administration, 30*(3), 352–377.

Jones, L., Bellis, M. A., Wood, S., Hughes, K., McCoy, E., Eckley, L., ... Shakespeare, T. (2012). Prevalence and risk of violence against children with disabilities: A systematic review and meta-analysis of observational studies. *The Lancet, 380*(9845), 899–907. Retrieved from https://doi.org/10.1016/S0140-6736(12)60692-8.

Kehn, M. E., Ho, P.-S., & Kroll, T. (2013). Identifying the health service needs of homeless adults with physical disabilities. *Public Health, 127*(8), 785–787. Retrieved from https://doi.org/10.1016/j.puhe.2013.01.011.

Koutsogeorgou, E., Leonardi, M., Bickenbach, J.-E., Cerniauskaite, M., Quintas, R., & Raggi, A. (2014). Social capital, disability, and usefulness of the International Classification of Functioning, Disability and Health for the development and monitoring of policy interventions. *Disability & Society, 29*(7), 1104–1116.

Krahn, G. L., Walker, D. K., & Correa-De-Araujo, R. (2015). Persons with disabilities as an unrecognized health disparity population. *American Journal of Public Health, 105*(Suppl 2), S198–S206. Retrieved from https://doi.org/10.2105/AJPH.2014.302182.

Kroll, T., Jones, G. C. G. C., Kehn, M., & Neri, M. T. M. T. (2006). Barriers and strategies affecting the utilization of primary preventive services for people with physical disabilities: A qualitative inquiry. *Health and Social Care in the Community*, *14*(4), 284–293. Retrieved from https://doi.org/10.1111/j.1365-2524.2006.00613.x.

Lafortune, G., & Balestat, G. (2007). Trends in severe disability among elderly people: Assessing the Evidence in 12 OECD Countries and the Future Implications, No 26, OECD Health Working Papers, OECD Publishing. Retrieved from https://doi.org/10.1787/217072070078

Lamichane, K. (2013). Disability and barriers to education: Evidence from Nepal. *Scandinavian Journal of Disability Research*, *15*(4), 311–324.

Loeb, M., Eide, A. H., & Mont, D. (2008). Approaching the measurement of disability prevalence: The case of Zambia. *ALTER-European Journal of Disability Research/Revue Européenne de Recherche Sur Le Handicap*, *2*(1), 32–43.

Lollar, D. J., & Andresen, E. M. (2011). *Public health perspectives on disability*. New York, NY: Springer. Retrieved from https://doi.org/10.1007/978-1-4419-7341-2.

Mannan, H., MacLachlan, M., & McVeigh, J. (2012). Core concepts of human rights and inclusion of vulnerable groups in the United Nations Convention on the Rights of Persons with Disabilities. *ALTER: European Journal of Disability Research*, *23*(3), 159–177.

Marks, B. A., & Heller, T. (2003). Bridging the equity gap: Health promotion for adults with intellectual and developmental disabilities. *The Nursing Clinics of North America*, *38*(2), 205–228. Retrieved from https://doi.org/10.1016/s0029-6465(02)00049-x.

McGuire, C. A. (2019). The categorisation of hearing loss through telephony in inter-war Britain. *History and Technology*, *35*(2), 138–155. Retrieved from https://doi.org/10.1080/07341512.2019.1652435.

Mikton, C., & Shakespeare, T. (2014). Introduction to special issue on violence against people with disability. *Journal of Interpersonal Violence*, *29*(17), 3055–3062. Retrieved from https://doi.org/10.1177/0886260514534531.

Mitra, S., & Sambamoorthi, U. (2014). Disability prevalence among adults: Estimates for 54 countries and progress toward a global estimate. *Disability and Rehabilitation*, *36*(11), 940–947. Retrieved from https://doi.org/10.3109/09638288.2013.825333.

Mitra, S., Posarac, A., & Vick, B. (2013). Disability and poverty in developing countries: A multidimensional study. *World Development*, *41*(1), 1–18. Retrieved from https://doi.org/10.1016/j.worlddev.2012.05.024.

Palmer, M., Nguyen, T., Neeman, T., Berry, H., Hull, T., & Harley, D. (2011). Health care utilization, cost burden and coping strategies by disability status: An analysis of the Viet Nam National Health Survey. *The International Journal of Health Planning and Management*, *26*(3), e151–e168.

Parens, E., & Asch, A. (1999). Special supplement: The disability rights critique of prenatal genetic testing reflections and recommendations. *The Hastings Center Report*, *29*(5), S1–S1. Retrieved from https://doi.org/10.2307/3527746

Roll, A. E. (2018). Health promotion for people with intellectual disabilities—A concept analysis. *Scandinavian Journal of Caring Sciences*, *32*(1), 422–429. Retrieved from https://doi.org/10.1111/scs.12448

Schroeder, R. (2010). Mobile phones and the inexorable advance of multimodal connectedness. *New Media and Society*, *12*(1), 75–90. Retrieved from https://doi.org/10.1177/1461444809355114.

Sen, A. (2005). Human rights and capabilities. *Journal of Human Development*, *6*(2), 151–166.

Shakespeare, T., & Watson, N. (2001). The social model of disability: An outdated ideology? *Research in Social Science and Disability*, *2*, 9–28. Retrieved from https://doi.org/10.1016/S1479-3547(01)80018-X.

Sherlock, P. L., & Barrientos, A. (2002). Nussbaum, capabilities and older people. *Journal of International Development*, *14*(3), 1163–1173.

Shogren, K. A., & Turnbull, H. R. (2014). Core concepts of disability policy, the Convention on the Rights of Persons with Disabilities, and public policy research with respect to developmental disabilities. *Journal of Policy and Practice in Intellectual Disabilities, 11*(1), 19–26.

Silvers, A., & Francis, L. (2013). Human rights, civil rights: Prescribing disability discrimination prevention in packaging essential health benefits. *Journal of Law, Medicine and Ethics, 41*(4), 781–791. Retrieved from https://doi.org/10.1111/jlme.12089.

Steinbach, R. J., Allyse, M., Michie, M., Liu, E. Y., & Cho, M. K. (2016). "This lifetime commitment": Public conceptions of disability and noninvasive prenatal genetic screening. *American Journal of Medical Genetics, Part A, 170*(2), 363–374. Retrieved from https://doi.org/10.1002/ajmg.a.37459.

Stiker, H.-J. (2019). *A history of disability*. Ann Arbor, MI: University of Michigan Press.

Terzi, L. (2005). A capability perspective on impairment, disability and special educational needs: Towards social justice in education. *Theory and Research in Education, 3*(2), 197–223.

Terzi, L. (2006). Beyond the Dilemma of Difference: the capability approach to disability and special educational needs. In. R Cigman (Ed.), *Included or Excluded?: The Challenge of the Mainstream for some SEN Children, with a foreword by Mary Warnock*. Routledge: Taylor & Francis Group.

Terzi, L. (2007). Capability and educational equality: The just distribution of resources to students with disabilities and special educational needs. *Journal of Philosophy of Education, 41*(4), 757–774.

Threats, T. (2015). *Communication disorders and the ICF*. Retrieved from http://www.asha.org/uploadedFiles/slp/AboutICFandCD.pdf.

Trani, J.-F., & Loeb, M. (2012). Poverty and disability: A vicious circle? Evidence from Afghanistan and Zambia. *Journal of International Development, 24*(S1), S19–S52.

Trani, J.-F., Bakhshi, P., Noor, A. A., & Mashkour, A. (2009). Lack of a will or of a way? Taking a capability approach for analysing disability policy shortcomings and ensuring programme Impact in Afghanistan. *European Journal of Development Research, 21*(2), 297–319.

Trani, J.-F., Bakhshi, P., Bellanca, N., Biggeri, M., & Marchetta, F. (2011). Disabilities through the capability approach lens: Implications for public policies. *ALTER: European Journal of Disability Research, 5*, 143–157.

Trochim, W. M., Cabrera, D. A., Milstein, B., Gallagher, R. S., & Leishow, S. J. (2006). Practical challenges of systems thinking and modeling in public health. *American Journal of Public Health, 96*(3), 538–546.

Turner, D. M., & Blackie, D. (n.d.). *Disability in the Industrial Revolution: Physical impairment in British coalmining 1780-1880*. Manchester: Manchester University Press. www.manchesteruniversitypress.co.uk

The Union of the Physically Impaired. (1975.) *The History of ADA*. Berkeley, California, USA. Retrieved from https://dredf.org/about-us/publications/the-history-of-the-ada/.

United Nations. (1948). *The Universal Declaration of Human Rights*. New York: United Nations Department of Public Information.

United Nations. (2006). *Convention on the Rights of Persons with Disabilities (CRPD)*. New York, United Nations. Retrieved from https://www.un.org/development/desa/disabilities/convention-on-the-rights-of-persons-with-disabilities.html.

United Nations. (2019). Disability and Development Report: Realizing the Sustainable Development Goals by, for and with persons with disabilities. New York. Retrieved from: https://social.un.org/publications/UN-Flagship-Report-Disability-Final.pdf

Vizard, P., Fakuda-Parr, S., & Elson, D. (2011). Introduction: The capability approach and human rights. *Journal of Human Development and Capabilities, 12*(1), 1–22.

Wei, W., Findley, P. A., & Sambamoorthi, U. (2006). Disability and receipt of clinical preventive services among women. *Women's Health Issues*, *16*(6), 286–296. Retrieved from https://doi.org/10.1016/j.whi.2006.09.002.

World Health Organization. (1986). The Ottawa Charter for Health Promotion. First International Conference on Health Promotion, Ottawa, 21 November 1986. http://www.who.int/healthpromotion/conferences/previous/ottawa/en/

World Health Organization. (2001) . *International classification of functioning, disability and health*. Geneva, ICF: World Health Organization.

World Health Organization. (2018). *WHO global disability action plan 2014–2021*. Geneva: World Health Organization. Retrieved from https://www.who.int/disabilities/actionplan/en/.

World Health Organization. (2019). *International Classification of Functioning, Disability and Health (ICF)*. Geneva: World Health Organization. Retrieved from https://www.who.int/classifications/icf/en/.

World Health Organization. (2011). *World report on disability*. Geneva: World Health Organization. Retrieved from https://apps.who.int/iris/handle/10665/44575

17
How Can Systems-Thinking Address the Barriers to Implementing the Right to Health and Rehabilitation in South Africa

Meghan Hussey, Malcolm MacLachlan, and Gubela Mji

Introduction

The World Health Organization (WHO) (2011) estimates that over 1 billion people worldwide, about 15% of the global population, have a disability, the majority of whom live in low- or middle-income countries. Persons with disabilities remain one of the most marginalized and under-studied groups in the areas of global health and development (World Health Organization, 2011). The right to health and access to healthcare for persons with disabilities are widely ignored and violated. People with disabilities are three times more likely than people without disabilities to report being denied access to healthcare, and even when they do receive it they are four times more likely to report receiving substandard care (United Nations General Assembly, 2018).

The United Nations Convention on the Rights of Persons with Disabilities (UN CRPD) (United Nations, 2006) was a milestone for international disability rights. Adopted in 2007, the goal of this international treaty is to protect and promote the full and equal rights and inherent dignity of persons with disabilities. This is the first document that specifically enshrines the rights of persons with disabilities as a vulnerable group and a group that has specific concerns that must be protected. A number of specific rights of persons with disabilities are laid out in the treaty. With regard to health, Article 25 of the CRPD specifically focuses on the right to health for persons with disabilities. It states:

> States Parties recognize that persons with disabilities have the right to the enjoyment of the highest attainable standard of health without discrimination on the basis of disability. States Parties shall take all appropriate measures to ensure access for persons with disabilities to health services that are gender-sensitive, including health-related rehabilitation. In particular, States Parties shall:
>
> (a) Provide persons with disabilities with the same range, quality and standard of free or affordable health care and programmes as provided to other persons, including in the area of sexual and reproductive health and population-based public health programmes;
>
> (b) Provide those health services needed by persons with disabilities specifically because of their disabilities, including early identification and intervention as

Meghan Hussey, Malcolm MacLachlan, and Gubela Mji, *How Can Systems-Thinking Address the Barriers to Implementing the Right to Health and Rehabilitation in South Africa* In: *Systems Thinking for Global Health*. Edited by: Fiona Larkan, Frédérique Vallières, Hasheem Mannan, and Naonori Kodate, Oxford University Press. DOI: 10.1093/oso/9780198799498.003.0017

appropriate, and services designed to minimize and prevent further disabilities, including among children and older persons;

(c) Provide these health services as close as possible to people's own communities, including in rural areas;

(d) Require health professionals to provide care of the same quality to persons with disabilities as to others, including on the basis of free and informed consent by, inter alia, raising awareness of the human rights, dignity, autonomy and needs of persons with disabilities through training and the promulgation of ethical standards for public and private health care;

(e) Prohibit discrimination against persons with disabilities in the provision of health insurance, and life insurance where such insurance is permitted by national law, which shall be provided in a fair and reasonable manner;

(f) Prevent discriminatory denial of health care or health services or food and fluids on the basis of disability.

As of 2016, the CRPD has been ratified by 181 countries (United Nations, 2020). However, barriers to its implementation remain. For the majority of persons with disabilities, the promise and vision of the rights enshrined in the CRPD globally has still not been fully realized. The commitment of countries to the CRPD and disability rights demonstrated by signature and ratification will only prove to be meaningful if it moves from policy to practice (Pinto, 2011).

This chapter will focus on the use of systems thinking to understand the context of these barriers to CRPD and how they relate to one another, providing insight that can be used as a basis for action toward implementation. A systems-thinking approach is key to working through strategies to overcome the barriers to implementing CRPD (McVeigh et al., 2016). A mere listing and understanding of what the barriers to implementation are is, however, insufficient. In order to address these barriers effectively, one needs to have an understanding of how they are connected to and influence each other, and how they are put into operation in context.

The authors will draw on experiences from South Africa to illustrate this. The first section of this chapter will delve into theoretical models of understanding disability and their application to global health and disability rights. In particular, we will look at the social model of disability which calls for an understanding of the social and environmental factors that are disabling for persons with physical or mental impairments. In the second section of this chapter, we will turn to the CPRD, its theoretical foundations, and its implementation. In the third section, we will focus on the example of South Africa. In South Africa, the types of barriers to the implementation of health and rehabilitation sections of the CRPD include attitudes, political priorities, available finances, organizational structures, physical environments, and communication practices within the health system.

We will explain how systems thinking can be applied to understanding and addressing the barriers to the implementation of the CPRD in South Africa. By adopting a systems-thinking approach, one can examine the context in which these barriers arise and how they influence each other. In South Africa, it is necessary to look at structural inequality and how these historical legacies perpetuate disparities in the health system that make it difficult to implement the right to health and rehabilitation for persons with disabilities. Furthermore, we illustrate how underlying negative personal and social attitudes toward persons with disabilities influence and drive barriers within the health system. Finally, we present examples from the African Network for Evidence to Action on Disability (AfriNEAD) and the United Nations Partnership for the Rights of People with Disability (UNPRPD), which illustrate that collective action and structural reform in South Africa can contribute to strengthening the health system for people with disabilities.

Theoretical Models of Disability

Disability has a complex relationship with health. Scholarship in the field of disability studies has provided a theoretical basis on which to draw from when analyzing disability, particularly the distinction between the "medical" and "social" models of disability. The "medical" model focuses primary on the biological or physical deficits of the individual and particular diagnoses, and emphasizes treatment or correction through medical procedures (Brisenden, 1998). This model locates the "problem" of disability within individual bodies or minds that differ from the "norm" (Pooran & Wilkie, 2005); and can in fact be extended to all forms of individualization, including some psychological perspectives on disability.

By contrast, the "social model" approaches disability as a social and cultural construction (Pothier, 1992). It differentiates between "impairment," the physical or mental difference, and the social conditions that keep the person from being able to participate in society fully and thus renders them "disabled" (Oliver, 1996). This places the locus of the problem within society and its inability to be inclusive of a diversity of abilities rather than a person's inability to function in society due to their particular impairments (Silvers, 1998) The social model of disability has become the basis for much disability activism, policy advocacy, and academic inquiry (Campbell & Oliver, 1996; Charlton 1998; Handley 2003; Gabel & Peters 2004; Watermeyer, 2006).

These two basic theoretical frameworks have been criticized as imperfect and unrealistic simplifications of the challenges faced by persons with disabilities in their daily lives. It has been pointed out that the social model of disability tends to put the entire onus on social barriers, particularly built environments (Shakespeare, 2013). What the social model struggles with is how to acknowledge and consider the real pain or restriction that people with disabilities can face because of their impairments that cannot be ameliorated by changing social conditions alone (French, 1993; Crow, 1996; Shakespeare, 2013). These critics claim that the diversity of lived experiences of disability call for a more nuanced inquiry into the relationship between the medical and social models and the development of new frameworks of understanding.

Other critics have pointed out that the social model has failed to be applied in a way that changes the social landscape for people with disabilities (Samaha, 2007). Some have claimed that though the social model theory provides a clear picture of the societal construction of disability, it does not provide a coherent agenda for disability equality (Stein, 2007). Weber (1998) calls for social model advocates to move beyond corrective justice and move toward a dual approach of proactively meeting the needs of persons with disabilities in order to enable their inclusion, while at the same time deconstructing barriers. In essence, while the social model has been valuable for being critical of social structures, greater focus on it being crucial for revising existing, or developing new, social structures that empower people with disability would be welcome.

The theoretical distinctions between "impairment" and "disability" have important implications for the field of health and may lead us to ask is, "is disability a health problem?" (MacLachlan & Mannan, 2013). The answer is quite complex. Many persons with disabilities do in fact have certain health problems that are a result of their particular impairments or diagnoses. For example, some people that use wheelchairs may have pressure sores or urinary tract infections and some with epilepsy may need pharmaceuticals in order to control their seizures. This has led some researchers to argue that the global health response to disability should emphasize training more specialized health professionals and establishing medical rehabilitation facilities (Haig, 2013). This would follow the traditional medical model of disability.

In contrast, others assert that the social determinants of health for persons with disabilities deserve more attention (Tomlinson et al., 2009; Mannan & MacLachlan, 2013). Poor health outcomes for persons with disabilities are also the result of social exclusion and lack of access (World Health Organization, 2011). As such, this approach focuses on the reforming health policies to be more equitable and include measures that protect the human rights of marginalized groups such as persons with disabilities (Mannan, MacLachlan, & McVeigh, 2012). It also is more focused on promoting models such as Community Based Rehabilitation (CBR), a holistic model that aims to address a variety of needs of persons with disabilities including health, education, livelihood, social, and empowerment (World Health Organization, 2004). This view has led the WHO to form the International Classification of Functioning Disability and Health (ICF), "in order to provide a coherent view of different perspectives of health from a biological, individual, and social perspective," which has also become known as the biopsychosocial model (World Health Organization, 2001: 20).

As will be discussed below, this move toward the social model has become the basis for the disability rights movement and the formulation and reform of disability policy internationally, particularly the CRPD. It also presents significant challenges to, and opportunities for, systems thinking in health services.

Disability Rights and the CRPD

Persons with disabilities come under the protection of several different international agreements that safeguard human rights, among them the Universal Declaration of Human Rights (1945), the International Covenant on Economic, Social and Cultural Rights, and the Convention on the Rights of the Child. However, due to a historic negative attitude toward impairments, persons with disabilities have often been excluded from mainstream society and been subjugated to the position of beneficiaries of charity, rather than the bearers of rights (Waddington & Diller, 2002; Quinn, 2009). Harpur (2011) asserts that the large room for interpretation is one reason that existing human rights mechanisms have not sufficiently protected persons with disabilities, as it leaves rights open to implementation that could be inclusive or exclusive of vulnerable groups.

The international disability rights community lauded the passage of the CRPD in 2008 as a critical turning point. The CPRD is strongly aligned with the social model of disability, making it the first human rights accord to protect persons with disabilities against discrimination in multiple domains, including healthcare (Stein & Lord, 2009; Lord et al., 2010). Megret (2008: 263) argued that the CRPD challenges traditional human rights discourse because the lives of persons with disabilities "typically require a much more complex social, political, economic and institutional set-up to enjoy rights on an equal basis than their able-bodied counterparts." It has also been said to raise the profile of disability in international policy to an unprecedented level of importance (Lang 2009). As such, hopes were staked on the ability of the CRPD to prompt national legislation and policy reform domestically in countries that have ratified the convention (Dimopoulus, 2010). Finally, it has been said that the CRPD represents a paradigm shift away from a welfare model of disability policy, toward a human rights approach, and therefore can be used by advocates to create real change (Harpur, 2012).

However, the CRPD must be successfully implemented. Quinn (2009) posits that a critical element of the CRPD is the triangulation between governments, independent human rights monitoring institutions, and civil society, which can provide increased accountability for its implementation. From a health systems perspective this can greatly increase the range of stakeholders who have a legitimate engagement with the health system on a regular basis and thus the sort of monitoring and evaluation criteria needed (see e.g., Huss & MacLachlan, 2016) These types of studies with a combination of monitoring measures are relatively rare, but they could be a promising tool to understanding human rights instruments and progress (Landman, 2004). Others have pointed out that quantitative indicators can serve as useful proxies for the measurement of a state's commitment to disability rights implementation (Pinto, 2011). Flynn (2011: 198–200) further identifies eight success factors to implementing disability policy in line with the CRPD, each of which could be seen as important components of systems thinking in regard to disability and health: leadership, consultation and participation of people with disabilities, integration of national disability strategies with implementation of the CRPD, positive legal obligations and funding programs, transparency and accountability, mainstreaming disability into general public policy, independent monitoring and review, and indicators and data.

Disability in South Africa

South Africa is among the states that has both signed and ratified both the CRPD and the optional protocol, yet much work remains to be done in terms of reforming policies and systems that will bring it into full compliance (United Nations Country Team South Africa, 2013). The number of South Africans over age five that are classified as disabled is around 2.8 million (Statistics South Africa, 2010). South Africans with disabilities face significant challenges in the areas of health and rehabilitation. It has been estimated that from 2002 to 2008, children with disabilities were 2.5 times more likely to be ill or injured than their non-disabled counterparts (Department of Social Development, Department of Women, Children and People with Disabilities, and United Nations Children's Fund, 2012).

In South Africa, the disability rights movement has its historical roots intertwined with the country's struggle for democracy and human rights in the face of the institutionalized racism of the apartheid state (Howell, Chalklen, & Alberts, 2006). The country's democratic transition in 1994 ushered in a new constitution and legal order that was based on the values of fundamental human rights for all citizens, including persons with disabilities (Heap, Lorenzo, & Thomas, 2009). Unfair discrimination on the basis of disability is explicitly prohibited in the South African Bill of Rights (Government of South Africa, 1996). Rights of persons with disabilities are included under the mandate of the South African Human Rights Commission (SAHRC) (Bhabha, 2009). Furthermore, persons with disabilities are included within the scope of legislation to promote equality and outlaw discrimination in South Africa, including the Employment Equity Act and the Promotion of and Prevention of Unfair Discrimination Act 4 of 2000. Finally, South Africa's ratification of the CRPD is important, as the South African Constitution requires courts to take international law into account when interpreting the Bill of Rights (Bhabha, 2009). Flynn (2011: 110) sees South Africa as an important contributor to global disability strategy development by being one of the first countries to incorporate disability policy in the country's broader society transformation. However, Flynn and others have acknowledged that there are many practical difficulties with the implementation of disability policy in South Africa (Dubem, 2005; Flynn, 2011: 108).

Due to the positive developments in disability rights in South Africa, the country therefore represents a good case study of the challenges of intersecting disability rights and health systems strengthening. Previous research on the health situation of persons with disabilities in the Southern Africa region has identified some categories of barriers that are useful to our understanding of the implementation of the health and rehabilitation articles of the CRPD. The first consistent theme is attitudinal barriers and stigma toward persons with disabilities in South Africa (Hanass-Hancock, 2008; Hussey, MacLachlan, & Mji, 2016). An assessment by the South African Human Rights Commission has found that "prejudice remains the greatest disability" and factors in exclusion from all areas of South African society (South African Human Rights Commission, 2002: 62). Attitudes around sexuality and disability have posed a particular barrier in the context of the HIV/AIDS epidemic in South Africa. Many health professionals and policy-makers still hold the incorrect notion that persons with disabilities are asexual, and thus are widely excluded them from prevention and treatment programs (Hanass-Hancock, 2009;Rohleder, Braathen, Swartz, & Eide, 2009; Groce, Rohleder, Eide, MacLachlan, & Swartz, 2013).

Poor attitudes also have an effect on the communication between patients with disabilities and healthcare providers. Physicians are reported to often speak to family members accompanying the patient with a disability rather than to the patient themselves (Smith, 2009; Hussey et al., 2016). This can lead to a substantial decrease in the quality of health services for persons with disabilities, who report feeling that they are not treated with respect. This violates the provision in Article 25 of the CRPD, which calls for raised awareness among health professions of the need for persons with disabilities to be treated with "dignity and autonomy."

Poverty is another significant barrier to the implementation of the CRPD in South Africa (Maistry & Vasi, 2010; Grut, Mji, Braathen, & Ingstad, 2012; Hussey et al., 2016;) and thus its impact on health systems. Poverty and income inequality is a major social determinant of access to healthcare and eventual health outcomes (Farmer, 1999; Wagstaff, 2002; Marmot, 2005; Wilkinson & Pickett, 2006). Persons with disabilities in developing countries are more likely to be poor and thus more vulnerable in the health system (Yeo & Moore, 2003; Braathen & Loeb, 2011). South Africa provides a form of social security for persons with disabilities in the form of disability grants (Department of Social Development, 2015). Means-tested disability grants are available to persons with disabilities who are over the age of 18 and Care Dependency grants are available for parents of children with disabilities (Department of Social Development, 2015). Currently, 1.1 million South Africans receive these grants, with many using them as their primary source of income (Statistics South Africa, 2007). While government assistance prevents complete destitution, it is still insufficient to keep persons with disabilities and their families from living in poverty (Maistry & Vasi, 2010). One study of the effects of disability grants on poverty among persons with disabilities in the Eastern and Western Cape regions of South Africa found disability grants did have a notable effect in equalizing the monthly incomes of persons with and without disabilities (Loeb, Eide, Jelsma, Toni, & Maart, 2008). However, a case study of access to healthcare in rural Eastern Cape South Africa suggests that poverty-related barriers still exist. A person born at home and unregistered at birth, for example, remains ineligible for a disability grant (Grut et al., 2012).

Research has also found that social grants for persons with disabilities have not always been effective, with some studies citing that the money was used by the whole family, rather than the health needs of the individual with a disability (Hussey et al., 2016, Grut et al., 2012). These researchers all stress the need to understand the historical suffering and burden of poverty that is a driving force behind such resource allocations. The South African philosophical concept of "*ubuntu*" means that people are defined by their relationship with other people. Ingstad (1997), has rightly pointed out that this concept and the stigma associated with disability means that, in this context, it is important to not only look at a "disabled person" but rather "disabled families" or "disabled communities." For a family living in poverty that includes a member with a disability, the South African Disability Grant may be one of the few means of social assistance available (East, 2012). This may lead to the calculation that it would be a poor "investment" to spend limited resources on the health of the family member with a disability (Yeo, 2001). Ashton (1999) has argued that in such situations of poverty, this should be seen as "a desperate but rational decision" rather than simply the reflection of ignorance.

Physical barriers are another often-cited category to the right to health for persons with disabilities. South Africa and neighboring countries, such as Namibia, have large populations of persons with disabilities in rural areas, where clinics are often geographically isolated (Van Rooy et al., 2012). An estimated 52% of all South Africans and 75% of poor South Africans live in rural areas (Reid & Vogel, 2006). Article 25c of the CRPD calls for health services to be provided as close as possible to an individual's community, including those in rural areas. A major physical barrier involves the distance between many people and health facilities and the lack of accessible transportation. Transportation costs are major barriers to realizing the right to health in South Africa (Gaede & Versteeg, 2011). Options for public transportation available for people with physical disabilities, especially wheelchair users, remain extremely limited (Gaede & Verteeg, 2011). Taxis often reportedly will refuse service for those with disabilities and the minibus taxis often used as public transportation are often not able to carry wheelchairs (Vergunst et al., 2015; Hussey et al., 2016). Attitude barriers or lack of sensitization can make other transport modes inaccessible for those with sensory disabilities who may not be able to see or hear their stop (Hussey et al., 2016). Studies in rural parts of South Africa and neighboring countries have found the concern about transportation even more pronounced due to the large distances and poor road infrastructure (Law, 2008; Visagie, Scheffler, & Schneider, 2013). While this problem is especially exacerbated for those in rural areas, even those in disadvantaged parts of urban areas such as Cape Town report transport as a major problem to accessing healthcare services (Maart & Jelsma, 2013). This physical barrier is connected to the barrier posed by poverty. Saloogee et al. (2007) found that in a peri-urban area one return trip for rehabilitation therapy at a hospital 30 kilometers away consumed as much as 5% of a family's monthly income. Distance to existing infrastructure and limited transportation therefore constitute significant environmental barriers.

Other barriers to health are found in the quality of care for persons with disabilities in health facilities. Inadequate staffing levels, lack of drugs, and lack of specialized equipment for persons with disabilities such as accessible toilets and rehabilitation devices are cited as recurring issues (Van Rooy et al., 2012). The lack of capacity to meet the demand for health services for both the general population and persons with disabilities has resulted in reported long waiting times at facilities or long waiting lists for equipment such as wheelchairs (Hussey et al., 2016; Vergunst et al., 2015). Health services and health education are often not adapted to meet accessibility needs of persons with disabilities. A study of use of health services by deaf people in South Africa found that lack of sign language interpreters was a major barrier for deaf patients in health facilities (Kritzinger, Schneider, Swartz, & Braathen, 2014). Similarly, research on HIV prevention programs in South Africa found that persons with visual impairments were frustrated by the lack of education materials provided in Braille (Philander & Swartz, 2006; UN Committee on the Rights of Persons with Disabilities, 2014; Philander and Swartz, 2006).

Systems Thinking

The "systems-as-cause" approach focuses on the internal actors that manage the health system. This is critical in understanding the barriers to implementing the CRPD in South Africa. Lack of understanding of the social model of disability or prejudicial attitudes held by the internal actors who manage and carry out health policies are an underlying cause of other types of barriers. For example, attitude barriers are an influencing factor on political barriers and financial barriers. When actors in charge of writing health policy and legislations have negative attitudes toward persons with disabilities or are ignorant of the challenges particular to this community, they will fail to address these proactively in policy documents. Some researchers have, for instance, found that that politicians have inadequate understanding of disability, particularly from a human rights perspective (Lang et al., 2011). While barrier removal is an undertaking that involves technical and financial solutions, it is also a question of policies (Amin et al., 2011; Mannan, Amin, MacLachlan, 2011) and the attitudes that influence these policies (Tomlinson et al., 2009). This is the case both for policy and design of the health system directly, but also of other areas that influence the health system, such as transportation. Attitudes therefore also influence financial barriers.

Budget allocations for rehabilitation services, community based rehabilitation programs, accessible facilities, and adaptive equipment are often made by those who may view them as less of a priority than other possible expenditures (Yeo, 2001; Banks & Polak, 2014). Previous research on wheelchair provision in South Africa found that a combination of budgetary measures and insufficient knowledge among provincial managers about the practical challenges was the major cause of the lack of implementation of the assistive device mandates of the CRPD as well as the South African Department of Health Guidelines (Visagie et al., 2013). Politicians will not put value on an issue they do not understand or a population they do not know or value. For this reason, some have noted that a major challenge to the actual implementation of the CRPD may still lie in overcoming barriers of attitude and culture (Hoefmans & De Beco, 2014).

In order to put policy into practice, the attitudes of health professionals and providers must also change. A training component on disability sensitization and inclusive health service provision should be included in training curricula for all cadre of clinicians. Input from Disabled Persons Organizations (DPOs)s is essential when reviewing and developing such training to ensure that it addresses needs of persons with disabilities and learns from their experiences.

Finally, operational thinking causes us to think about the context in which these barriers arise. The barriers of geography and poverty are interrelated and must be understood in light of the history of South Africa. The apartheid state created a situation in which some communities were systematically underdeveloped and disadvantaged. Although the post-Apartheid era ushered in decades of robust economic growth, this has been uneven (Leibbrandt & Woolard, 2010). South Africa's GINI coefficient, a measure of economic inequality, increased from 0.6 to 0.7 in 2009, making it among the most unequal societies in the world (Statistics South Africa, 2010). This poverty is distributed unevenly among provinces, as well as among racial groups. It has been cited as a major cause of the inequitable deployment of health personnel and resources in South Africa, which researchers have found has a health system that is skewed in favor of the rich (Ataguba & McIntyre, 2012). Statistics show that although South Africa is slightly above the benchmark of core personnel set by the WHO, these personnel vary markedly in their geographic distribution (Day & Gray, 2012).

The compounding influence of disadvantage in terms of race, class, geographical location, and disability creates a particular challenge in South Africa. A deeper understanding of how these barriers arose and have been perpetuated in South Africa compels us to view any strategy to overcome them as part of a more mainstream development effort that addresses the systematic inequalities within South African society and to consider how these play out in access to the health system and the sort of treatment available once it is accessed.

Systems thinking can also be a remedy for what Collins (2008) sees as the flaws of linear approach to monitoring of human rights. A single-issue focus leaves out the examination of context and other factors relevant to understanding the rights situation. The "circular monitoring" approach that she advocates is much closer to the "forest thinking" of a systems thinking approach, collecting all information about the human rights status of the group under analysis as well as contextual information in order to analyze and report on the situation. The CRPD must be integrated in the larger process of achieving human rights for vulnerable and disadvantaged groups in South Africa, if its impact on health systems is to be truly felt. The implementation of the CRPD is thus incumbent on converting rights into right-based approaches to development and global health. As such, some authors have suggested that the disability grant or care dependency grant be repackaged in a way that provides specifically for services that would enhance the functioning of the person with the disability, such as assistive devices, rehabilitation, or skills training, thus allowing for persons with disabilities to contribute to the collective needs of the family and ensuring that they are the recipients of the benefit intended from the grants (Loeb et al., 2008; Grahem et al., 2013).

While the prospect of developing health systems thinking that truly benefits people with disability in South Africa may seem daunting, much has been achieved and much is being done that can pave the road to greater achievements. We end by noting two of these initiatives: the AfriNEAD and the UNPRPD in South Africa.

The AfriNEAD is a regional African disability research network that was established in 2007. AfriNEAD aimed at establishing a diverse "community of practice" to provide evidence and ways of collating evidence to improve the lives of disabled people in Africa. The goal was to be an inclusive network, drawing on the best skills, expertise, and goodwill of researchers, disability activists, government, and civil society. Some AfriNEAD members are prominent researchers; others bring their insider knowledge of what it takes to effect changes for marginalized people in difficult contexts. While the majority of members celebrate in this diversity, the gulf in lived experience among members brings its own tensions and dynamics and requires flexibility to accommodate different perspectives. One of the key roles for the leadership is to help people who may feel far apart from one another, to have a common sense of purpose, and to value what each brings to the greater project of improving lives. This is easier said than done and AfriNEAD is a long-term project, the outcome of which is by no means certain. What is clear is that integral to the process of developing sustainable networks within an African cosmology is the need to pay close attention to the relationships among all participants with sometimes contrasting view, and it is in this context that the concept of *ubuntu* is especially relevant

The cultural principle of *ubuntu* (as used in South Africa, or other linguistic variations used throughout Africa) refers to a social system of interconnectedness and interrelatedness whereby people's humanity is determined not only by their personal qualities, but in terms of how they relate to each other and all in their community (Boon, 1996). The idea that "a person is a person through other persons" encapsulates the essence of the *ubuntu* philosophy, contrasting sharply with more individualized

Western views. In this regard, the notion that disabled people should strive for "independence" is called into question; instead, the integration of the disabled person within the family and community is seen as an important goal. *Ubuntu* is a more interconnected way of being which locates people not as independent individuals. This is one of the elements that sustains AfriNEAD and keep the membership glued together as there is a common focus which is about facilitation of the use of research evidence to improve the lives of PWDs in Africa. Health systems within the South African context should see *ubuntu* as a resource and an asset that could enhance healthcare delivery.

In 2013 the UNPRPD project, "Accelerating the Implementation of the UNCRPD in South Africa," sought to articulate a CRPD-compliant policy framework, develop a framework for disability-sensitive budgeting, and strengthen monitoring capacity in the area of disability rights (United Nations Partnership for the Rights of People with Disability, 2016). To focus just on the first of these targets, the program saw a White Paper on the Rights of Persons with Disabilities, along with an Implementation Matrix, approved by Cabinet on December 9, 2015. This work drew on the analytical framework provided by EquiFrame (Amin et al., 2011) and other approaches, to create structural reform, changing the structures through which society operates. For instance, regarding the influence on health of this high-level White Paper, South Africa has now revised several policies regarding disability and rehabilitation and made them more rights-focused and systems-orientated. Two important features of the South African experience were the importance of cross-sectoral working, for instance, between the Department of Social Development and the Department of Health, and the critical role of civil society working in unison with government (United Nations Partnership for the Rights of People with Disability, 2016). This illustrates how the health system is often more expansive, and needs to be more porous, if it is to work well, than is often appreciated. This helps use realize that health systems thinking often need to be more inclusive, more complex—not simpler—if it is going to really work for the most marginalized.

Conclusion

The purpose of this chapter is to explain how systems thinking can be a lens through which to view barriers to the implementation of the health and rehabilitation articles of the CRPD. These barrier span the realms of politics, finances, the health system, the physical environment, and communication. Persistent underlying negative attitudinal barriers within South African society, that stigmatize and exclude persons with disabilities, influenced all these barriers. This indicates that a first step toward addressing the technical issues that impede the CRPD is addressing the attitudes of key decision-makers and society at large about persons with disabilities and mainstreaming consideration of disability into the overall development framework. While these tasks are certainly challenging, there are some positive indications that through the use of collective action and structural change, the health system in South Africa can indeed be made more inclusive of, and useful to, people with disabilities, and in so doing allow them to contribute fully to South African society.

References

Amin, M., MacLachlan, M., Mannan, H., El Tayeb, S., El Khatim, A., Swartz, L, … Schneider, M. (2011). EquiFrame: A framework for analysis of the inclusion of human rights and vulnerable groups in health policies. *Health & Human Rights, 13*(2), 1–20.

Ashton, B. (1999). *Promoting the rights of disabled children globally disabled children become adults: Some implications*. Action on Disability & Development, Somerset.

Ataguba, J. E., & McIntyre, D. (2012). Paying for and receiving benefits from health services in South Africa: Is the health system equitable? *Health Policy and Planning, 27*(suppl 1), i35–i45.

Banks, L. M., & Polack, S. (2014). *The economic costs of exclusion and gains of inclusion of people with disabilities.* Cambridge: CBM/International Centre for Evidence in Disability, London School of Hygiene and Tropical Medicine.

Bhabha, F. (2009). Disability equality rights in South Africa: concepts, interpretation and the transformation imperative. *South African Journal on Human Rights, 25*(2), 218–245.

Boon, M. (1996). *The African way—The power of interactive leadership.* Struik Publishers, Johannesburg, South Africa.

Braathen, S. H., & Loeb, M. E. (2011). "No disabled can go here … ": How education affects disability and poverty in Malawi. *Disability and poverty: A global challenge* (pp. 71–93). Bristol, UK: Policy Press.

Brisenden, S. (1998) Independent living and the medical model of disability. In T. Shakespeare (Ed.), *The disability reader: Social science perspectives* (pp. 20–27). London: Cassel.

Campbell, J., & Oliver, M. (1996). *Disability politics*. London: Routledge.

Charlton, J. I. (1998). *Nothing about us without us: Disability oppression and empowerment.* Berkeley, CA: 380.

Collins, T. M. (2008). The significance of different approaches to human rights monitoring: A case study of child rights. *The International Journal of Human Rights, 12*(2), 159–187.

Crow, L. (2010). Including all of our lives: Renewing the social model of disability. In *Equality, Participation and Inclusion 1* (pp. 136–152). Routledge.

Day, C., & Gray, A. (2012). Health and related indicators: Health information. *South African Health Review,* Vol 2012-2013 No.1 207–329.

Department of Social Development. (2015). *White Paper on The Rights of Persons With Disabilities.* Pretoria: Department of Social Development.

Department of Social Development, Department of Women, Children and People with Disabilities, and United Nations Children's Fund. (2012). *Children with disabilities in South Africa: A situation analysis: 2001–2011.* Pretoria: Department of Social Development/ Department of Women, Children and People with Disabilities/UNICEF.

Dimopoulos, A. (2010). *Issues in human rights protection of intellectually disabled persons (Medical Law and Ethics).* Ashgate Publishing Group.

Dube, A. K. (2005). The role and effectiveness of disability legislation in South Africa. *Samaita Consultancy and Programme Design,* 1–89. https://assets.publishing.service.gov.uk/media/57a08c5ce5274a27b2001155/PolicyProject_legislation_sa.pdf

East, C. J. (2012). *An investigation of the lived reality of the disjuncture between policy and practice in the implementation of South Africa's disability grant.* (Masters' thesis. University of Cape Town).

Farmer, P. (1999). Pathologies of power: Rethinking health and human rights. *American Journal of Public Health, 89*(10), 1486–1496.

Flynn, E. (2011). *From rhetoric to action: Implementing the UN Convention on the Rights of Persons with Disabilities*. Cambridge: Cambridge University Press.

French, S. (1993). Disability, impairment or something in between. In J. Swain, S. French, C. Barnes, & C. Thomas (Eds.), *Disabling barriers, enabling environments* (pp. 17–25). London: Sage.

Gabel, S., & Peters, S. (2004). Presage of a paradigm shift? Beyond the social model of disability toward resistance theories of disability. *Disability & Society, 19*(6), 585–600.

Gaede, B., & Versteeg, M. (2011). The state of the right to health in rural South Africa. *South African Health Review*, 99–106.

Government of South Africa. (1996). Constitution of the Republic of South Africa, no. 108. *Government Gazette, 378*(17678). Retrieved from https://www.gov.za/sites/default/files/images/a108-96.pdf

Graham, L., Moodley, J., & Selipsky, L. (2013). The disability–poverty nexus and the case for a capabilities approach: Evidence from Johannesburg, South Africa. *Disability & Society, 28*(3), 324–337.

Groce, N., Rohleder, P., Eide, A.H., MacLachlan, M., & Swartz, L. (2013). Disability and HIV/AIDS: A review and agenda for research. *Social Science & Medicine, 77*, 31–40.

Grut, L., Mji, G., Braathen, S. H., & Ingstad, B. (2012). Accessing community health services: Challenges faced by poor people with disabilities in a rural community in South Africa. *African Journal of Disability, 1*(1), 1–7.

Haig, A. J. (2013). Disability policy must espouse medical as well as social rehabilitation. *Social Inclusion, 1*(2), 136–138.

Hanass-Hancock J. (2009). Disability and HIV/AIDS—a systematic review of literature on Africa. *Journal of the International AIDS Society, 12*, 34. https://doi.org/10.1186/1758-2652-12-34.

Hanass-Hancock, J., & Nixon, S. A. (2009). The fields of HIV and disability: Past, present and future. *Journal of the International AIDS Society, 12*(1), 1.

Handley, P. (2003). Theorising disability: Beyond "common sense". *Politics, 23*(2), 109–118.

Harpur, P. (2011). Time to be heard: How advocates can use the Convention on the Rights of Persons with Disabilities to drive change. *Valparaiso University Law Review, 45*(3), 1271–1296.

Harpur, P. (2012). Embracing the new disability rights paradigm: the importance of the Convention on the Rights of Persons with Disabilities. *Disability & Society, 27*(1), 1–14.

Heap, M., Lorenzo, T., & Thomas, J. (2009). "We've moved away from disability as a health issue, it's a human rights issue": Reflecting on 10 years of the right to equality in South Africa. *Disability & Society, 24*(7), 857–868.

Hoefmans, A., & De Beco, G. (2014). *The UN Convention on the Rights of Persons with Disabilities: An integral and integrated approach to the implementation of disability rights*. Brussels: European Commission.

Howell, C., Chalklen, S., & Alberts, T. (2006). A history of the disability rights movement in South Africa. *Disability and social change: A South African Agenda*, 46–84.

Huss, T., & MacLachlan, M. (2016). *Equity and Inclusion in Policy Processes (EquIPP): A framework to support equity & inclusion in the process of policy development, implementation and evaluation*. Dublin: Global Health Press.

Hussey, M., MacLachlan, M., & Mji, G. (2017). Barriers to the implementation of the health and rehabilitation articles of the United Nations convention on the rights of persons with disabilities in South Africa. *International Journal of Health Policy and Management, 6*(4), 207–218.

Ingstad, B. (1997). *Community-based rehabilitation in Botswana: The myth of the hidden disabled*. Lewiston, NY: Edwin Mellen Press.

Kritzinger, J., Schneider, M., Swartz, L., & Braathen, S. H. (2014). "I just answer 'yes' to everything they say": Access to health care for deaf people in Worcester, South Africa and the politics of exclusion. *Patient Education and Counseling, 94*(3), 379–383.

Landman, T. (2004). Measuring human rights: Principle, practice, and policy. *Human Rights Quarterly, 26*, 906.

Lang, R., Kett, M., Groce, N., & Trani, J. F. (2011). Implementing the United Nations Convention on the rights of persons with disabilities: Principles, implications, practice and limitations. *Alter, 5*(3), 206–220.

Lang, R. (2009). The United Nations Convention on the right and dignities for persons with disability: A panacea for ending disability discrimination? *ALTER-European Journal of Disability Research/Revue Européenne de Recherche sur le Handicap, 3*(3), 266–285.

Law, F. B. (2008). *Developing a policy analysis framework to establish level of access and equity embedded in South African health policies for people with disabilities.* (Doctoral dissertation, Stellenbosch: Stellenbosch University). 52

Leibbrandt, M., Woolard, I., Finn, A., & Argent, J. (2010). Trends in South African income distribution and poverty since the fall of apartheid. *OECD Social, Employment and Migration Working Papers*, No. 101, OECD Publishing.

Loeb, M., Eide, A. H., Jelsma, J., Toni, M. K., & Maart, S. (2008). Poverty and disability in Eastern and Western Cape Provinces, South Africa. *Disability & Society, 23*(4), 311–321.

Lord, J., Posarac, A., Nicoli, M., Peffley, K., McClain-Nhlapo, C., & Keogh, M. (2010). *Disability and international cooperation and development: A review of policies and practices.* Washington, DC: World Bank.

Maart, S., & Jelsma, J. (2013). Disability and access to health care—A community based descriptive study. *Disability & Rehabilitation, 36*(18), 1489–1493

MacLachlan, M., & Mannan, H. (2013). Is disability a health problem? *Social Inclusion, 1*(2), 139–141.

Maistry, M., & Vasi, S. (2010). *Social development, including social grants. The Eastern Cape Basic Services Delivery and Socio Economic Trends Series: 12.* East London: Fort Hare Institute of Social and Economic Research (FHISER).

Mannan, H., Amin, M., MacLachlan, M., & The EquitAble Consortium. (2011). *The EquiFrame Manual: An analytical tool for evaluating and facilitating the inclusion of core concepts of human rights and vulnerable groups in policy documents.* Dublin: The Global Health Press.

Mannan, H., MacLachlan, M., McVeigh, J., & EquitAble Consortium. (2012). Core concepts of human rights and inclusion of vulnerable groups in the United Nations Convention on the Rights of Persons with Disabilities. *ALTER-European Journal of Disability Research/Revue Européenne de Recherche sur le Handicap, 6*(3), 159–177.

Marmot, M. (2005). Social determinants of health inequalities. *The Lancet, 365*(9464), 1099–1104.

McVeigh, J., MacLachlan, M., Gilmore, B., McClean, C., Eide, A.H., Mannan, H., ... Normand, C. (2016). Promoting good policy for leadership and governance of health related rehabilitation: a realist synthesis. *Globalization & Health, 12*, 49.

Mégret, F. (2008). The disabilities convention: Towards a holistic concept of rights. *The International Journal of Human Rights, 12*(2), 261–278.

Oliver, M. (1996). *Understanding disability: From theory to practice.* New York, NY: St Martin's Press.

Philander, J. H., & Swartz, L. (2006). Needs, barriers, and concerns regarding HIV prevention among South Africans with visual impairments: A key informant study. *Journal of Visual Impairment & Blindness, 100*(2), 111–115.

Pinto, P. C. (2010). Monitoring human rights: A holistic approach. In *Critical perspectives on human rights and disability law* (pp. 451–477). Brill Nijhoff.

Pooran, B. D., & Wilkie, C. (2005). Failing to achieve equality: Disability rights in Australia, Canada, and the United States. *Journal of Law and Social Policy, 20*, 1.

Pothier, D. (1992). Miles to go: Some personal reflections on the social construction of disability. *Dalhousie Law Journal, 14*, 526.

Quinn, G. (2009). The United Nations Convention on the Rights of Persons with Disabilities: Toward a new international politics of disability. *Texas Journal on Civil Liberties & Civil Rights, 15*(1), 33.

Reid, P., & Vogel, C. (2006). Living and responding to multiple stressors in South Africa—Glimpses from KwaZulu-Natal. *Global Environmental Change, 16*(2), 195–206.

Rohleder, P., Braathen, S. H., Swartz, L., & Eide, A. H. (2009). HIV/AIDS and disability in Southern Africa: A review of relevant literature. *Disability and Rehabilitation, 31*(1), 51–59.

Saloojee, G., Phohole, M., Saloojee, H., & IJsselmuiden, C. (2007). Unmet health, welfare and educational needs of disabled children in an impoverished South African peri-urban township. *Child: Care, Health and Development, 33*(3), 230–235.

Samaha, A. M. (2007). What good is the social model of disability? *University of Chicago Law Review, 74.*

Shakespeare, T. (2013). *Disability rights and wrongs revisited.* New York, NY: Routledge.

Silvers, A., Wasserman, D. T., Mahowald, M. B., & Mahowald, M. B. (1998). *Disability, difference, discrimination: Perspectives on justice in bioethics and public policy* (Vol. 94). Rowman & Littlefield.

Smith, D. L. (2009). Disparities in patient–physician communication for persons with a disability from the 2006 Medical Expenditure Panel Survey (MEPS). *Disability and Health Journal, 2*(4), 206–215.

South African Human Rights Commission. (2002). *Towards a barrier-free society: A report on accessibility and built environments.* Cape Town: South African Human Rights Commission. Retrieved from https://www.westerncape.gov.za/text/2004/11/towards_barrier_free_society.pdf.

Statistics South Africa. (2007). *Community Survey, 2007, Revised version*, Statistical release P0301, Pretoria, 01 June 2012, from http://www.statssa.gov.za/publications/P0301/P0301.pdf

Statistics South Africa. (2010). *General household survey.* Pretoria: Statistics South Africa. 53.

Stein, M. A. (2007). Disability human rights. *California Law Review, 95.*

Stein, M. A., & Lord, J. E. (2009). *Future prospects for the United Nations Convention on the Rights of Persons with Disabilities.* Paper presented at the UN Convention on the Rights of Persons with Disabilities: European and Scandinavian Perspectives.

Tomlinson, M., Swartz, L., Officer, A., Chan, K. Y., Rudan, I., & Saxena, S. (2009). Research priorities for health of people with disabilities: an expert opinion exercise. *The Lancet, 374*(9704), 1857–1862.

United Nations. (2006). *The Convention on the Rights of Persons with Disabilities.* New York, NY: United Nations. Retrieved from: http://www.un.org/disabilities/default.asp?id=61.

United Nations. Treaty Series, vol. 2515, p. 3. Retrieved from https://treaties.un.org/doc/Publication/MTDSG/Volume%20I/Chapter%20IV/IV-15.en.pdf.

United Nations Committee on the Rights of Persons with Disabilities. (2014). *Consideration of reports submitted by States parties under article 35 of the Convention Initial reports of State parties due in 2009 South Africa.* CRPD/C/ZAF/1.

United Nations Country Team South Africa. (2013). *Accelerating the implementation of the UNCRPD in South Africa.* Pretoria: UN Partnership for the Rights of Persons with Disabilities.

United Nations Enable. (2015). *UN Enable—promoting the rights of persons with disabilities.* Retrieved from http://www.un.org/disabilities/.

United Nations General Assembly. (2018). *United Nations 2018 flagship report on disability and development: realization of the Sustainable Development Goals by, for and with persons with disabilities, UN Doc. A/73/220.* New York, NY: United Nations General Assembly.

United Nations Partnership on the Rights of Persons with Disabilities. (2016). *Connections: Building partnerships for disability rights.* New York, NY: United Nations Development Program.

Van Rooy, G., Amadhila, E. M., Mufune, P., Swartz, L., Mannan, H., & MacLachlan, M. (2012). Perceived barriers to accessing health services among people with disabilities in rural northern Namibia. *Disability & Society, 27*(6), 761–775.

Vergunst, R., Swartz, L., Mji, G., MacLachlan, M., & Mannan, H. (2015). "You must carry your wheelchair"–barriers to accessing healthcare in a South African rural area. *Global Health Action, 8*(1), 29003.

Visagie, S., Scheffler, E., & Schneider, M. (2013). Policy implementation in wheelchair service delivery in a rural South African setting: original research. *African Journal of Disability,* (2), 1. Retrieved from http://www.ajod.org/index.php/ajod/article/view/63/105The.

Waddington, L. B., & Diller, M. (2002). Tensions and coherence in disability policy: The uneasy relationship between social welfare and civil rights models of disability in American, European and international employment law. *Disability Rights Law and Policy, International and National Perspectives,* 241–280.

Wagstaff, A. (2002). Poverty and health sector inequalities. *Bulletin of the World Health Organization, 80*(2), 97–105.

Watermeyer, B. (2006). *Disability and social change: A South African agenda.* Cape Town: HSRC Press.

Weber, M. C. (1998). Beyond the Americans with Disabilities Act: A national employment policy for people with disabilities. *Buffalo Law Review, 46,* 123.

Wilkinson, R. G., & Pickett, K. E. (2006). Income inequality and population health: A review and explanation of the evidence. *Social Science and Medicine, 62*(7), 1768–1784.

World Health Organization. (2001). International classification of functioning, disability and health: ICF. Geneva: World Health Organization.

World Health Organization. (2004). *CBR: A strategy for rehabilitation, equalization of opportunities, poverty reduction and, social inclusion of people with disabilities.* Geneva: World Health Organization.

World Health Organization. (2011). *World report on disability.* Geneva: World Health Organization.

Yeo, R. (2001). *Chronic poverty and disability.* Chronic Poverty Research Centre Working Paper (4). Action on Disability and Development Somerset, United Kingdom.

Yeo, R., & Moore, K. (2003). Including disabled people in poverty reduction work: "Nothing about us, without us." *World Development, 31*(3), 571–590.

18
Systems Thinking for Global Health Initiatives (GHIs) in Sub-Saharan Africa

Amanuel Kidane and Lillian Mwanri

Introduction

The unprecedented suffering caused by HIV/AIDS and other epidemics gave rise to the creation and expansion of Global Health Initiatives (GHIs) (Chima & Homedes, 2015). With their emergence in 2000 (World Health Organization, 2009), the GHIs are global partnerships which were formed to reverse the course of HIV/AIDS and other diseases. They are characterized by tackling an issue of international concern and run programs of sizable scope and funding in multiple countries (Mwisongo, Soumare, & Nabyonga-Orem, 2016). Three GHIs that are considered to be the largest, accounting for two-thirds of the external funding resourced for HIV/AIDS are, the United States President's Emergency Plan for AIDS Relief (PEPFAR), the Global Fund to Fight AIDS, Tuberculosis and Malaria (GFTAM), and the World Bank's Multi-country AIDS Programme (MAP) (Hanefeld, 2010).

This chapter details the positive and negative effects of GHIs and the lessons that are drawn from their implementation in Sub-Saharan Africa (SSA). While GHIs have created significant access to HIV/AIDS treatment and other services, and improved quality of care, they have negatively impacted the health systems of SSA countries mainly in the areas of health workforce, leadership and governance, financing, and health information systems. This primarily resulted from a failure to embrace systems thinking. For instance, in several African countries including Uganda, Tanzania, and Zambia, the migration of health workers from the public sector to better paying HIV/AIDS programs has disrupted the health workforce market and created dissatisfaction among those left behind in public facilities (Hanefeld, 2010; Eunice, Mwanri, & Ward, 2017; Lohman et al., 2017).

The first section of this chapter briefly defines GHIs and lists the major GHIs which have been implemented in SSA countries, with a focus on those that have been financing HIV/AIDS programs. The second section provides a detailed analysis of the positive and negative effects of GHIs on the health systems of SSA countries using the six elements in the World Health Organization's (WHO) health system framework (health workforce, leadership and governance, financing, service delivery, medicines and technologies, and information system). The final section identifies the major lessons learnt from the implementation of GHIs.

Amanuel Kidane and Lillian Mwanri, *Systems Thinking for Global Health Initiatives (GHIs) in Sub-Saharan Africa* In: *Systems Thinking for Global Health.* Edited by: Fiona Larkan, Frédérique Vallières, Hasheem Mannan, and Naonori Kodate, Oxford University Press. DOI: 10.1093/oso/9780198799498.003.0018

Global Health Initiatives (GHIs)

GHIs are a form of global health financing and governance mechanisms that emerged following the rapid spread of HIV/AIDS pandemic and other infectious diseases (Hanefeld, 2010; Chima & Homedes, 2015). They are characterized by mobilizing and resourcing a significant amount of funds with a focus on addressing health problems of international concern involving a plethora of partnerships and direct finances to targeted countries. It is reported that over 100 GHIs were developed and implemented in several low- and medium-income countries, particularly in the hard-hit SSA countries (Mwisongo et al., 2016).

The major known GHIs are PEPFAR, GFTAM, MAP, the Global Alliance for Vaccines and Immunisation, the United States President's Malaria Initiative, the Roll Back Malaria partnership, Stop TB Partnership, and the Global Leprosy Programme (Mwisongo et al., 2016). Since the emergence of the HIV pandemic, the first three GHIs are the largest GHIs accounting for two-thirds of the external funding resourced for HIV/AIDS (Hanefeld, 2010).

The GHIs covered in this chapter are mainly those which have been financing HIV/AIDS programs in SSA countries.

Impact of Global Health Initiatives on Health Systems of SSA Countries

Implementation of the GHIs, particularly the GFTAM, the MAP, and the PEPFAR have yielded great social and economic returns. Between 2000 and 2015, there was a reduction of 35% and 70% for new HIV infections among adults and children, respectively. Similarly, in 2016, over 18.2 million people living with HIV/AIDS were on treatment, a 95% increase from less than 1 million in 2000 (Biesma, Brugha, Harmer, Walsh, Spicer, & Walt, 2009; Joint United Nations Programme on HIV/AIDS, 2016).

While these achievements have been encouraging, examining the impact of GHIs through a health system lens reveals more complex and at times grave unintended effects of the initiatives. In this chapter, we use the WHO's health system framework to describe both the positive and negative effects of GHIs on SSA countries' health systems (World Health Organization, 2007).

Positive and Negative Effects of GHIs

(i) Health workforce

GHIs have supported several health workforce development initiatives in SSA. Hundreds of thousands of health workers were trained and their skills in the management of diseases improved (Craveiro & Dussault, 2016). Further to this, GHIs have contributed to the retention of health workers. In Kenya, GHIs covered salaries of additional 2,000 health workers until the government became capable of bearing the cost and running the program. Similarly, GHIs provided incentives for health workers to work in remote areas (Yu, Souteyrand, Banda, Kaufman, & Perriëns, 2008) and they have reduced external brain drain of health workers as they created more jobs for health workers to work in their country (Cohn et al., 2011).

The other and more promising contribution of GHIs has been task-shifting initiatives where non-health professionals were trained to take roles and assist health workers. GHIs have supported the development of policies and guidelines on task-shifting and one study reported that out of seventy-eight low- and middle-income countries, twenty-eight had the policy in place in the earlier stages of the AIDS pandemic (Yu et al., 2008).

The improved access to anti-retroviral treatment (ART) is also reported to have lessened the effect of the pandemic on health workers, where HIV-positive health workers were able to receive treatment sufficient to be able to return to work. Malawi is an example, where 250 HIV-positive health workers received ART and rejoined the health workforce in the fight against the pandemic (Yu et al., 2008), improving this nation's human resource for health.

While GHIs have significantly contributed to building the capacity of health workers through training, mentorship, and supportive supervisions, their focus has been on short-term gains. As a result, they have insufficiently addressed the health workforce shortage and retention in many SSA countries (Chima & Homedes, 2015). This has resulted in several negative effects. One of the commonly reported effects of such an approach is an internal brain drain of qualified health personnel. Reports from Rwanda, for instance, indicated that medical doctors working in non-governmental organizations (NGOs) were receiving six times the salaries of their public-sector counterparts. This inequity in renumeration has motivated many in the human health workforce, including doctors and nurses, to leave their routine health service delivery roles and join AIDS care, disproportionately affecting the human resource for health needed to address the myriad issues in the health systems (Yu et al., 2008). For example, in Kenya and Malawi, GHIs' support for health workforce development to work in HIV/AIDS programs created a vacuum of staff in the public sector (Hanefeld, 2010). In countries such as Nigeria, maldistribution of health workers was created as a result of the influence of GHIs forcing the government to redistribute health workers from facilities not targeted by the program to those identified by GHIs to help the projects succeed (Chima & Homedes, 2015).

Similarly, in several African countries including Uganda, Tanzania, Zambia, Rwanda, and South Africa, a significant number of qualified health workers were reported to have migrated from the public sector to better paying HIV/AIDS-related jobs at different international NGOs and multilateral and UN agencies (Yu et al., 2008; Hanefeld, 2010; Mwisongo et al, 2016; Lohman et al., 2017). In a 2016 study, half of the medical graduates from Uganda's Mbarara University joined NGOs working on HIV/AIDS. Similarly, in Zambia, nine out of fifteen interviewees from GHIs who participated in a study about the impact of GHIs on a health system were recent recruits from the public sector (Hanefeld, 2010).

The migration of health workers from public facilities to NGOs affected more than the distribution of health workforce and has led to dissatisfaction by health workers left behind in public facilities due to high differences in both salaries and other opportunities such as training and *per diem* benefits. The effect of these on regular public health system duties led to forcing district health offices to make significant adjustments, including spending additional time and resources to fill vacant positions (Eunice et al., 2017; Lohman et al., 2017).

The scale-up of HIV services both in terms of scope of service and number of facilities offering the services has further burdened the workload of an already constrained health workforce. In Angola, for instance, collecting additional data and indicators have added more work to the daily assignments of health workers (Craveiro & Dussault, 2016). In Ethiopia, HIV/AIDS programs had reportedly imposed excessive workload on public sector health workers until the government decided to make some adjustments to their entitlements (Yu et al., 2008).

In addition to all this, some studies have revealed that the different training offered by GHIs have created a training workload demanding the trainees to be absent from their job and creating tensions with those who didn't get the opportunity to train. Some of the training was also not evaluated for its impact (Atun, Pothapregada, Kwansah, Degbotse, & Lazarus, 2011; Chima & Homedes, 2015; Craveiro & Dussault, 2016).

As some studies hinted, the above problems have resulted in distorting the health workforce market and caused fragmentation and instability of the health systems in the affected countries (Mwisongo et al., 2016; Lohman et al., 2017).

(ii) Leadership and governance

GHIs have brought important benefits to health system governance of beneficiary countries. In crude terms, GHIs programs, particularly GFTAM, were reported to be in alignment with health policy, strategies, and national priorities of several fund-recipient countries (Yu et al., 2008; Lohman et al., 2017). This is particularly true in the case of HIV/AIDS, tuberculosis, and malaria programs as these diseases were the focus of many partnerships established between GHIs and SSA countries. The alignment and integration of GHIs programs into national health plans was more pronounced in countries with strong government leadership (Yu et al., 2008; Atun et al., 2011). As part of this process, some GHIs stimulated the formulation of national health strategies, leading to strengthened capacity of government leadership teams. PEPFAR, for instance, has supported capacity building of health leaders at the sub-national level in Tanzania to mitigate weaknesses in health governance (Craveiro & Dussault, 2016; Mwisongo et al., 2016).

GHIs, particularly the GFTAM, has further improved the involvement of non-state actors such as non-governmental organizations, civil society, and faith-based organizations in national decision-making and coordinated responses to HIV/AIDS. The creation of the Country Coordinating Mechanism (CCM) in SSA countries, which brought all actors to one table, played a pivotal role in giving voice to non-state actors and previously neglected community members such as drug users, men who have sex with men, and sex workers (Yu et al., 2008; Chima & Homedes, 2015).

Despite the above positive contributions, GHIs have had significant counterproductive effects on the leadership and governance of targeted countries' health systems. The first and commonly reported challenge has been the coordination of stakeholders. The proliferation of stakeholders including donors and implementing partners with often varying interests, particularly in the global response to HIV/AIDS, made it difficult for countries to coordinate them (Hanefeld, 2010; Mwisongo et al., 2016). The situation, however, varies from country to country and it has been observed to be influenced by the extent to which a country is dependent on a donor or the GHI, and the strength of a country's leadership. In Angola, for example, GHIs have integrated well into the country's health system as the country was less dependent on external aid, which helped it to take the upper hand in leading the response. Variations between implementation of different GHIs are reported. The GFTAM, for example, has been perceived as more responsive to countries' needs, and has been more participatory in the design of its programs compared to PEPFAR. However, competition among the different partners was reported which affected harmonization of the different programs (Hanefeld, 2010; Craveiro & Dussault, 2016). In other countries such as Nigeria, the lack of proper stewardship from the Ministry of Health was reported to have left GHIs to decide on the most appropriate direction they wished to take independently (Chima & Homedes, 2015).

Countries' weak political leadership and dependency on GHIs have negatively impacted their broader national strategies and policies. GHIs were observed to set their priorities at their headquarters and define fund-recipient countries' health systems based on predetermined objectives. One of such cases was observed in Zambia where the national HIV/AIDS treatment targets and priorities were set based on GHIs' targets and priorities (Hanefeld, 2010).

The other challenge has been the duplication of structures. Different GHIs instituted their structures and coordinating mechanisms, implemented different planning cycles, and designed reporting timetables to suit their own interests. The additional structures created by GHIs were reported to be counterproductive, leading to inefficiencies. The CCM which has been active in almost all beneficiary countries, for instance, was found to be unnecessary and a duplication of an already existing structure which could have been used and further strengthened by the GFTAM and other GHIs (Atun et al., 2011). In several SSA countries such as Tanzania and Zambia, a joint donor–government health coordination mechanism called the Sector-wide Approach was established and is still active. However, it was reported that no GHI utilized this structure at least until 2016, as they preferred to establish their own structures and committees (Mwisongo et al., 2016).

(iii) Financing

GHIs have introduced innovative financing mechanisms and contributed to reducing treatment costs (Palen et al., 2012). Co-financing and fund matching strategies have encouraged governments to allocate additional resources to support HIV/AIDS and other health services. While the increase in domestic financing through such initiatives has been reported to be modest, there are countries where this has seen a steady and encouraging move over the GHI years. In Nigeria the Government's co-financing for HIV/AIDS increased from 7% in 2008 to 50% in 2012 (Atun et al., 2011; Chima & Homedes, 2015). Technical efficiencies such as improved supply chain systems and standardization of clinical monitoring mechanisms have further brought cost savings to GHIs. Such improved processes reduced the annual per-patient ART cost to PEPFAR by 70% from $1,100 in its early phase to $335 by 2012 (Palen et al., 2012).

On the other hand, it has been reported that the GHIs have weakened financial systems of fund-recipient countries. Given the limited absorptive capacity of SSA countries and GHIs' inflexible requirements on fund utilization, most of the funding has been channeled through international NGOs with very limited resources going directly to governments. This process has favored the application of GHIs' financial systems over countries' financial systems resulting in continued weaknesses in the system (Mwisongo et al., 2016; Lohman et al., 2017). While there are reports that some GHIs have made efforts to improve the financial management system of SSA countries, this movement remained limited at the national level without any cascade to sub-national levels (Mwisongo et al., 2016).

Despite GHIs' significant country budget allocations for HIV, which was estimated at 80% or more of a country's entire health sector budget, funding to non-HIV programs has been very limited (Craveiro & Dussault, 2016; Lohman et al., 2017). This has led to changes in priorities and neglect of other health programs. As mentioned earlier, co-financing initiatives and some health system strengthening funds have tried to address the challenge, but the problems remain largely unresolved (Atun et al., 2011).

The other negative effect of GHIs is a dependency on foreign aid. It has been consistently reported that the programs that GHIs introduced in SSA countries became a race for short-term gain without due consideration to the long-term financial sustainability of the programs. The programs, particularly HIV/AIDS treatment, are expensive for SSA countries to carry out by themselves in the absence of donor funding (Hanefeld, 2010; Chima & Homedes, 2015; Mwisongo et al., 2016).

(iv) Service delivery

One of the most significant contributions of GHIs is an enormous increase in access to services and treatment and care of HIV/AIDS and other priority diseases (Cohn et al., 2011). The Joint United Nations Programme on HIV/AIDS 2019 report showed that 23.3 million of the 37.9 million people living with HIV globally were on treatment at the end of 2018, a three-fold increase from 2010 (Joint United Nations Programme on HIV/AIDS, 2016). Services have rapidly expanded, and the quality and standard of care significantly improved over the years since the emergence of the HIV pandemic. Similarly, the number of providers, both government and non-government institutions, has significantly increased, enabling diversification of providers and expansion of services (Chima & Homedes, 2015; Mwisongo et al., 2016).

The rapid scaling up of care and treatment services has brought impressive achievements. The incidence and prevalence of priority diseases, particularly HIV, tuberculosis, and malaria have significantly reduced. At a population level mortality from HIV has reduced resulting in a notable increase to life expectancy in several SSA counties. Best care and treatment practices from HIV services have also positively impacted other primary healthcare services including child vaccinations, family planning and health promotion activities (Yu et al., 2008; Cohn et al., 2011; Cohen, Li, Giese, & Mancuso, 2013; Chima & Homedes, 2015).

The achievements are, however, shadowed by some negative effects. GHI supported programs including HIV have hampered non-HIV programs including maternal and child health services (Chima & Homedes, 2015). Two reasons are usually mentioned for this. The first is the lack of adequate funding to support these programs and the second is a shift in attention and prioritization to HIV programs from all other health services (Atun et al., 2011). In some SSA countries, this has caused a shortage of service providers, resulting in a reduction and unavailability of antenatal care and reproductive health services (Yu et al., 2008), which has raised claims that HIV programs might have widened inequity gaps (Mwisongo et al., 2016).

The other major concern is sustainability of HIV services. While GHIs have enabled successful scaling up of HIV, tuberculosis, and malaria services, the programs are reported still to be dependent on donor funding and their continuation in the absence of external funding would be difficult for many SSA countries, although few economically better-off countries like South Africa might be able to manage the challenge (Hanefeld, 2010; Mwisongo et al., 2016).

(v) Medicines and technologies (supply chain)

The procurement and distribution of drugs and medical equipment for HIV/AIDS and other diseases form a big part of GHIs' work. GHIs have increased the availability of medicines through direct purchase of drugs, strengthening supply management systems, and supporting strategies to reduce stockouts (Mwisongo et al., 2016). Some of the system strengthening tools and frameworks including drug development, pricing, distribution, and use were replicated to supply chain of other diseases. In South Africa, for instance, new tools which were developed to decentralize ART drugs were applied to medicines of other chronic diseases such as mental illness (Embrey, Hoos, & Quick, 2009).

For the sake of efficient and real-time availability of the supplies, GHIs implemented an autonomous supply chain management system often managed by foreign experts and logistic companies and this approach has compromised the growth of country-owned institutions which are created to serve the same purpose (Chima & Homedes, 2015). While some studies have indicated that GHIs procurement systems have gradually been integrated into beneficiary countries' procurement systems, this effort has not extended far enough, with bulk procurements still made through parallel systems putting the sustainability of the approach at stake (Chima & Homedes, 2015; Mwisongo et al., 2016). Ethiopia is a good example where the Ministry of Health outsourced the procurement of drugs and medical supplies from international companies through the United Nations Children's Fund (Yu et al., 2008).

(vi) Information system

Digitization of the health information system of several SSA countries, particularly in HIV/AIDS services, is one of GHIs' legacies. Different health information technology elements have been implemented to improve real-time data collection, reporting, and utilization. Electronic ART patient tracking is one of such initiatives. The support has further ignited a culture of proper record keeping and data gathering, and improved availability of good quality of data using population surveys (Yu et al., 2008; Chima & Homedes, 2015; Mwisongo et al., 2016).

However, similar to the above-mentioned challenges, GHIs implemented a parallel structure of data gathering and reporting across all tiers of a health system from district to national levels (Yu et al., 2008; Hanefeld, 2010; Craveiro & Dussault, 2016). The main reason for such structures has been the difference between GHIs partners and fund-recipient countries in the frequency and timeliness of reporting and the number and type of indicators required. In some instances, there has been an issue of trust of government reports by donors and implementing partners, and as a result, partners were observed to be reluctant even when they were asked to integrate their information systems with countries data collection and reporting systems (Atun et al., 2011; Craveiro & Dussault, 2016). The existence of parallel information systems is generally reported to have paralyzed countries' information systems and burdened their staff as they try to report on both government and partner reports. As a result, the use of data for planning and decision-making remains weak in many SSA countries (Hanefeld, 2010; Atun et al., 2011; Craveiro & Dussault, 2016' Mwisongo et al., 2016).

Table 18.1 offers a summary table of our findings.

Table 18.1 Summary of positive and negative effects of GHIs on health systems of SSA countries

Ser No	Health System Building Block	GHIs' Effects	
		Positive Effects	**Negative Effects**
1	Health Workforce	• Health workers' disease management knowledge and skills improved • Retention of health workers through salaries and incentives improved • Creation of more jobs reduced external brain drain • Task-shifting policies improved access to services and reduced burden on health workers	• Internal brain drain from government to non-state actors created a vacuum in the public sector • Work burden and dissatisfaction among constrained health workers increased • Maldistribution of health workers • Training workload resulting in more absenteeism from work • Distortion of the health workforce market

(continued)

Table 18.1 Continued

Ser No	Health System Building Block	GHIs' Effects: Positive Effects	GHIs' Effects: Negative Effects
2	Leadership and Governance	• General alignment of GHIs to countries' priorities • Stimulated formulation of national policies and strategies • Participation of non-state actors improved	• Duplication of efforts and weak coordination among actors • Duplication of GHIs' structures to governments' structures • GHIs influence in setting priorities and targets
3	Financing	• Introduction of innovative financing mechanisms brought a modest increase in domestic financing • Cost savings as a result of technical efficiencies	• GHIs financial procedures weakened countries' financial systems • Limited non-HIV funding created neglect of other health services • Dependency on foreign aid
4	Service Delivery	• Improved access to and quality of services of priority diseases • Rapid scaling up of HIV/AIDS, tuberculosis, and malaria services • Decreased morbidity and mortality and increased life expectancy	• Crowding out of non-HIV services • Donor dependency of service approach and scale-up
5	Medicines and Technologies	• Increase in availability of drugs and medical equipment for priority diseases • Modest improvements in countries' supply chain management capacity	• GHIs' autonomous supply chain management systems weakened countries' supply chain systems
6	Information System	• Digitization of countries' health information systems improved real-time collection and reporting of information • Improved record-keeping and data gathering	• GHIs' parallel data collection and reporting systems weakened and burdened countries information systems

Lesson Learned from the Implementation of GHIs in SSA

(vi) Short-term results at the expense of long-term health system effects

The unprecedented challenges brought by HIV/AIDS pandemic and other diseases demanded GHIs to implement flagship programs that are disease-specific, vertically oriented, and results-focused. While this approach has registered impressive achievements in reducing disease incidence and prevalence as well as reducing morbidities and mortality (Yu et al., 2008; Cohn et al., 2011; Cohen et al., 2013; Chima & Homedes, 2015), it has produced significant consequences to health systems of fund recipient countries including dependency on aid, unsustainable intervention models, and disrupted health workforce market (Hanefeld, 2010; Chima & Homedes, 2015; Mwisongo et al., 2016; Lohman et al., 2017). GHI donors and implementing partners have gradually realized the negative effects of the programs and thus started providing some support for building the capacity of health systems. However, this support has been limited in both scope and size of funding and has come late toward the phasing-out stage of the programs. More health systems strengthening support could have been provided in the very early stage of the flagship programs so that disease-specific achievements can be realized in parallel to building health systems. As such, the latter could also have had a synergetic effect to GHIs' primary objectives.

(vii) The interdependence of health system elements was not appreciated and leveraged

The unintended effects of GHIs outlined earlier show that GHIs did not leverage the interdependence and complex nature of health system elements as they focused on achieving disease-specific targets. The positive contribution of an intervention or an input in one health system element, has possibly had one or more positive or negative effects as an output in another health system element. A high level of complexity of health system elements was ignored or was not anticipated or understood. Consequently, specific remedies to tackle the unintended effects of each intervention have not been timely implemented.

(viii) Country leadership's role in health system strengthening

The implementation of GHIs showed that alignment and integration of GHI programs with countries' strategies and plans were comparatively more pronounced in countries who exercised strong leadership or those who were economically better-off and less dependent on foreign aid. While the purpose of GHI partnership was to design and implement programs that match recipient countries' priorities and plans, this was not the case in some of the major GHIs. In countries with weak leadership, such as Nigeria and Zambia, GHI partners had an upper hand and they influenced priorities according to their own interests, program philosophy, and targets, which had its negative ramifications on these nations' health systems.

(ix) Chronic HIV and the double burden of diseases

GHIs have rapidly expanded the scaling up of ART and as a result, HIV/AIDS has gradually become a chronic disease. The prevalence of comorbidities associated with HIV/AIDS is also increasing. For instance, one study in South Africa reported that close to 30% of older adults with HIV had two or more chronic conditions (Negin et al., 2012). This is further aggravated by the increasing trend in non-communicable diseases. Of the 56 million deaths that occurred globally in 2012, 68% were reported to be due to non-communicable diseases, mainly cardiovascular disease, cancers, diabetes, and chronic lung diseases (World Health Organization, 2014). The burden of non-communicable diseases along with chronic HIV/AIDS is a more complex problem that requires a comprehensive understanding of how health systems could adequately and sustainability respond to the challenge.

Conclusion

In the last three decades, GHIs have transformed access to and quality of care and treatment for HIV/AIDS and other high-priority diseases. However, despite the benefits and the good intentions they bring, during this period, they have missed the opportunity to transform the health system of SSA countries to sustain and support themselves. These initiatives have generated several unintended effects on the health system of these countries due to the vertical, short-term, and disease-specific orientation of the programs. The lessons learnt from these programs need to be considered in the design and implementation of similar initiatives in the future and an opportunity exists to use the lessons in the current response to chronic HIV/AIDS and the double burden of diseases in SSA countries.

References

Atun, R., Pothapregada, S. K., Kwansah, J., Degbotse, D., & Lazarus, J. V. (2011). Critical interactions between the Global Fund-supported HIV programmes and the health system in Ghana. *Journal of Acquired Immune Deficiency Syndrome, 57,* Suppl 2, S72–76.

Biesma, R., Brugha, R., Harmer, A., Walsh, A., Spicer, N., & Walt, G. (2009). The effects of global health initiatives on country health systems: A review of the evidence from HIV/AIDS control. *Health Policy and Planning, 24,* 239–252.

Chima, C. C., & Homedes, N. (2015). Impact of global health governance on country health systems: The case of HIV initiatives in Nigeria. *Journal of Global Health, 5*(1), 1–13.

Cohen, R.L., Li, Y., Giese, R., & Mancuso, J.D. (2013). An evaluation of the President's Emergency Plan for AIDS Relief effect on health systems strengthening in sub-Saharan Africa. *Journal of Acquired Immune Deficiency Syndrome, 62*(4), 471–479.

Cohn, J., Russell, A., Baker, B., Kayongo, A., Wanjiku, E., & Davis, P. (2011). Using global health initiatives to strengthen health systems: A civil society perspective. *Global Public Health, 6*(7), 687–702.

Craveiro, I., & Dussault, D. (2016). The impact of global health initiatives on the health system in Angola. *Global Public Health, 11*(4), 475–495.

Embrey, M., Hoos, D., & Quick, J. (2009). How AIDS funding strengthens health systems: Progress in pharmaceutical management. *Journal of Acquired Immune Deficiency Syndrome, 52*(Suppl 1), S34–37.

Eunice, O., Mwanri, L., & Ward, P. (2017). Is task-shifting a solution to the health workers' shortage in northern Ghana? *PloS One, 12,* 1–22(3).

Hanefeld, J. (2010). The impact of Global Health Initiatives at the national and sub-national level—A policy analysis of their role in the implementation processes of antiretroviral treatment (ART) roll-out in Zambia and South Africa. *AIDS Care, 22*(Suppl 1), 93–102.

Joint United Nations Programme on HIV/AIDS. (2016). *AIDS by numbers.* Geneva: UNAIDS.

Joint United Nations Programme on HIV/AIDS. (2019). *Global AIDS update 2019.* Geneva: UNAIDS.

Lohman, N., Hagopian, A., Luboga, S. A., Stover, B., Lim, T. W., Makumbi, F., Kiwanuka, N., Lubega, F., Ndizihiwe, A., Mukooyo, E., Barnhart, S., & Pfeiffer, J. (2017). District health officer perceptions of PEPFAR's influence on the health system in Uganda, 2005–2011. *International Journal of Health Policy Management, 6*(2), 83–95.

Mwisongo, A., Soumare, A. N., & Nabyonga-Orem, J. (2016). An analytical perspective of global health initiatives in Tanzania and Zambia. *BMC Health Service Research, 16*, Suppl 4, 256–264.

Negin, J., Martiniuk, A., Cumming, R. G., Naidoo, N., Phaswana-Mafuya, N., Madurai, L., Williams, S., & Kowal, P. (2012). Prevalence of HIV and chronic comorbidities among older adults. *AIDS, 26*(1), 55–63.

Palen, J., El-sadr, W., Phoya, A., Imtiaz, R., Einterz, R., Quain, E., Blandford, J., Bouey, P., & Lion, A. (2012). PEPFAR, health system strengthening, and promoting sustainability and country ownership. *Journal of Acquired Immune Deficiency Syndrome, 60*, Suppl 3, S113–119.

World Health Organization Maximizing Positive Synergies Collaborative Group. (2009). An assessment of interactions between global health initiatives and country health systems. *The Lancet, 373*(9681), 2137–2169.

World Health Organization. (2007). *Everybody's business—strengthening health systems to improve health outcomes: WHO's framework for action.* In. Geneva: World Health Organization.

World Health Organization. (2014). *Global status report on noncommunicable diseases 2014.* Geneva: World Health Organization.

Yu, D., Souteyrand, Y., Banda, M.A, Kaufman, J., & Perriëns, J. (2008). Investment in HIV/AIDS programmes: Does it help strengthen health systems in developing countries? *Global Health,4,* 1–10.

19

Systems Thinking for Pastoral Health

Challenges and Prospects in Ethiopia

Mirgissa Kaba

Introduction

Ethiopia is the second most populous country in Africa. With over eighty cultural groups, the country is known to have some of the region's poorest development indicators. The country has different ecological characteristics, with the largest land mass being lowland, marked by an arid and semi-arid geographic profile, bordering with Somalia in the east, Kenya in the south, and Sudan and South Sudan in the south-west. Most Ethiopian pastoralists live in Somali, Afar, Oromia, and Southern Region states, with others living in Gambella and Benishangul-Gumuz regions. Although more recent figures are lacking, estimates show that two-thirds of the land mass of Ethiopia and 10–12 million people in Ethiopia are considered pastoral (Desta, 2006).

Early definitions conceptualize pastoralism as a production system with prominence of livestock as means of livelihood. Focusing on the Nuer, Evans-Pritchard indicated that cattle are "dearest possessions and sources of life necessities" (1940: 10) although the tribe may practice horticulture as well. Criticisms of this definition, however, were that it excludes pastoral ways of life that are not dependent on livestock rearing but which otherwise fully adhere to pastoral culture in arid and semi-arid settings. Currently, pastoralism is widely regarded as a livelihood whereby sociocultural norms, beliefs, and values, and traditional knowledge revolve around livestock. Pastoralists' health is thus linked to their livelihood and their adaptive capacity to cope with prevailing contexts (Davies, Niamir-Fuller, Kerven, & Bauer, 2010).

Systems thinking and its associated approaches are widely recognized as a means to address complex problems in order to maximize desired outcomes. Specifically, systems approaches are about proactive adaptations to contexts, bridging boundaries and forging opportunities to operate together against common problem of interest. Launched in 2004/2005, Ethiopia's flagship community Health Extension Program (HEP) aimed to improve access to health services for communities including pastorals. As part of HEP, women who had completed high school at grade 10 were trained as health extension workers (HEWs) to provide promoted, preventive, and selected curative services, with special attention to catering to women and children in rural areas. Today, there are more than 42,000 HEWs deployed throughout the country (Banteyerga, 2018).

Mirgissa Kaba, *Systems Thinking for Pastoral Health* In: *Systems Thinking for Global Health.* Edited by: Fiona Larkan, Frédérique Vallières, Hasheem Mannan, and Naonori Kodate, Oxford University Press.
DOI: 10.1093/oso/9780198799498.003.0019

In addition to the training of HEWs, the HEP also resulted in other health system strengthening investments, including the building of health facilities, improving health sector governance, training providers at different levels, and improving logistics and information management. Consequently, the HEP is credited with propelling the country toward having met most of the Millennium Development Goals (MDGs) commitments. Correspondingly, the country has recorded a 67% reduction in under-five mortality, a 71% decline in maternal mortality ratio, a 90% decline in new HIV infections, a decrease in malaria-related deaths by 73%, and a more than 50% decline in mortality due to tuberculosis (Federal Ministry of Health and United Nations, 2014). Nonetheless, inequities in health services provision between rural and urban, and between agrarian and pastoral settings prevail. Specifically, health service delivery within pastoral settings of Ethiopia has suffered from an inadequate number of trained health providers, limited health infrastructure, and a shortage of financing, equipment, and supplies (Federal Ministry of Health and United Nations, 2014).

Health and Pastoral Life

Defending the lack of service provision to pastoral communities, some groups have argued that pastoral livelihoods are obsolete, non-productive, and full of risks, with no or limited contribution to the national economy. For these groups, settlement, whereby pastoral communal land could be transformed into commercial farms, is considered as a solution (Rettberg, 2010). Conversely, others argue that pastoral livelihoods are the best coping and survival strategy to those who live in a rather harsh climate (Devereux, 2010), as pastoralist production systems maximize what the climate offers and promote resource sharing at household and clan level (Behnke & Kerven, 2013). Moreover, complex health and livelihood risk scenarios are continuously evaluated within pastoralist communities such that decisions are not only about preserving human life but also about the lives of animals, while considering the importance of preserving the physical environment. Furthermore, evidence supports that in addition to meeting the needs of their own household, pastoral economies further supply food from animal byproducts (i.e., meat and milk) to highlanders, thus contributing to the country's economy (Devereux, 2010).

The health implications of pastoral living, however, are less recognized. Given their close interaction with harsh environments and the livestock that serve as the source of their livelihood, pastoralists are at an increased risk of zoonotic disease transmission. Indeed, zoonotic diseases such as brucellosis and bovine tuberculosis are common health problems in pastoral setting due to raw milk consumption and animal–human connection in pastoral settings (Gumi et al., 2012). The harsh and inconsistent physical environments also serve as a breeding grounds for disease-causing pathogens. Consequently, improving prevention, early detection, preparedness, and routine healthcare in settings where animals and humans are in constant contact remains a major area of attention.

A shortage of supplies and limited number and mix of skilled human resources for health are typical features in pastoral settings with poor infrastructure. Despite weak health service distribution, supplies, human resources, and infrastructure, and their resultant poor health indicators being well recognized by the Federal Ministry of Health however, there have as yet been no viable measures taken to improve pastoral health service delivery commensurate to pastoral ways of life (Federal Ministry of Health and United Nations, 2014). Accordingly, a health service delivery package that pays attention to the context of pastoral settings should be designed, introduced, and institutionalized to meet service needs of pastoral communities (Wild et al., 2020).

Systems Thinking and Pastoral Life

Recognizing that pastoral life is characterized by an inextricable relationship between humans, animals, and the environment is key to improving health service delivery in pastoral communities. Akin to systems thinking, pastoral understanding of health and prevention measures therefore rests on an understanding of pastoral health across the human, animal, and climate spectrum. Although, on the surface, the words system and pastoralism may appear to be at odds with each other, on the contrary, and given the dynamic nature and complexity of pastoral life, consideration of systems thinking as an analytical framework could greatly contribute to a better understanding of the pastoral way of life. Moreover, systems thinking for pastoral development provides opportunities to engage pastoral communities as stakeholders in the design and redesign of interventions that speak to the local context (Zinsstag et al., 2011). Similarly, the "One Health" principle offers a useful framework to understand the inextricable linkage of human, livestock, wildlife, and the physical environment (Zinsstag et al., 2011). The One Health is a strategy that calls for collaboration between disciplines of different perspectives and approaches, and development sectors in addressing prevailing health problems. The strategy recognizes that humans, animals, and the environmental health problems cannot be understood and addressed in isolation, particularly in pastoral settings offering prominence to systems approach.

Lack of Systems Thinking in Pastoral Health Service Provision

Ethiopian national health plans, including the twenty-year Health Sector Development Program (HSDP) and the subsequent Health Sector Transformation Plan (HSTP), all failed to describe a strategy or package of health interventions that take into account the unique needs of pastoral life. This is likely to have been as a result of the government's lack of engagement with pastoral communities in the design and delivery of essential health programs, including the HEP. Consequently, the design of hospitals and health center infrastructure, maternal and child health education, and public health communication programs are all informed by the same package of intervention and approaches, regardless of whether implementation takes place in an agrarian or urban setting. Similarly, other health packages such as hygiene and environmental sanitation, family health, disease prevention and control, and health education and communication—all developed for other parts of country—continue to be implemented within pastoral settings.

As pastoral communities were not engaged in the design and delivery of the HEP, recruitment of HEWs consequently adopted the same criteria as were used for agrarian settings (Teklehaimanot, Tolera, Michael, & Teklehaimanot, 2019). Specifically, it turned out that the requirement of HEWs being females who completed education up to grade 10 was not feasible at the beginning, and services are instead entrusted to males who completed grade 8, undermining acceptability of service, particularly for maternal and child health.

Second, the standardization of the design of hospital, health centers, and community health post buildings across the country means that these designs are largely inappropriate for arid and semi-arid contexts. Materials and equipment used in the construction of health facilities, for example, are not suited to pastoral contexts. Similarly, hospital beds, mattresses, sheets, and blankets are difficult to use in arid and semi-arid settings. Accordingly, calls for more "appropriate" beds made from cement and under shaded areas where patients can lie comfortably instead of in a sweltering room were observed by the author in the Afdher zone of Somali region. Provision of supplies, storage of supplies, and timing of service provision for pastoral regions in Ethiopia also present a problem. Likewise, availability of electricity and cold chains for vaccines remain critical challenges for service delivery.

Third, current evidence suggests limited health service utilization among pastoral communities, particularly maternal health services (Federal Ministry of Health and United Nations, 2014). Analysis of evidence from the Ethiopian Demographic and Health Survey of 2019 suggests that women in regions characterized as pastoral (Afar and Somali) are reluctant to use basic maternal health services, including attending at least four antenatal care (ANC) visits during pregnancy, and there are poor rates of institutional delivery, and low uptake of postnatal care (PNC) services within two days after birth (ICF, 2019) (Figure 19.1).

Another study also suggests weak service uptake for emergency obstetric and neonatal care among pastoral communities, even where such services have been

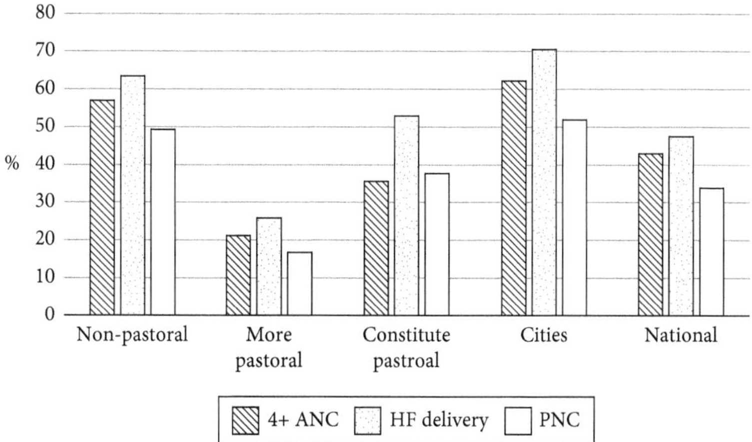

Figure 19.1 Key indicators of women who received maternal health services during pregnancy, delivery and postnatal

introduced. In addition, poor iron and folic acid intake during pregnancy has been documented in pastoral settings (Gebre, Debie, Berhane, & Redddy, 2017).

Finally, health messaging for pastoral communities fails to take cultural, social, economic, and physical environmental contexts into consideration. Studies on HIV among pastoral communities indicated that health messages were generic developed for agrarians and urban settings. A study from the Borana pastoral community reveals that the generic HIV prevention message of Abstinence, Be faithful, and Condom (ABC) did not take the communities sexual life into consideration. Among the Borana community, abstinence until marriage is observed, while faithfulness was difficult to ensure after marriage, at least when the study was carried out between 2008 and 2010 (Kaba, 2013).

Opportunities to Improve Pastoral Health

More recent strategic approaches by the Health Systems Directorate of the Ministry of Health and Pastoral Community Development Program suggest a recognition of the health challenges existing within pastoral communities and the need to adopt more systems-thinking approaches to address these challenges (Esayas, Gebremeskel, Desta, & Kassa, 2019). For example, the Food and Agriculture Organization of the United Nations (FAO) in Ethiopia has collaborated with the Ministries in charge of Agriculture, Health and Environment to start health programs to combat zoonotic diseases and address their impact on the human–animal ecosystem. Likewise, the initiative and Memorandum of Understanding signed between the health, agriculture, and environmental sectors called for policies and investments that take into account the dynamics of pastoral society and changing climates, thereby facilitating pastoral development (Little, Behnke, McPeak, & Gebru, 2010). Likewise, One Health research initiatives launched by various institutions and universities including the FAO, International Livestock Research Institute, Ohio State University, and the University of Liverpool, in collaboration with local universities and the Ministry of Health, are useful initiatives in recognition of the need for alignment to improve pastoral health. Such initiatives are outcomes from growing understanding of the intricate interactions between human and animal health, as well as the physical environment, and how this understanding could contribute to preventing, detecting, and responding to conventional and emerging health problems.

Key Recommendations and Conclusion

- **Communities as a resource for healthcare:** Pastoral communities have established wisdom, skills, and resources to respond to animal and human health problems in harsh physical environments. Pastoral resources are under-explored, underdeveloped, and insufficiently applied to improve the health system of pastoral communities, including their awareness about health.
- **Development of pastoral livelihood-informed healthcare package:** Pastoral livelihood is dynamic. Accordingly, pastoral health systems could operate well

when/if health packages accommodate animal health as well as mobility patterns of the community in response to changing climates. Such a service delivery structure needs to be informed by the climate informed livelihood structure of pastoral settings.

- **Stronger research and documentation:** Evidence on pastoral livelihood and health is quite limited. Despite the interface between animal, human, and climate, there is a dearth of evidence offering a holistic picture of pastoral health. Strengthening collaboration between stakeholders and improving in-country capacity for holistic interdisciplinary and multi-sectoral research that applies systems thinking or One Health approaches are critical.

Pastoralism is an important form of livelihood in arid and semi-arid lowlands of Ethiopia, characteristic of a signification portion of the Ethiopian population spread across a large land mass. Previous attempts to settle pastoralist have included the provision of basic services such as education, health, and water. However, the failure to recognize the holistic feature of pastoral health means that these initiatives have been met with little success, with a lack acceptable supplies and limited numbers and skill mix of human for health resources still common among pastoral communities. Implementation of health programs following the same national strategy and tools do not appear to benefit pastoral communities, who continue to demonstrate poorer key health indicators. Strengthening health systems within pastoral communities therefore calls for a tailored approach and greater understanding of pastoral ways of life, their mobility patterns, networks, and clan-based social structures, rather than impose fixed/static service delivery proven effective in agrarian settings.

References

Banteyerga, H. (2018). Ethiopia's health extension program: Improving health through community involvement. *MEDICC Review, 2011 Jul;13*(3), 46–9. doi: 10.1590/s1555-7960201100030001 1. PMID: 21778960

Behnke, R. H., & Kerven, C. (2013). Counting the costs: Replacing pastoralism with irrigated agriculture in the Awash Valley. In A. Catley, J. Lind, & I. Scoones (Eds.), *Pastoralism and development in Africa: Dynamic change at the margins* (pp. 57–70). Abingdon: Routledge.

Davies, J., Niamir-Fuller, M., Kerven, C., & Bauer, K. (2010). Extensive livestock production in transition: The future of sustainable pastoralism. In H. Steinfeld, H. A. Mooney, F., & Schneider, L. E. Neville (Eds.), *livestock in a changing landscape, Volume 1: Drivers, consequences, and responses* (pp. 285–308). Washington, DC: Island Press.

Desta, S. (2006). Pastoralism and development in Ethiopia. *Ethiopian Economic Association, 9*(3), 12–20.

Devereux, S. (2010). Better marginalised than incorporated? Pastoralist livelihoods in Somali Region, Ethiopia. *European Journal of Development Research, 22*, 678–695. doi:10.1057/ejdr.2010.29

Esayas, N, Gebremeskel, S., Desta, G., & Kassa, K. (2019). *Pastoral development in Ethiopia: Trends and the way forward.* Washington, DC: World Bank and IFAD.

Ethiopian Public Health Institute and ICF. (2019). *Ethiopia mini demographic and health survey 2019: Key indicators.* Rockville, MD: EPHI and ICF.

Evans-Pritchard, E. E. (1940). *The Nuer. A description of the modes of livelihood and political institutions of a Nilotic people*. Oxford: Clarendon Press.

Federal Ministry of Health and United Nations. (2014). *Accelerated action plan for reducing maternal mortality*. Addis Ababa: Federal Ministry of Health and United Nations.

Gebre A., Debie A., Berhane A., & Redddy P. S. (2017). Determinants of compliance to iron-folic acid supplementation among pregnant women in pastoral communities of Afar region: The cases of Mille and Assaita Districts, Afar, Ethiopia-2015. *Medico Res. Chronicles, 4*, 352–362.

Gumi, B., Schelling, E., Berg, S., Firdessa, R., Erenso, G., Mekonnen, W., ... Zinsstag, J. (2012). Zoonotic transmission of tuberculosis between pastoralists and their livestock in South-East Ethiopia. *Ecohealth, 9*(2), 139–149. doi:10.1007/s10393-012-0754-x

Kaba, M. (2013). Tapping local resources for HIV prevention among the Borana pastoral community. *Ethiopian Journal of Health Development, 27*(1), 33–39.

Little, P. D., Behnke, R., McPeak, J., & Gebru, G. (2010). Future scenarios for pastoral development in Ethiopia, 2010–2025: Report number 2 on pastoral economic growth and development policy assessment. Addis Ababa, Ethiopia.

Rettberg, S. (2010). Livelihoods within the Afar Region of Ethiopia. In C. Altare (Ed.), *Ethical sugar. Sugar cane and indigenous people* (pp. 7–12). Montpellier: SupAgro.

Teklehaimanot, H. D., Tolera, B., Michael, G., & Teklehaimanot, A. (2019). *Improving immunisation coverage in Ethiopia: A formative evaluation in pastoral communities, 3ie Formative Evaluation Report*. New Delhi: International Initiative for Impact Evaluation (3ie). Available at: https://doi.org/10.23846/TW10FE03

Wild, H., Mendonsa, E., Trautwein, M., Edwards, J., Jowell, A., Gebre, A., ... Barry, M. (2020). Health interventions among mobile pastoralists: a systematic review to guide health service design. *Tropical Health and International Health, 25*(11), 1332–1352.

Zinsstag, J., Schelling, E., Waltner-Toews, D., & Tanner, M. (2011). From "one medicine" to "one health" and systemic approaches to health and well-being. *Preventive Veterinary Medicine, 101*(3–4), 148–156. Retrieved from http://dx.doi.org/10.1016/j.prevetmed.2010.07.003.

20

Systems Thinking in the Implementation of the Framework Convention on Tobacco Control

Lessons from ASEAN

Tikki Pang and Gianna Gayle Herrera Amul

Introduction

The Framework Convention in Tobacco Control (FCTC) is the most widely embraced global health treaty and has recently gained status as a Sustainable Development Goal target. Tobacco is the leading risk factor in the rise of non-communicable diseases, with tobacco-related diseases causing 8.1 million deaths (14.5% of global deaths), and 213.4 million disability-adjusted life years (DALYs) (8.55% of global DALYs) in 2017 alone (Institute of Health Metrics and Evaluation, 2020). Systems thinking has been promoted to strengthen health systems, with the core argument that health systems are composed of dynamic, interrelated, and interacting nested building blocks (de Savigny & Adam, 2009) with people at the center of the system. Previous work on systems thinking for tobacco control has primarily focused on specific tobacco control sub-systems such as healthcare services through smoking cessation programs, and on governance of regulatory networks (National Cancer Institute 2007; Borland, Young, Coghill, & Zhang, 2010; Young, Borland, & Coghill, 2012; Battle-Fisher, 2015). Few studies, however, have addressed the dynamics of three critical building blocks of health systems for the future success of tobacco control: governance, financing, and information.

This chapter will thus examine how a more holistic, systems-thinking approach can improve governance, financing, and information as the most relevant health system building blocks to successful FCTC implementation. Using a case study approach, it emphasizes the relationships among the various actors and stakeholders involved in the implementation of the FCTC in South East Asia, particularly among member states of the Association of Southeast Asian Nations (ASEAN). It has a specific focus on how the interaction between intergovernmental organizations, philanthropic foundations, and non-governmental organizations (NGOs) involved in tobacco control, and unrelenting tobacco industry interference influence the state of FCTC implementation in the region.

Tikki Pang and Gianna Gayle Herrera Amul, *Systems Thinking in the Implementation of the Framework Convention on Tobacco Control* In: *Systems Thinking for Global Health.* Edited by: Fiona Larkan, Frédérique Vallières, Hasheem Mannan, and Naonori Kodate, Oxford University Press. © Oxford University Press 2023. DOI: 10.1093/oso/9780198799498.003.0020

Dynamics of Tobacco Control in ASEAN

The core issue for tobacco control in ASEAN is that the four growing economies of ASEAN—Indonesia, the Philippines, Thailand, and Vietnam—are considered among the top twenty markets for cigarettes globally (Euromonitor International, 2017). Given the varying stages of socio-economic development among member states of ASEAN, the progress of implementation of the FCTC in the region is similarly wide-ranging. All ASEAN member states (AMS) are party to the FCTC, except Indonesia. With Singapore's stringent tobacco control measures to Indonesia's deficit in tobacco control policies, there is not only a policy gap but also an implementation gap among AMS. Most of the AMS with developing economies and developing health systems have relatively weak tobacco control policies, not only in comparison with the strong tobacco control measures of Singapore but also in the wider context of the Asia Pacific, with Australia pioneering plain tobacco packaging measures globally.

Governance

Governance in tobacco control involves, among other functions, dealing with political and economic pressures from different sectors and interference from the tobacco industry brought about by policy proposals to reduce tobacco use. Moreover, leadership as a dimension of governance is vital not only in bringing key stakeholders to the table but also in strengthening the implementation of existing tobacco control measures.

The FCTC covers a range of governance functions that, when implemented at the national level, can contribute to the prevention and control of tobacco use and consumption, and in the long term, the protection and promotion of public health. For example, protecting public health policies from the commercial and vested interests of the tobacco industry (Article 5.3) and the adoption and implementation of smoke-free policies (Article 8) reinforce leadership. Additionally, the development, implementation, updating, and review of comprehensive multisectoral national tobacco control strategies through establishing, reinforcing and financing a national coordinating mechanism or focal points for tobacco control (Articles 5.1 and 5.2) sustain governance and financing.

At the global level, the World Health Organization (WHO) and the FCTC Secretariat provides policy guidance and direction in the implementation of the FCTC. WHO regional offices have their own regional action plans to implement the FCTC under the Tobacco Free Initiative, most of which are focused on building national capacities, developing legislation for tobacco control, and enabling regional cooperation (WHO Western Pacific Regional Office, 2015; WHO Southeast Asia Regional Office, 2017). On the other hand, the FCTC Secretariat serves as the enabling platform for monitoring FCTC implementation, coordination, and international cooperation.

From a systems point of view, much of the progress in tobacco control in the region was driven by civil society organizations (CSOs) and decisive political leaders confronting tenacious interference and opposition from the tobacco industry, both local and multinational. Attempts in introducing FCTC-compliant or WHO-recommended tobacco control policies by governments, both sub-national and national, are constantly being undermined by stealthy and powerful tobacco industry lobby groups. Most of the local tobacco industry lobby groups are supported by multinational tobacco companies who have acquired local tobacco companies and who support local tobacco growers in a number of AMS, except for Brunei and Singapore.

The Dynamics of Governance and Tobacco Industry Interference

It is within this dynamic that the legislation and strict implementation of FCTC Article 5.3 that seeks to protect public policy from tobacco control interference should thus be the primary policy goal for tobacco control advocacy to prevent further interference from tobacco companies. For those who have policies specific to implementing Article 5.3, weak versions have created problems in many AMS, with a high degree of tobacco industry interference during the policy-making process for Article 5.3 (Assunta & Dorotheo, 2016). This in turn opens up policy loopholes and leads to the watering down of subsequent tobacco control measures. The policy-making process is just the tip of the iceberg in this dynamic since even with a good policy, effective implementation without legal challenges brought about by tobacco companies is rare. Tobacco companies operating in AMS have commonly challenged governments in court about the legality of the tobacco taxes, and tobacco advertising, promotion, and sponsorship (TAPS) restrictions. There are cases when tobacco control policies are left not implemented because of the legal challenges that force governments to delay implementation until the legality of the policies are affirmed or verified in local and international courts.

Globally, the tobacco industry has a long history of challenging and interfering in the formulation and implementation of tobacco control policies, not only at the national level but also at the international level by exploiting specific provisions of trade and investment agreements among countries where they operate (Lee, Ling, & Glantz, 2012). With global trade and foreign direct investment, multinational tobacco companies found new markets in low- and middle-income countries (LMICs). Over the past decade or so, multinational tobacco companies have been acquiring local tobacco companies in LMICs.

The shift from high-income countries (where tobacco control is currently at their strongest) to LMICs (where tobacco control is at their weakest) is also reflected in the transition of multinational tobacco companies shifting their resources toward influencing and lobbying LMICs to oppose stronger tobacco control policies in the local and international arena. From a systems point of view, tobacco industry interference influences policy among AMS in three ways: (i) watering down of tobacco control policies in countries that are party to the FCTC; (ii) influencing FCTC Convention of Parties' (COP) delegations to oppose stronger FCTC guidelines; and (iii) influencing countries' delegations to prioritize trade over health at other intergovernmental platforms (see Figure 20.1).

The first kind of interference is local—a strategy which involves multinational tobacco companies co-opting tobacco farmers, agriculture, finance and trade ministries, and local tobacco companies to highlight their concerns in ongoing policy deliberations and most often, even after legislation of a tobacco control measure. Cases of such interference are evident whenever Indonesia's health ministry proposes strong tobacco

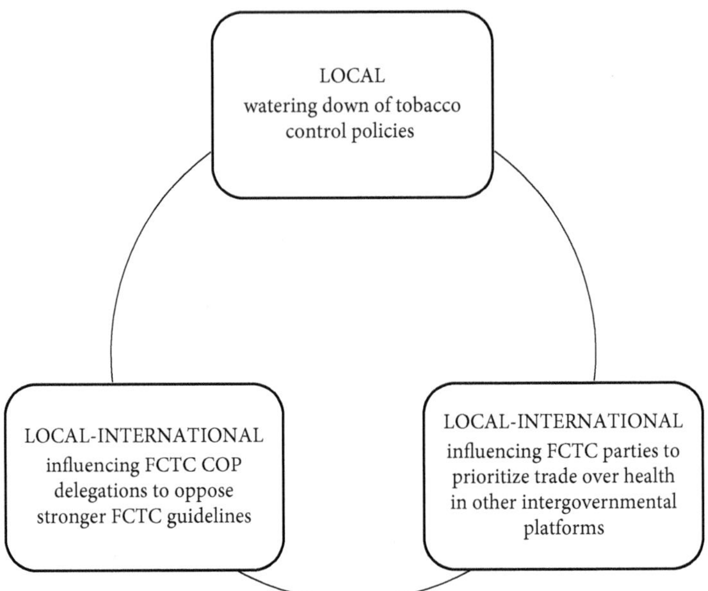

Figure 20.1 Tobacco industry interference in LMICs

control policies and finds itself being opposed by trade and economic ministries to the extent that Indonesia remains the only AMS yet to ratify the FCTC. This is also evident in Laos where a twenty-five-year license agreement (2001–2026) between the Lao government and Imperial Tobacco Limited prevented the government increasing tobacco taxes (Doward, 2014). In 2016, the Lao Ministry of Health reported that the agreement also prevented the implementation of a Prime Ministerial decree which earmarks tobacco taxes for a tobacco control fund (Lao PDR FCTC Report, 2016).

The second kind of interference is both local and international, involving both co-option and indirect interference to weaken the FCTC. This was evident in a recent Reuters' exposé of Philip Morris International's influence over Vietnam's delegation at the FCTC COP in Moscow in 2014 (Kalra et al., 2017). Such a case points to a systemic challenge, one that involves complexity at the domestic level. Although the multisectoral nature of tobacco control necessitates the involvement of finance and trade ministries alongside health ministers in the FCTC COP, it also introduces the complex ties of finance and trade ministries with the tobacco industry, especially in countries where there is no adequate protection of public health policies from tobacco industry interference.

The third kind of interference is particularly observable at the Technical Barriers to Trade (TBT) Committee and the Trade-Related Aspects of Intellectual Property (TRIPS) Council in the World Trade Organization (WTO) (Eckhardt, Holden, & Callard, 2016). Some of the AMS have lodged complaints at the WTO: Indonesia against the United States (2010) on clove cigarettes, against Australia (2013) on plain packaging, and the Philippines against Thailand (2008) on its customs valuation of cigarettes. As of December 2016, Vietnam, Indonesia, Laos, Philippines, Thailand, Myanmar, and Malaysia all have cases against them by investors through the investor–state dispute settlement (ISDS) mechanism amounting to US$ 9.5 billion (Ong, 2016).

These cases illustrate the complexity of AMS' participation in the WTO, their free trade agreements, and their obligations as parties to the FCTC (Hsu, 2014).

In sum, tobacco industry interference is a coherent strategy and pattern of industry behavior focused on the relationships it has with government ministries and their links to the local tobacco industry. These relationships are critical for the tobacco industry in its goals to undermine the FCTC and the prevention of implementation or weakening tobacco control policies in LMICs at various levels of policymaking.

The Dynamics of Governance and the Intermediary Channels for Information and Financing

Although there is no formal regional health governance mechanism in ASEAN, the ASEAN Focal Points on Tobacco Control (AFPTC), through collaboration with the Southeast Asia Tobacco Control Alliance (SEATCA), form part of the regional health framework based on the health goals of the ASEAN Socio-Cultural Community, one of the pillars of the ASEAN Community. On the one hand, the interministerial AFPTC serve as a platform for developing mutually beneficial strategic tobacco control measures to strengthen and support tobacco control implementation in line with the FCTC as well as to develop, implement, monitor, review progress, and evaluate regional cooperation on tobacco control. On the other hand, the regional civil society network SEATCA functions primarily as a tobacco control advocacy organization that also acts as an information clearing house, monitoring the progress in tobacco control among AMS and generating input and feedback for evidence-based tobacco control policy in AMS. SEATCA also serves as an intermediary channel for financing tobacco control campaigns and evidence-based tobacco policy research in AMS (see Figure 20.2).

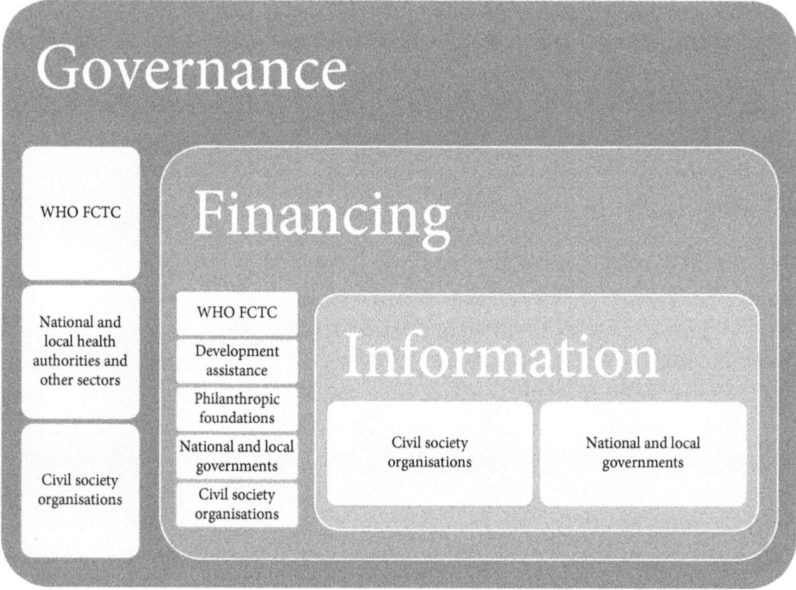

Figure 20.2 The systemic interaction between governance, financing, and information in tobacco control

Although not considered a high priority compared to pandemics and emerging and re-emerging infectious diseases, tobacco control is a recurrent component of the ASEAN health agenda (Caballero-Anthony & Amul, 2015). Tobacco control is embedded in the ASEAN Socio-Cultural Community Blueprints (2016–2030) and the ASEAN post-2015 health development agenda (2016–2020). The ASEAN health agenda includes promoting healthy lifestyles that would prioritize the prevention and control of noncommunicable diseases, and the reduction of tobacco consumption and harmful use of alcohol, and the strengthening of health systems and access to care that are geared toward universal health coverage, among others. The regional health agenda aims to strengthen health systems to incorporate universal health coverage toward the early detection, prevention, and management of NCDs, and to adopt the *Health in All Policies* approach to promote healthy lifestyles and reduce NCD burden in ASEAN.

Financing

Financing mainly enables implementation of various articles of the Convention but may also include innovations in financing tobacco control, in the form of a "sin tax" on tobacco which can be directed to a dedicated tobacco control fund. Such a fund can support not only health promotion campaigns toward healthier lifestyles, but also smoking cessation programs. Only a few of the AMS have dedicated tobacco control funding and most AMS do not allot enough funds to meet the optimal tobacco control expenditure per person. Most of the current and recent financing for information campaigns particularly for tobacco control advocacy and promotion of healthy lifestyles (often in collaboration with tobacco control CSOs) in many AMS are funded through the support of philanthropic foundations, namely Bloomberg Philanthropies with the Bloomberg Initiative to Reduce Tobacco Use, and the Bill and Melinda Gates Foundation with its Global Health Grants. Other sources of funding through development assistance for health (DAH) are channeled to the FCTC Secretariat which then allocates funding for the advocacy, legislation, and implementation of the FCTC in LMICs. With FCTC implementation included as an SDG target, more development funding is channeled to LMICs through the FCTC Secretariat (World Health Organization, 2017).

Linking Governance and Financing: The Role of Philanthropic Foundations

From a systems point of view, the financing sub-system is dense with the interaction and collaboration between two main funders that serve as a critical node in the tobacco control network, Bloomberg and the Gates Foundation. Philanthropic foundations have been increasingly recognized as global health actors, supporting not only tobacco control policies in LMICs but also tobacco control advocacy, research, and evidence-based tobacco control. The involvement of major philanthropic foundations in tobacco control started when the Rockefeller Foundation

(2003a; 2003b; 2004) committed about US$ 7 million, for tobacco control in South East Asia through the Trading Tobacco for Health Initiative from 2000 to 2004. When the Rockefeller Foundation shifted its focus to funding urban resilience, Bloomberg Philanthropies took its place as the main philanthropic foundation involved in tobacco control. Since it began in 2006 with US$ 375 million as a six-year investment, the Bloomberg Initiative to Reduce Tobacco Use has been funding the implementation of the MPOWER package in fifty-nine LMICs, including some AMS, supporting governments, intergovernmental organizations, local authorities, and NGOs. By 2016, the foundation has contributed almost US$ 1 billion to support tobacco control (Bloomberg Philanthropies, 2016). The foundation funded the WHO's data collection and analysis for the first country assessments of the tobacco epidemic and tobacco control measures which was published as the *WHO Report on the Global Tobacco Epidemic* (Bloomberg Philanthropies 2011). The report launched the MPOWER package of demand reduction measures. In ASEAN, the Bloomberg Initiative focuses on Indonesia, the Philippines, Vietnam and Thailand, four of the 15 countries where two-thirds of the global smoking population lives. In addition to the MPOWER initiative that focuses on demand-reduction measures, Bloomberg Philanthropies with the Bill and Melinda Gates Foundation are co-funding a USD4 million Anti-Tobacco Trade Litigation Fund, administered by the US-based Campaign for Tobacco-Free Kids, to support countries facing legal challenges from tobacco companies in international trade tribunals to hinder strong tobacco control (Bloomberg Philanthropies, 2015).

With a cumulative US$ 210 million commitment since 2008, the Bill and Melinda Gates Foundation linked up with Bloomberg Philanthropies to support tobacco control policies in LMICs, specifically in building capacities and the policy evidence base for governments and NGOs in Africa, China, and South East Asia (Bill and Melinda Gates Foundation, 2017). The Gates Foundation supports policy interventions (education and advocacy) on tobacco taxation, bans on tobacco advertising, graphic health warning labels and plain packaging, and smoke-free indoor environments, as well as social marketing, both traditional and innovative, and targeted campaigns to shift perceptions related to tobacco use, and building the evidence base for local and global tobacco control. Furthermore, together with Bloomberg Philanthropies, the Bill and Melinda Gates Foundation contributes to a trust fund for the operation and implementation of the World Bank's Tobacco Control Program (World Bank, 2017). Since the World Bank published the seminal report on *Curbing the epidemic—governments and the economics of tobacco control* in 1999 which contributed to the FCTC, it has been campaigning for tobacco taxation as the most cost-effective tobacco control strategy. As early as 1991, the World Bank enforced a policy not to lend, invest in, or guarantee investments or loans for tobacco production, processing, or marketing.

Information

Another vital health system building block that supports both governance and financing is information. In the FCTC, the obligation to establish a national system for the epidemiological surveillance of tobacco consumption and exposure to tobacco smoke, and related social, economic, and health indicators that can be integrated into national, regional, and global health surveillance systems for analysis and comparison (Articles 20.2 and 20.3) contributes to the improvement of the health information system.

Information goes both ways, as an output in health promotion programs for smoking cessation; campaigns for smoke-free areas and plain packaging of cigarettes; comprehensive bans on tobacco advertising, promotion, and sponsorship; and as input and feedback for policy on the monitoring and surveillance of tobacco use and the epidemiology of smoking-related diseases. The former is often linked to and identified with governance rather than the information building block, but evidence-based information is not only critical for policy-making but also for strategic health promotion and raising the awareness of the public. With the ubiquity of misleading information in various media platforms that the tobacco industry can manipulate, it is important that adequate, reliable information about tobacco use as a determinant of health is available not only for policymakers in the health and non-health sectors but also properly disseminated and communicated toward the education of the public.

The role of non-state actors in tobacco control especially in health promotion should not be undermined. Civil society organizations were instrumental in both the negotiations for the FCTC and in its implementation when it entered into force. SEATCA and locally based CSOs have a larger role in monitoring the implementation of the FCTC among the AMS, often working in collaboration with governments in surveillance. SEATCA started out from a number of research programs toward regional capacity building for tobacco control advocacy funded by the Rockefeller Foundation through the Action on Smoking and Health (ASH Thailand) and the Thai Health Promotion Foundation. As the core regional tobacco control policy advocacy network, SEATCA has strong links with the ASEAN Secretariat and is involved with almost all the activities of the AFPTC. SEATCA also supported the AFPTC in preparing the first ASEAN Tobacco Control Report (2012) with the Vietnam Steering Committee on Smoking and Health, with support from the International Union against Tuberculosis and Lung Disease (the Union). The report served as the first comparative report of tobacco control implementation in ASEAN. Since 2013, SEATCA has been publishing the ASEAN Tobacco Control Atlas to monitor the progress of tobacco control in ASEAN. The 2016 edition was also published in five ASEAN languages, including Khmer, Bahasa Indonesia, Laotian, Burmese, and Vietnamese (Southeast Asia Tobacco Control Alliance, 2016). The translation of the report into these languages enables SEATCA to reach out to a wider audience, not only to the English proficient among the AMS but also to those at grassroots level working on health promotion. In addition, SEATCA's website hosts the image bank of copyright-free pictorial health warnings of AMS in collaboration with the AFPTC.

SEATCA also acts as a regional node in the global tobacco control network, as an active member of the Framework Convention Alliance (FCA). The FCA, a global alliance that contributed to the development and negotiation of the FCTC, was also instrumental in the development of the implementing guidelines of the FCTC which set the benchmark for FCTC implementation (Mamudu & Glantz, 2009; Lee, 2010). The FCA acts as the core global tobacco control network that lobbies, pressures, monitors, and assists governments and mobilizes civil society toward FCTC implementation. The FCA was also responsible for advocating the integration of the FCTC in the SDGs. The FCA collaborates with and is strongly supported by HealthBridge Canada, Action on Smoking and Health USA, Campaign for Tobacco-Free Kids (CTFK), Canadian Cancer Society, Cancer Council Australia, Norwegian Cancer Society, and Vital Strategies. These civil society actors perform a range of functions from policy research to tobacco control advocacy, to financial and technical support for policy-making, implementation, and litigation, to monitoring implementation (Gneiting, 2016).

Conclusion

Strong governance mechanisms, underpinned by commitment, political will, reliable and timely data, innovative financing, and grassroots support through civil society are critical for the successful implementation of the FCTC. Ensuring strong governance is particularly important in many countries in the region that, due to the power and resources of the tobacco industry, face major challenges in effective implementation of the FCTC as a means of addressing a major risk factor in the increase seen in the prevalence and incidence of non-communicable diseases in the region.

The primary lesson that other regions can learn from ASEAN is the need to monitor the activities of the tobacco industry constantly and identify the industry's inconsistencies and infringements, not only of the FCTC but also of domestic tobacco control laws. This can be done through sufficiently financed and independent civil society groups and monitoring initiatives. A second lesson is that the increasing evidence that supports taxation measures to fund not only health promotion programs but also universal healthcare goals in several ASEAN member states (e.g., Thailand and the Philippines) should help countries in other regions to formulate effective evidence-based tobacco control policies. There is concrete evidence for real-world investment cases for tobacco control. Last but not the least, the importance of political will and good governance shows that the system dynamics that are at play, from policy formulation to implementation to evaluation, need to take into account system interference from the tobacco industry which will constantly assert their perceived role and responsibility to influence tobacco control policies globally. Governments need to be able to protect their policies from industry strategies that help the tobacco industry preserve their political and economic power.

References

ASEAN Focal Points on Tobacco Control and SEATCA. (2012). *The ASEAN Tobacco Control Report*. Jakarta and Bangkok: ASEAN Focal Points on Tobacco Control and SEATCA.

Retrieved from http://asean.org/storage/images/rotating_banner/the%20asean%20tobacco%20control%20report.pdf.

Assunta, M., & Dorotheo, E. U. (2016). SEATCA Tobacco industry interference index: a tool for measuring the implementation of WHO Framework Convention on Tobacco Control Article 5.3. *Tobacco Control, 25*(3), 313–318.

Battle-Fisher, M. (2015). *Application of systems thinking to health policy and public health ethics.* Heidelberg/New York/Dordrecht/London: Springer International Publishing.

Bill and Melinda Gates Foundation. (2017). *Tobacco control, What we do.* Retrieved from http://www.gatesfoundation.org/What-We-Do/Global-Policy/Tobacco-Control.

Bloomberg Philanthropies. (2011). *Accelerating the worldwide movement to reduce tobacco use.* New York: Bloomberg Philanthropies. Retrieved from https://www.bbhub.io/dotorg/sites/2/2014/04/BloombergPhilanthropies2011TobaccoReport.pdf.

Bloomberg Philanthropies. (2015, March 18). Bloomberg Philanthropies and the Bill & Melinda Gates Foundation launch anti-tobacco trade litigation fund. Press Release. Retrieved from https://www.bloomberg.org/press/releases/bloomberg-philanthropies-bill-melinda-gates-foundation-launch-anti-tobacco-trade-litigation-fund/, accessed June 8, 2017.

Bloomberg Philanthropies. (2016, December 5). Michael R Bloomberg commits $360 million to reduce tobacco use—Raising total giving on tobacco control efforts to nearly $1 billion. Press release. Retrieved from https://www.bloomberg.org/press/releases/michael-r-bloomberg-commits-360-million-reduce-tobacco-use-raising-total-giving-tobacco-control-efforts-nearly-1-billion/.

Borland, R., Young, D., Coghill, K., & Zhang, J. Y. (2009). The tobacco use management system: Analyzing tobacco control from a systems perspective. *American Journal of Public Health, 100*(7), 1229–1236.

Carey, G., Malbon, E., Carey, N., Joyce, A., Crammond, B., & Carey, A. (2015). Systems science and systems thinking for public health: A systematic review of the field. *BMJ Open, 5,* e009002.

Cavana, R. Y., & Cliffod, L. V. (2009). Integrative system dynamics: Analysis of policy options for tobacco control in New Zealand. *Systems Research and Behavioral Science, 25,* 675–94.

de Savigny, D., & Adam, T. (Eds.). (2009). *Systems thinking for health systems strengthening.* Geneva: World Health Organization.

Doward, J. (2014, October 5). UK cigarette firm criticised over Laos tobacco tax deal. *The Guardian.* https://www.theguardian.com/world/2014/oct/05/imperial-tobacco-laos-cigarette-tax-deal, accessed October 1, 2017.

Eckhardt, J., Holden, C., & Callard, C. D. (2016). Tobacco control and the World Trade Organization: Mapping member states' positions after the Framework Convention on Tobacco Control. *Tobacco Control, 25,* 692–698. doi:10.1136/tobaccocontrol-2015-052486

Euromonitor International. (2017). *Global tobacco: Key findings part I—Cigarettes. Passport.*

Framework Convention Alliance. (n.d.). *Our accomplishments, About us.* Retrieved from http://www.fctc.org/our-accomplishments/.

Framework Convention Alliance. *About us.* Retrieved from http://www.fctc.org/about-us/.

Framework Convention on Tobacco Control (FCTC) Secretariat. (2017, April 4). Convention Secretariat announced FCTC 2030 selected parties. Press Release, http://www.who.int/fctc/mediacentre/news/2017/fctc2030-parties-announced/en/, accessed June 8, 2017.

Gneiting, U. (2016). From global agenda-setting to domestic implementation: successes and challenges of the global health network on tobacco control. *Health Policy and Planning, 31,* i74–i86, doi:10.1093/heapol/cvz001

Hsu, L. (2014). Tobacco control in ASEAN. In A. D. Mitchell & T. Voon (Eds.), *The global tobacco epidemic and the law* (pp. 142–165). Cheltenham: Edward Elgar Publishing

Institute of Health Metrics and Evaluation. (2020). *Global burden of disease study 2017 results.* Seattle, WA: Institute for Health Metrics and Evaluation (IHME). Retrieved from http://ghdx.healthdata.org/gbd-results-tool?params=gbd-api-2017-permalink/2446aec958f8e3398954cdc5e7a49fb0.

Kalra, A., Bansal, P., Wilson, D., & Lasseter, T. (2017, July 13). Part 1: Inside Philip Morris' campaign to subvert the global anti-smoking treaty. *Reuters Investigates: The Philip Morris Files.* Retrieved from https://www.reuters.com/investigates/special-report/pmi-who-fctc/#article-part-1-treaty-blitz

Lao PDR FCTC Report. (2016). Core Questionnaire of the Reporting Instrument of WHO FCTC: Lao PDR. *WHO Framework Convention on Tobacco Control Secretariat.* Geneva: World Health Organization. Retrieved from https://untobaccocontrol.org/impldb/wp-content/uploads/Lao_PDR_2018_report.pdf

Lee, K. (2010). Civil society organizations and the functions of global health governance: What role within intergovernmental organizations. *Global Health Governance, 3*(2). Retrieved from http://blogs.shu.edu/ghg/files/2011/11/Lee_Civil-Society-Organizations-and-the-Functions-of-Global-Health-Governance_Spring-2010.pdf.

Lee, S., Ling, P. M., & Glantz, S. A. (2012). The vector of the tobacco epidemic: tobacco industry practices in low and middle-income countries. *Cancer Causes and Control, 23*(Suppl 1), 117–129. doi:10.1007/s10552-012-9914-0

Luke, D. A., Wald, L. M., Carothers, B. J., Bach, L. E., & Harris, J. K. (2013). Network influences on dissemination of evidence-based guidelines in state tobacco control programs. *Health Education & Behavior, 40*, 33S–42S.

Mamudu, H. M., & Glantz, S. A. (2009). Civil society and the negotiation of the Framework Convention on Tobacco Control. *Global Public Health, 4*(2), 150–168. doi:10.1080/17441690802095355

Marcus, S. E., Leischow, S. J., Mabry, P. L., & Clark, P. I. (2010). Lessons learned from the application of systems science to tobacco control at the National Cancer Institute. *American Journal of Public Health, 100*(7), 1163–1165.

Caballero-Anthony, M., & Amul, G. G. H. (2015). Health and human security: Pathways to advancing a human-centered approach to health security in East Asia. In S. Rushton & J. Youde (Eds.), *Routledge handbook of global health security* (pp. 32–47). London: Routledge.

National Cancer Institute. (2007). *Greater than the sum: Systems thinking in tobacco control. National Cancer Institute Tobacco Control Monograph 18.* Bethesda, MD: US Department of Health and Human Services, National Institutes of Health. NIH Pub. No. 06-6085.

Ong, T. (2016, December 8). Multinationals launch 50 lawsuits worth $31b against Asian nations. *ABC News.* Retrieved from http://www.abc.net.au/news/2016-12-08/report-shows-hidden-costs-of-rcep-trade-deal/8103602.

The Rockefeller Foundation. (2003a). *Annual report 2001.* Retrieved from https://assets.rockefellerfoundation.org/app/uploads/20150530121728/Annual-Report-2001.pdf.

The Rockefeller Foundation. (2003b). *Annual report 2002.* Retrieved from https://assets.rockefellerfoundation.org/app/uploads/20150530121729/Annual-Report-2002.pdf.

The Rockefeller Foundation. (2004). *Annual report 2003.* Retrieved from https://assets.rockefellerfoundation.org/app/uploads/20150530121731/Annual-Report-2003.pdf

Smith, K. E. (2013). Understanding the influence of evidence in public health policy: What can we learn from the "tobacco wars?" *Social Policy and Administration, 47*(4), 382–398.

Southeast Asia Tobacco Control Alliance (SEATCA). (2016, November 10). *SEATCA's new and expanded The Tobacco Control Atlas launched at COP7.* Press Release. Retrieved from http://seatca.org/?p=10182.

Weishar, H., Amos, A., & Collin, J. (2015). Capturing complexity: mixing methods in the analysis of a European tobacco control policy network. *International Journal of Social Research Methodology, 18*, 175–92.

World Bank. (2017, August 15). Tobacco Control Program. Last updated August 15, 2017. Retrieved from http://www.worldbank.org/en/topic/health/brief/tobacco.

World Health Organization. (2007). *Everybody's business: Strengthening health systems to improve health outcomes: WHO's framework for action*. Geneva: World Health Organization.

World Health Organization. (2017, April 4). Convention Secretariat announces FCTC 2030 selected parties. *WHO Framework Convention on Tobacco Control*. Retrieved from http://www.who.int/fctc/mediacentre/news/2017/fctc2030-parties-announced/en/.

World Health Organization Southeast Asia Regional Office (WHO SEARO). (2017). *Accelerating WHO FCTC implementation in the WHO South-East Asia region—A practical approach*. Geneva: World Health Organization.

World Health Organization Western Pacific Regional Office (WHO WPRO). (2015). *Regional action plan for the tobacco free initiative in the Western Pacific (2015–2019)*. Geneva: World Health.

World Trade Organization. Australia—Certain Measures Concerning Trademarks, Geographical Indications and Other Plain Packaging Requirements Applicable to Tobacco Products and Packaging. Dispute DS 467. Retrieved from https://www.wto.org/english/tratop_e/dispu_e/cases_e/ds467_e.htm.

World Trade Organization. Thailand—Customs and Fiscal Measures on Cigarettes from the Philippines. Dispute DS371. Retrieved from https://www.wto.org/english/tratop_e/dispu_e/cases_e/ds371_e.htm.

World Trade Organization. United States—Measures Affecting the Production and Sale of Clove Cigarettes. Dispute DS406. Retrieved from https://www.wto.org/english/tratop_e/dispu_e/cases_e/ds406_e.htm.

Young, D., Borland, R., & Coghill, K. (2012). Changing the tobacco use management system: Blending systems thinking with actor-network theory. *Review of Policy Research, 29*(2), 251–279.

21
The Planetary Health Imperative to Eradicate Nuclear Weapons

Tilman Ruff

> " ... from a health perspective—a proper understanding of what nuclear weapons will do invalidates all arguments for continued possession of these weapons and requires that they urgently be prohibited and eliminated as the only course of action commensurate with the existential danger they pose." (UN General Assembly, 2016)

Existential Threats to Survival and Health

Among the myriad causes of death, illness, and suffering, it is those with potential to cause not only individual or mass death but disrupt the ongoing chain of life itself which can jeopardize the possibility of life for future generations that most demand priority and attention. Consequences of such cataclysmic proportions make intolerable the mere existence of danger that is preventable.

Until our sun expands into a red giant star in 6 billion or so years and makes the earth inhospitable, there are three existential challenges we must navigate collectively.

The first is collision of the earth with a celestial body, such as a large meteorite. Such collisions have been the main cause of previous major extinctions, like that of the dinosaurs. We may now be able to anticipate and avoid some such catastrophic collisions and should work collectively to improve these capabilities.

The second is environmental disruption, with degradation and depletion of vital resources and ecosystems; inadequately mitigated global heating posing the greatest such threat.

The third, more acute and less potentially reversible, is the danger of nuclear war. The World Health Assembly in 1983 identified nuclear weapons as "the greatest immediate threat to the health and welfare of mankind" (World Health Organization, 1983). Preventing use of nuclear weapons, by accident or design, necessitates their eradication; a necessary, urgent, and feasible precondition for securing planetary and human survival, health, and sustainability.

The latter two of these existential challenges are of recent and human origin, needing human solutions. Those of us alive since 1945 when nuclear weapons were first exploded, and more recently since evidence of human-induced climate disruption became unequivocal, are in all human evolutionary history the first generations

Tilman Ruff, *The Planetary Health Imperative to Eradicate Nuclear Weapons* In: *Systems Thinking for Global Health.* Edited by: Fiona Larkan, Frédérique Vallières, Hasheem Mannan, and Naonori Kodate, Oxford University Press. DOI: 10.1093/oso/9780198799498.003.0021

to face existential threats of our own collective making. While the enormous and unprecedented responsibility we bear is a daunting challenge and burden, it is also a precious gift. No people in all human history have had as great an opportunity as those alive now to avert harm and do good for humanity, and for all the current and potential future denizens with whom we share planet earth.

For each of these existential threats, the severity and pervasiveness of the potential impacts make the broader ecosystem frame of planetary health more appropriate than one limited to human health, even if viewed globally.

Health evidence and health professionals have played and continue to play a central role in work to control nuclear weapons. This work involves mobilization and coalition building within the health sector, and also necessitates expertise and wide collaborations well beyond the health sector. The health systems building blocks most germane to this work are information/evidence, resources (especially human), and governance/leadership. A number of elements of a systems approach have proven useful to the health contribution toward freeing our world from nuclear weapons, in particular dynamic, big-picture thinking, a broad ecological perspective of positive and resisting forces and actors, an understanding of the non-linearity of political and social change, and the roles of focused interventions, critical mass, and tipping points. Applying the lessons of what has worked in efforts to control and eliminate other indiscriminate and inhumane weapons has also been key. This chapter discusses approaches and lessons useful in what has become known as the Humanitarian Initiative on nuclear weapons developed over the last decade, and especially the first international legal instrument to prohibit nuclear weapons and provide a framework for their elimination: the 2017 UN Treaty on the Prohibition of Nuclear Weapons.

Nuclear Weapons and Fissile Materials

Nuclear weapons are by far the most destructive, indiscriminate, persistently toxic weapons ever invented.

The nuclear fission processes inside an atomic weapon and a nuclear reactor are fundamentally similar, and both increase the radioactivity present in the starting materials millions of times. In a thermonuclear (or hydrogen) bomb, highly enriched uranium (HEU) and/or plutonium undergoes fission, producing immense heat and pressure which enable isotopes of hydrogen (deuterium and tritium) to fuse, releasing vast, essentially limitless amounts of energy. This is the main process driving the sun. Single nuclear weapons have been detonated with more than four times the destructive power of all explosives used in all wars throughout human history.

Fissile materials are both toxic and weapons-usable over geological periods that make the time frames of human institutions irrelevant. Therefore, a sound approach is based on primary prevention and the inherent dangers of nuclear weapons and fissile materials. The custodial political leaders, their intentions, policies, and personalities, alliances, and governments, the areas within their jurisdiction, the functioning of governance and regulatory institutions, on the other hand, can transform overnight.

The current global stockpile of HEU is estimated at 1,330 tons, and for plutonium already separated from spent reactor fuel, 536 tons (International Panel on Fissile

Materials, 2021). With modern US nuclear weapons known to contain an average of 4 kilograms (kg) of plutonium (or 12 kg of HEU), current fissile material stocks are sufficient to reconstitute the current global nuclear arsenal of 13,100 weapons many times over (Kristensen & Korda, 2021). Hence, ending production of weapons-usable materials, eliminating them wherever possible, and storing the rest as securely as humanly possible are key to achieving and sustaining a world free of nuclear weapons.

The Effects of Nuclear Weapons

An understanding of the effects of nuclear weapons is a crucial underpinning for all considerations and policy relating to them. Evidence of the true extent of the effects of nuclear weapons has frequently not been collected, or has been covered up, misrepresented, or disregarded by governments, victim to the myths that nuclear weapons are just weapons like any other, only larger, and can be used to serve legitimate military purposes and enhance security. The reality is vastly different. No humanitarian response, reconciliation, or recovery is possible after a nuclear war. The concept of "winners" would be meaningless; there would be only losers.

(i) Acute effects

Nuclear weapons produce an enormous blast wave that causes trauma both directly (such as lung trauma and ear drum rupture) and indirectly through powerful winds which can turn objects, including people, into missiles. Intense heat causes direct vaporization, incineration, and burns and ignites anything flammable over a large area. A defining feature of nuclear weapons is the release of huge amounts of radioactivity in the initial pulse as well as through radioactive fallout, containing hundreds of different radioisotopes with half-lives ranging from fractions of a second to millions of years. Fallout is dispersed by wind and water over great distances, eventually worldwide. Ionizing radiation causes acute multi-organ toxicity (acute radiation sickness) at high acute doses, and in the long term any level causes dose-related genetic damage and lifelong subsequent increased risk of cancer and chronic diseases. Genetic damage may be inherited by future generations, who would also be at further risk through living in a radioactively contaminated environment.

The electromagnetic pulse (EMP) from a single high-altitude nuclear explosion would cover a continental size area with voltage a million times greater than lightning. This would disrupt the vast array of not specifically protected electrical and electronic equipment on which the infrastructure of modern societies is highly dependent, including water and electricity supply, telecommunications, computer systems, transport networks, medical equipment, traffic lights, banking, and most commerce and trade (Ruff, 2013).

While the average size of the weapons in the global nuclear arsenal is 200 kilotons (kt) high explosive equivalent, thirteen times the size of the Hiroshima bomb, the largest currently deployed nuclear weapons contain 5 million tons (Mt) of high explosive equivalent for blast. Within a thousandth of a second, conditions akin to the center of the sun would be produced: 100 million °C and 100 million atmospheres of pressure in a fireball which would rapidly expand to 1.8 kilometers (km) across. Within 4.7 km in every direction, winds of 750 km/h and a blast wave over 140 kPa would destroy all buildings and vaporize the upper layer of the earth. To 7.5 km in every direction, winds of 460 km/h and blast pressures of 80 kPa would break apart concrete and steel buildings and vaporize aluminum. For 12.3 km in every direction, asphalt would melt and windows fragment into more than 4,000 projectile glass shards per square meter (m^2). Stretching 22.6 km in every direction, over an area of 1605 km^2, everything flammable would ignite—wood, vegetation, paper, cloth, plastics, petrol, oil from ruptured tanks, and cars; further fueled by ruptured gas pipes, downed electricity lines, and leaking chemicals. Within half an hour, hundreds of thousands of fires would coalesce into a giant firestorm 45 km across, with temperatures of more than 800 °C, sucking in air and creating winds of more than 320 km/h, consuming all available oxygen (Ruff, 2013). Shelters would become crematoria and every living thing would die within this fire zone.

Streets would be impassable. There would be no ambulances, fire engines, or police, no power or communications or functioning hospitals. The vast majority of injured and burnt people would die alone without any human comfort or relief from their agonizing pain (World Health Organization, 1987).

(ii) Climate impacts and nuclear famine

There have been important new findings regarding ionizing radiation health effects in recent years, in the direction of greater health consequences than previously estimated (Ruff, 2017). However, it is in relation to the impacts of nuclear war on climate, agriculture, and nutrition that scientific advances of the greatest moment have been made in the past fourteen years. It is not just large-scale nuclear war between Russia and the United States that poses a global threat. A series of studies have shown that a localized, regional nuclear war utilizing a tiny fraction of the global nuclear arsenal would also have catastrophic worldwide effects.

Nuclear weapons are extremely efficient at igniting simultaneous fires over large areas, which would rapidly coalesce and loft large volumes of sooty smoke into the stratosphere. The scenario most frequently studied and recently updated (Toon et al., 2019) is nuclear war between India and Pakistan. These countries have fought four wars and many skirmishes since their partition in 1947. The most recently studied scenario assumes that in 2025, each country will possess 250 nuclear weapons, and 250 are used in a war between them. This number constitutes less than 2% of the current global nuclear arsenal and less than 1% of its explosive power. The direct effects in South Asia are catastrophic. Depending on whether the weapons used had yields of fifteen (Hiroshima-size), 50 or 100 kt, between 50 and 125 million people would die from the early direct effects of the explosions, fires, and local radiation.

The global consequences would, however, be far more devastating. Cities ignited by the nuclear explosions would loft dark smoke containing between 16.1 million tons (for 15 kt warheads) and 36.6 million tons (for 100 kt warheads) of black carbon high into the upper atmosphere. Previously, three teams of climate scientists using three different climate models and making conservative assumptions each showed significant drops in average surface temperature, sunlight, and precipitation across the globe, with the effects lasting for over a decade for a smaller scenario involving 100 15kt nuclear explosions (Mills, Toon, Lee-Taylor, & Robock, 2015). While the fuel density of modern cities and industrial areas varies, there is nothing specific to India/Pakistan about such a scenario, and urban populations and fuel densities are tending to rise worldwide. In the Toon 2019 study, average global land temperatures decline by as much as 4–8C. By comparison, the Last Glacial Maximum 20,000 years ago saw a decline in temperatures of 3–8C. Following nuclear war, ice-age conditions would develop within a few weeks.

This climate disruption would in turn profoundly reduce food production. For a scenario involving 100 15 kt explosions, producing 5 million tons of smoke, considering only the impact of colder temperatures, reduced sunlight, and precipitation decline, global grain crops would reduce by 20% for the first five years and 10–15% for the second five years (Toon et al., 2017), with much larger declines at higher latitudes.

Adequate human nutrition cannot be sustained in the face of widespread decline of food production of this magnitude. Total world grain reserves typically amount to 60–120 days of global consumption and would not begin to offset the shortfall over a decade or more (Toon et al., 2017). Furthermore, the United Nations Food and Agriculture Organization (FAO) estimates there were 768 million people in 2020 who are already chronically undernourished, and a rising number of people—2.37 billion—currently facing moderate or severe food insecurity (Food and Agriculture Organization, 2021). In addition, a further 300+ million people who receive adequate nutrition today live in countries highly dependent on food imports, which would quickly dry up following a nuclear war. Conservatively estimated, without taking account of land polluted by radiation and toxic chemicals, dramatically increased ultraviolet (UV) radiation harmful to plants and animals both on land and in water, disruption to trade and agricultural inputs including seed, fertilizer, fuel, pesticides, etc., or the disease epidemics and social conflict that inevitably accompany famine, around 2 billion people would starve, following a regional nuclear war involving 0.7% of the global arsenal and less than 0.1% of its total yield (Helfand, 2013).

A recent study (Toon et al., 2019) estimates reductions in net primary productivity (NPP) for the range of weapons yields already described. This is a measure of broad ecological health, reflecting the amount of carbon dioxide (CO_2) converted to plant matter, after accounting for plant respiration. It is therefore a proxy envelope for the maximum amount of food which could be harvested. NPP would decline by 15–30% on land and 10–20% in the oceans over several years. This is comparable to the total amount of food and fiber currently used by humans. In some densely populated regions of Europe, south and east Asia, humans appropriate 63–80% of NPP, and people in most of India, eastern China, parts of the Middle East, and equatorial Africa consume more than 100% of local NPP, with consequently little or no margin to cope with the multiyear productivity loss that would follow a regional nuclear war anywhere in the world.

Large-scale war between the United States and Russia would be far worse. A war involving the strategic (long range) weapons now deployed would put 150 million tons of black carbon in the upper atmosphere, and drop temperatures around the world by 8–10 °C. In the interior regions of North America and Eurasia, temperatures would fall by 25–30 °C for more than a decade. In temperate regions of the northern Hemisphere, temperatures would fall below freezing for part of every day for at least two years (Coupe, Bardeen, Robock, Toon, 2019). Food production would cease and the vast majority—perhaps all—of the human race would starve (Helfand et al., 2016).

This evidence of severe global impacts from even a limited regional nuclear war involving a tiny fraction of the world stockpile means that all nuclear arsenals, not only those of Russia and the United States, pose a global danger. During most of the Cold War it was argued that the risk of "mutually assured destruction" would keep the peace between rationally and reliably governed nuclear-armed rivals. However, we now know that use of nuclear weapons would be suicidal, even without highly probable nuclear escalation and retaliation, resulting in "self-assured destruction" (Toon et al, 2017). Nuclear weapons are effectively global suicide bombs.

The Growing Risk of Nuclear War

The current international security landscape is alarming. Relations between United States/NATO and Russia are at their lowest ebb since the end of the Cold War, with Russian annexation of Crimea, and an increase of aggressive threats, military exercises, and deployments. The arms control treaties that have helped prevent nuclear catastrophe for the last half century are being progressively dismantled. The signature disarmament treaty that ushered in the end of the Cold War, the Intermediate Nuclear Forces Treaty, was abandoned in 2019. The Anti-Ballistic Missile Treaty and Open Skies Treaty have also been abandoned. In early 2021, a new United States administration joined Russia in extending the New Strategic Arms Reduction (START) Treaty for five years, two days before the treaty would otherwise have expired. This is the only remaining constraint on Russian and US nuclear weapons, together possessing 90% of the global total. While exploratory Russian–US talks on nuclear weapons resumed in 2021, both sides are developing new nuclear weapons and lowering the threshold for nuclear war.

Tensions simmer between China, United States, Japan, and others in the South China Sea. Almost weekly skirmishes along their disputed border, a continuing nuclear arms race, weak security of nuclear weapons, and policies envisioning early use of nuclear weapons, highlight the real danger of armed conflict turning nuclear between India and Pakistan. The welcome signs in recent years of rapprochement and dialog replacing irresponsible escalating nuclear threats between DPRK (North Korea) and the United States are reversing. The landmark agreement which saw unprecedented and effectively verified constraints on Iran's nuclear program is unraveling after the United States walked away from the agreement. The danger of nuclear weapons detonations as a result of cyberattack is growing (Helfand et al., 2016). A climate stressed-world is already witnessing a sharp increase in the number of internationalized armed conflicts over the last decade (World Bank, 2018), many involving nuclear-armed states and thereby posing growing risks of nuclear escalation.

Meanwhile, all nine nuclear-armed states are committed not only to indefinite retention of their nuclear arsenals, but all are investing large sums—together over US$

105 billion annually—in modernizing them, developing new weapons with new capacities, making them more accurate and "usable."

No wonder then that the thirteen Nobel Laureates and other custodians of the Doomsday Clock, along with most authoritative others, assess the dangers of nuclear war to be as high as they have ever been, and growing. In January 2018 the hands of the Clock were moved forward to two minutes to midnight, as close to midnight as they have been since 1953, when both the United States and USSR in rapid succession tested thermonuclear bombs. The hands were kept there in 2019. In January 2020, they were moved to 100 seconds to midnight, closer than they have ever been (Science and Security Board, 2020). They said:

> Humanity continues to face two simultaneous existential dangers—nuclear war and climate change—that are compounded by a threat multiplier, cyber-enabled information warfare, that undercuts society's ability to respond....
>
> In the nuclear realm, national leaders have ended or undermined several major arms control treaties and negotiations during the last year, creating an environment conducive to a renewed nuclear arms race, to the proliferation of nuclear weapons, and to lowered barriers to nuclear war. Political conflicts regarding nuclear programs in Iran and North Korea remain unresolved and are, if anything, worsening. US–Russia cooperation on arms control and disarmament is all but nonexistent.

In 2021, the hands of the clock remain at 100 seconds to midnight.

Experience with Other Indiscriminate, Inhumane Weapons

Substantial progress has been made toward the control and elimination of other types of weapons with inevitably inhumane and indiscriminate effects: biological and chemical weapons, antipersonnel landmines, and cluster munitions. Although the histories differ, a common element which has proven effective can be summarized as stigmatize, prohibit, and eliminate. In each case, incontrovertible evidence that the respective weapons, however used, would have indiscriminate and inhumane effects provided the basis for codifying their rejection in an international treaty enshrining a consistent standard for all states. Prohibiting unacceptable weapons does not *per se* eliminate them, but it provides the necessary justification and basis for progressive work toward eliminating weapons deemed unacceptable under international law. Indeed, no other approach has proven effective; no weapon has been eliminated without first being prohibited.

While work remains to be done to eliminate each type of prohibited weapon, and setbacks occur, each type of prohibited weapon is now less often produced, deployed, traded, stockpiled, used, and justified.

Importantly, once established, norms become stronger over time and influence even states not formally signed up to the relevant treaty. For example, until President Trump in early 2020 signaled a return to the US use of landmines, the United States had in 2014 put in place prohibitions on landmine production and use and had been proudly declaring itself in international forums to essentially be in compliance with the landmines ban. It has also ceased production of cluster munitions, even though it opposed and hasn't signed either treaty.

When use of chemical weapons in Syria was confirmed by a UN investigation in 2013, Russia and the United States forced the Syrian regime to join the Chemical Weapons Convention, and Syria's declared stockpile of 1,260 tons of chemical weapons and precursors was destroyed in 2014.

All countries except for North Korea have stopped nuclear test explosions, even though the Comprehensive Test Ban Treaty negotiated in 1996 has not yet entered into force because key nuclear-capable countries have not yet joined.

Until recently, it was a gaping anomaly that this proven approach had not been applied to the last remaining weapon of mass destruction to be outlawed: nuclear weapons, the most destructive of all.

The Current Status of Nuclear Weapons and Disarmament

While the number of nuclear weapons has reduced from 70,300 in 1986 to an estimated 13,100 in August 2021, and with increasing accuracy explosive yields have trended downwards, their destructive potential is not significantly reduced. This is because of enormous redundancy in destructive capacity ("overkill"), increased understanding of the severity of their effects, and the fact that "smaller" nuclear weapons—in the tens to hundreds of kT range—distribute destruction more efficiently. In cities such weapons produce 100 times as many acute fatalities and 100 times as much smoke from fires per kt of explosive yield as mT-range weapons. (Toon et al., 2007).

The pace of nuclear reductions has slowed significantly since the 1990s, and China, India, North Korea, Pakistan, Russia and the United Kingdom are increasing their arsenals. Almost 4,000 warheads are operationally deployed, of which about 2,000 US, Russian, British, and French warheads are on high alert, ready for use within minutes (Kristensen & Korda, 2021).

The unprecedented threat posed by nuclear weapons was recognized in the very first resolution of the United Nations General Assembly (UNGA) in January 1946, calling for the elimination of atomic weapons. The preamble of the 1970 nuclear non-proliferation treaty (NPT) opens, "Considering the devastation that would be visited upon all mankind by a nuclear war and the consequent need to make every effort to avert the danger of such a war . . . ." The obligation to pursue effective measures toward nuclear disarmament enshrined in Article 6 is a shared responsibility of all 190 NPT signatory states and part of customary international law.

The International Court of Justice, the world's highest legal authority, in its 1996 Advisory Opinion on nuclear weapons confirmed that under the UN Charter, if the use of force in a given case is illegal then the threat to use such force will likewise be illegal, that is that the threat—the basis of policies of nuclear deterrence—and the use of nuclear weapons "stand together" legally. The Court unanimously ruled that there exists an obligation not only to pursue in good faith but to bring to a conclusion negotiations leading to nuclear disarmament.

Yet there are currently no negotiations underway or planned between nuclear-armed states to reduce warheads or curtail nuclear operations and modernizations, nothing to replace the erosion of the existing treaty constraints on nuclear proliferation described earlier, and between them there is no proposed or agreed process to fulfil their half-century-old binding legal obligation to disarm.

In this bleak landscape of nuclear modernization, failure of disarmament and growing risk of nuclear war, the negotiation and adoption in 2017 of the UN Treaty on the Prohibition of Nuclear Weapons by the majority of the world's states which neither possess nor assist in preparations for possible use of nuclear weapons stands as a beacon lighting the only currently defined pathway toward the eradication of nuclear weapons.

What's in the Treaty on the Prohibition of Nuclear Weapons (TPNW)?

The mandate provided in December 2016 by the UNGA was "to negotiate a legally binding instrument to prohibit nuclear weapons, leading toward their total elimination." The treaty was adopted at the UN in New York on July 7, 2017, by a vote of 122 to 1.

Drawing on other disarmament treaties, the treaty provides the first categorical and comprehensive prohibition of nuclear weapons and activities enabling their possession, deployment, and possible use (UN General Assembly, 2017). Its preamble articulates deep concern about the catastrophic humanitarian consequences of any use of nuclear weapons, the consequent need to eliminate them completely, and guarantee that they never again be used under any circumstances. It states that the risks posed by nuclear weapons threaten the security of all humanity and therefore all states share the responsibility to prevent any use. It recognizes that the consequences of nuclear weapons use cannot be adequately addressed, pose grave implications for human survival, the environment, socio-economic development, food security, and the health of current and future generations. For the first time in a nuclear disarmament instrument, tribute is paid to survivors of nuclear use (*hibakusha*) and testing, and the disproportionate impact of nuclear weapons on women and girls, and on indigenous peoples, are recognized.

The treaty commits each state party never under any circumstances to develop, test, produce, manufacture, otherwise acquire, possess, or stockpile nuclear weapons. It prohibits the transfer, use, or threat of use of nuclear weapons, and to assist, encourage, or induce, in any way, anyone to engage in any prohibited activity.

The treaty is crafted to enable states that own nuclear weapons, owned them previously, or have them stationed on their territory, to join. It requires that nuclear weapons, nuclear weapons programs and facilities be eliminated under verifiable, irreversible, and time-bound plans to be agreed with states parties. The details of these elimination regimes require the active participation of the states possessing the weapons, but the treaty provides a clear framework and non-discriminatory principles for these regimes.

Members of the North Atlantic Treaty Organization (NATO), Australia, Japan, and South Korea, which provide justification for threat of use and assist in military preparations for possible use of nuclear weapons, can join provided they cease such assistance. There is no requirement to end military cooperation with nuclear-armed states, provided such cooperation does not involve prohibited (nuclear weapons) activities. A number of states which cooperate militarily with the United States but don't claim protection from US nuclear weapons, such as New Zealand, Thailand and the Philippines, have ratified the treaty, with no disruption to their ongoing (non-nuclear) military cooperation with the United States.

The treaty provides for nuclear safeguards standards at least consistent with NPT obligations, and that these may change—hopefully strengthen—over time. No state can reasonably argue that this treaty undermines or contradicts the NPT, or that it could not join it.

States joining the treaty will need to take national legal, administrative, and other measures, including penal sanctions, to implement their commitments.

The treaty builds on humanitarian and human rights-based norms developed in the landmine and cluster munitions treaties, providing for needs-based assistance to victims and feasible clean-up of contaminated environments. This is the first treaty related to nuclear weapons which obliges states in a position to do so to assist people affected by the use or testing of nuclear weapons, without discrimination, including medical care, rehabilitation, and psychological support, as well as for their social and economic inclusion. Clearly much of the harm caused by nuclear weapons cannot be undone in the way traumatic injuries may be able to be treated, and that discrete munitions can be cleared, but these provisions should help ensure that the ongoing needs of survivors and for clean-up are not ignored or forgotten. The responsibility of states that have used or tested nuclear weapons draws specific mention.

States parties will meet at least every two years to review and promote treaty implementation. A two-thirds majority will be able to amend it or add protocols to it. The treaty is of unlimited duration and must be accepted *in toto* by joining states; they cannot opt out of any parts of it.

The treaty entered into legal force on 22 January 2021, after fifty governments had ratified it. As of January 26, 2022, eighty-six states have signed and fifty-nine have ratified.

The Process of Achieving the Ban Treaty Broke New Ground

The treaty is not only historic in substance; the process of its genesis also transformed the otherwise moribund nuclear disarmament landscape (Ruff, 2018b).

First, the process leading to the negotiation and adoption of this treaty was led by states without nuclear weapons. This changed the status quo of nuclear arms control and disarmament steps being almost solely in the hands of the states that claim a special right to possess nuclear weapons and thereby threaten all humanity with indiscriminate nuclear violence.

Second, this treaty, more than any other nuclear disarmament treaty, has an unequivocal basis in humanitarian evidence and norms. It builds directly on the evidence-based conclusions of the three first-ever intergovernmental Humanitarian Impacts of Nuclear Weapons conferences in Norway, Mexico, and Austria from 2013 to 2014 (Europe Integration, 2014a). At the end of the Vienna conference, attended by 158 states, Austria launched the Humanitarian Pledge to work to fill the legal gap for the prohibition and elimination of nuclear weapons (Europe Integration, 2014b). It was joined in this pledge by 126 other states. Health evidence on the catastrophic consequences of any use of nuclear weapons, the impossibility of any effective health and emergency response for the victims of nuclear weapons, and the imperative for prevention, as well as evidence from leading climate scientists on the nuclear winter and famine that would follow even a regional nuclear war was presented and updated at each of the humanitarian conferences. This evidence was unchallenged. It provided an authoritative evidence base for the process of securing a negotiating mandate and for the treaty negotiations themselves. Health evidence is central in the treaty's preamble, which outlines the basis and purpose of the treaty.

Third, the level of participation of civil society was unprecedented in the nuclear field. Academic and other civil society experts, including in public health and climate science, made important contributions to the negotiation of the treaty. The International Committee of the Red Cross (ICRC), with its status as partner to governments in humanitarian assistance and a key custodian of international humanitarian law (law regulating armed conflict), also made seminal contributions on behalf of the world's largest humanitarian organization to a strong final treaty.

Fourth, those directly harmed by nuclear weapons had prominence unprecedented in intergovernmental forums regarding nuclear weapons. Japanese *hibakusha* and nuclear test survivors grounded discussions in the lived experience of what nuclear weapons actually do, reminding diplomats why their work mattered, and why concluding the ambitious goal of an effective treaty by the end of the negotiating mandate on July 7, 2017 was of utmost importance. Their prominent participation lent the process legitimacy, moral weight, and humanity. Nuclear weapons can be daunting, difficult, and uncomfortable to grasp, remote from everyday human experience. The courageous testimony of survivors combined powerfully with scientific evidence to make clear what nuclear weapons do and the urgent imperative to eradicate them.

Fifth, the negotiation of the treaty through the UNGA was highly effective. This was the first time in twenty-one years that a nuclear disarmament treaty was negotiated in the United Nations. Crucially, its most inclusive and fundamental organ, the General Assembly, is able to decide substantive matters by two-thirds majority vote if consensus cannot be achieved. This is in contrast to the NPT review conferences and the UN Conference on Disarmament (CD), which are both shackled by a requirement for consensus, meaning lowest common denominator or no agreed outcomes (and explains why the CD has been unable to agree even on an agenda since 1996). In the UN Security Council, each of five nuclear-armed permanent members is able to veto any decision. Being adopted in the most inclusive global forum by such an overwhelming majority also affords the treaty moral and political credibility.

Not only was the UNGA negotiating process effective, it was efficient. This ambitious treaty was able to traverse from negotiating mandate to adopted text in just eight months, with only four weeks of face-to-face negotiations. This reflected both a lack of opposition in the room by nuclear-armed and nuclear-dependent states opposed to the treaty, which boycotted the negotiations, and a remarkable level of goodwill on the part of negotiating states.

The treaty in both process as well as substance thus represents a seismic shift in bringing global democracy to nuclear disarmament, and in asserting the interests of shared humanity. It bodes well for other negotiations that might be undertaken in the UNGA. This disruption of the dominance of nuclear-armed states is likely one of the reasons why they have opposed the treaty so vociferously.

Sixth, fierce political and economic pressure has been brought to bear on states supporting banning nuclear weapons by nuclear-armed states, particularly France, Russia, the United Kingdom, and the United States. A number of supportive states, particularly smaller and poorer nations in Africa, Latin America, South East Asia, and the South Pacific, were successfully pressured not to vote or to abstain. However, the majority supporting the treaty was so overwhelming that nuclear-armed states failed to derail its negotiation or adoption.

Seventh, the boycott of the negotiations by all nuclear-armed states, and all additional states that claim protection from US nuclear weapons except for the Netherlands (not supportive but forced to participate by public and parliamentary pressure), throws into sharp relief their current commitment to retaining, modernizing, and continuing to threaten use of their nuclear arsenals, rather than fulfilling their obligation to eliminate them. These governments claim to be good international citizens, to respect and promote human rights and the rule of law, to support disarmament, and have joined treaties that prohibit and provide for the elimination of other inhumane and indiscriminate weapons. Boycotting multilateral negotiations to ban the worst weapons of mass destruction and opposing the resultant international treaty, makes clear the shortfall in their sincerity and consistency to fulfill their NPT Article 6 obligation "to pursue negotiations in good faith on effective measures relating to cessation of the nuclear arms race at an early date and to nuclear disarmament."

Box 21.1 identifies measures supporting nuclear disarmament ripe for engagement of health professionals, which are relevant for the vast majority of the world's states which don't possess nuclear weapons.

Health Evidence and Global Health Partnership Played a Key Role in Achieving the Ban Treaty

Peak global health bodies have long identified the health imperative for eradication of nuclear weapons. The World Federation of Public Health Associations (WFPHA) General Assembly in 1993 recognized "that the continued existence of nuclear weapons poses an unacceptable risk to global health and the global environment," and in 1997 reaffirmed its call for the abolition of nuclear weapons.

The World Medical Association (WMA) in its Statement on Nuclear Weapons updated in 2018 "joins with others ... including the Red Cross and Red Crescent movement, International Physicians for the Prevention of Nuclear War, the International

Box 21.1 Selected measures to stigmatize, prohibit, and eliminate nuclear weapons which can be taken by the 184 UN member states without nuclear weapons

Promptly sign, ratify, or accede to, and implement the Treaty on the Prohibition of Nuclear Weapons. This includes measures to implement their treaty obligations, including through domestic law, regulation, and penal sanctions. National legislation should make it a criminal offence for anyone within their jurisdiction to engage in the development, production, testing, acquisition, stockpiling, transfer, deployment, threat of use, or use of nuclear weapons, as well as assistance, financing, encouragement, or inducement of these. They are obliged to cooperate with other states parties to facilitate implementation of the treaty, work for universal adherence of all states to the treaty and undertake feasible measures to assist the victims of nuclear use or testing and remediate environments so contaminated.

Adopt nuclear weapons-free military policies. The states which do not own nuclear weapons but claim protection from US or Russian nuclear weapons and collaborate in preparations for their possible use can adopt policies which preclude their participation in threat or use of nuclear weapons. This includes the twenty-seven non-nuclear-armed members of NATO, Australia, Japan, South Korea, Armenia and Belarus.

Adopt policies to preclude government and private investment in companies producing nuclear weapons.

End production of separated plutonium and highly enriched uranium (HEU), which can be used to build nuclear weapons. Any stocks of plutonium or HEU should where possible be eliminated or stored as securely as possible in centralized locations under international control.

Phase out nuclear power and accelerate building renewable energy systems and energy efficiency. Nuclear power in addition to its other hazards requires uranium enrichment and creates plutonium, both of which can be used for nuclear weapons.

Close or internationalize uranium enrichment plants (which can readily be used to produce HEU). Cease development of new uranium enrichment modalities (such as laser enrichment) which aggravate dangers of nuclear weapons proliferation.

Develop and deploy accelerators rather than nuclear reactors to produce radioisotopes for medical and scientific use.

Campaign to Abolish Nuclear Weapons, and a large majority of UN member states, in calling, as a mission of physicians, on all states to promptly sign, ratify or accede to, and faithfully implement the Treaty on the Prohibition of Nuclear Weapons; and Requests that all National Medical Associations join the WMA in supporting this

Declaration, ... educate the general public and to urge their respective governments to work urgently to prohibit and eliminate nuclear weapons ...."

In April 2016, International Physicians for the Prevention of Nuclear War (IPPNW), was joined by WFPHA, the WMA, and the International Council of Nurses (ICN) in submitting to a UNGA Working Group a joint Working Paper (UN General Assembly, 2016). It details the planetary health imperative to ban and eliminate nuclear weapons. This unified call by leading global health professional federations, reinforced by joint op-eds in international media and in-person testimony, proved influential in the Group recommending to the UNGA that a treaty prohibiting nuclear weapons and providing for their elimination would be the next best nuclear disarmament step the world could take. This led to the UNGA mandate for the treaty negotiations, supported by over 120 states, a voting majority of more than three to one. Every opportunity was taken to publish further op-eds and submit further joint submissions, commentaries, and working papers, and provide oral testimony to the UNGA and then the treaty negotiating conference, strongly supporting a ban treaty on public health grounds. This united and authoritative call and active engagement by the world's most prominent international health federations mattered. Key diplomats have made clear the value of these submissions, and some of the elements so proposed are reflected in the treaty text.

Responsibilities of Health Professionals in the Eradication of Nuclear Weapons

A Chatham House Research Paper by Lewis et al. (2017) describes nuclear disarmament as the missing link in multilateralism: a blind spot. They consider how in relation to many spheres of international concern and responsibility—including development, climate change, public health, humanitarian action, international law, gender issues, protection of cultural heritage, and cybersecurity—all that has been achieved toward a safer and more secure world is in jeopardy "owing to the international failure to address nuclear disarmament and non-proliferation effectively." This failure "puts everything else at risk." They argue that "all those who are concerned about the survival and the betterment of humanity need to be equally concerned about nuclear weapons and nuclear disarmament." They urge that "[p]rogress on nuclear disarmament should be factored into monitoring progress on the SDGs" (Sustainable Development Goals).

All other human achievements, progress and efforts including in health could come to naught if we do not succeed in eradicating nuclear weapons before they are again used. There is only one acceptable answer to the stark, binary choice humanity faces: will it be the end of nuclear weapons, or the end of us? Health evidence, collaboration, and advocacy helped deliver and inform the landmark UN Treaty on the Prohibition of Nuclear Weapons, and a campaign coalition initiated by a medical federation was the major civil society partner contributing to this achievement (see Case Study). These contributions continue a long and proud tradition of action by health professionals to encourage movement away from the nuclear precipice. Such work helped end nuclear test explosions in the atmosphere, and helped governments step back from the brink and end the Cold War (Helfand et al., 2016; Forrow, Ruff, & Thurlow, 2018).

Case study—The International Campaign to Abolish Nuclear Weapons (ICAN)

ICAN was born in 2006 in Melbourne, Australia, and launched in 2007, out of dismay and frustration at the continuing failure to progress nuclear disarmament, alongside the inspiration provided by the success of the International Campaign to Ban Landmines in working initially with a small number of governments of small and medium-sized countries, to achieve a treaty banning landmines five years after its formation. This occurred despite the opposition of large and powerful users and producers of these weapons, such as China, Russia, and the United States.

ICAN was founded and initially developed by the Medical Association for Prevention of War (MAPW) on behalf of and in close collaboration with the international medical federation International Physicians for the Prevention of Nuclear War (Nobel Peace Prize 1985), of which MAPW is the Australian affiliate. ICAN was conceived as an outreach and coordination vehicle for more unified work around a clear focus in the diverse civil society movement for nuclear disarmament. IPPNW took responsibility to host and build the campaign until it could flourish independently. IPPNW is now one of ten organizations comprising the ICAN International Steering Group. By mid 2021, ICAN had become a campaign coalition of 607 diverse partner organizations in 106 countries. It served as the civil society coordinator for each of the three international conferences on the humanitarian impacts of nuclear weapons (2013–2014). ICAN went on to be the main global civil society coordinating partner working with governments to achieve the Treaty on the Prohibition of Nuclear Weapons, and then for the treaty's entry into force and implementation (Ruff, 2018b).

ICAN's principles, formulated early, have served the campaign well:

- Building on the experience of the treaties banning biological and chemical weapons, landmines, and cluster munitions; a clear, compelling and simple vision—eradication of nuclear weapons through a treaty/treaties to prohibit and eliminate them;
- A flexible and organizationally simple and lean campaign coalition model, making it easy and without cost for organizations to join as partners; respectful of and building on rather than competing with or duplicating existing organizations;
- As globally inclusive as possible;
- Involving diverse people, especially including young people, whose consciousness is post-Cold War and awareness of nuclear weapons often low;

- Coordinated messages, strategies, and engaging materials to make it as easy as possible for organizations around the world to work in a cohesive way;
- Balancing horror, humor, and hope in focusing as the basis for ICAN's work on the unacceptable catastrophic humanitarian impacts of nuclear weapons and the urgent humanitarian imperative for their prohibition and elimination. Scientific including health and climate evidence and advocacy based on this evidence are thus central to ICAN's work;
- Giving prominence to the lived human experience and voices of survivors of the nuclear bombings in Japan (*hibakusha*) and nuclear test explosions worldwide;
- Working both with governments, and to mobilize the public.

A key shift in strategy emerged in 2009–2010 in recognition that there was foreseeably no prospect of success for nuclear disarmament measures which depend on nuclear-armed states, given that none of these states were (or are) currently serious about disarmament. Therefore, breaking the logjam in nuclear disarmament depends on states free from nuclear weapons. These cannot eliminate weapons they don't possess, but they could fill the "legal gap" by unequivocally making nuclear weapons illegal, if they utilized a process which could not be blocked or vetoed by nuclear-armed states or their nuclear-dependent allies. This approach is similar to that used successfully for the landmine and cluster munitions ban treaties, where negotiations (outside the UN) were led by states without the respective weapons, but was new in the nuclear field.

ICAN was awarded the Nobel Peace Prize for 2017 "for its work to draw attention to the catastrophic humanitarian consequences of any use of nuclear weapons and for its ground-breaking efforts to achieve a treaty-based prohibition of such weapons" (The Norwegian Nobel Committee, 2017).

The treaty provides a powerful new tool in the essential ongoing work to eradicate weapons which daily jeopardize our future by risking indiscriminate nuclear violence. Health evidence and advocacy by health professionals to remove this most acute existential threat to global health and survival is as vital as ever (Ruff, 2018a). Box 21.2 and Table 21.1 outline some relevant public health principles and opportunities for health action, needed both within and beyond the health sector. The tools and approaches described which helped to achieve the historic first treaty to outlaw the world's most dangerous weapons must now be built upon and extended to complete the urgent, feasible, and necessary task to eradicate nuclear weapons. Evidence, its implications, advocacy based on these, applying the lessons of history of what has worked, building broad civil society coalitions around focused goals, working effectively with enlightened governments—local, regional, and national—divestment from companies profiting from building the worst weapons of mass destruction (Snyder, 2022), persistent and dedicated health professionals thinking and acting outside the box, will all be needed to complete the task of stigmatizing, prohibiting and eliminating nuclear weapons.

Box 21.2 Some public health principles relevant to the eradication of nuclear weapons

Use evidence-based communication and advocacy in support of a clear, compelling goal

Build wide collaborations and coalitions between health professionals, and with other professions and spheres of activity

Find and nurture champions—diverse in culture, age, gender, location, expertise, natural constituencies

Give prominence to the voices and lived experience of those who have suffered most from nuclear weapons—survivors of Hiroshima and Nagasaki and nuclear test explosions worldwide

Seek to make universal vulnerability to nuclear weapons a basis for promoting nuclear weapons eradication as a shared responsibility; a necessary part of everyone/every organization's business, even if it is not their core business; and make it as easy as possible to contribute to a collective effort in a coordinated way

Norms and social acceptance or rejection of products and behavior can be influential

Legislation can be as much a step in a process as an end in itself

Use common criteria for health priorities to help overcome the continuing historic neglect of the existential threat posed by nuclear weapons:

- the magnitude of the problem/threat/consequences—for the most acute existential threat of human making to planetary health, no level of risk can be acceptable or sustainable
- the preventability of the threat
- the availability of opportunities and tools for action

Table 21.1 Selected opportunities for health professionals to progress the eradication of nuclear weapons

Field of activity	Examples of public health contributions	Opportunities for further contributions by health professionals
Building, updating, and communicating the evidence base on health impacts of nuclear weapons	Expert reports by WHO, national medical associations, the International Council of Scientific Unions, national academies of science, and other scientific bodies	Existing reports need updating and follow-up; very few have been updated since the 1980s, e.g., the last detailed WHO report on the effects of nuclear war on health and health services dates from 1987
		Urge governments and national expert bodies to examine effects on their population and region of the climatic and nutritional effects of nuclear war

(continued)

Table 21.1 Continued

		Promote understanding and action regarding the need to secure a stable and hospitable climate, by preventing runaway global heating as well as a precipitous ice age caused by nuclear war
Build collaborations among health professionals	2016–2017 joint op-eds and working papers submitted to UN Working Group on nuclear disarmament, UN General Assembly and ban treaty negotiations by International Physicians for the Prevention of Nuclear War (IPPNW), International Council of Nurses (ICN), World Federation of Public Health Associations WFPHA), and World Medical Association (WMA)	Engage additional national and international associations of health professions in policies, statements, submissions, articles, etc., and other educational and advocacy work regarding the planetary health imperative to eliminate nuclear weapons, and urging all governments to join the Treaty on the Prohibition of Nuclear Weapons
Health professional education	Extensive resources available at: http://www.ippnw.org/resources-abolition-nuclear-weapons.html; Resources on climate and famine effects of nuclear war compiled by Professor Alan Robock: http://climate.envsci.rutgers.edu/nuclear/; Medical Peace Work online courses and resources: http://www.medicalpeacework.org	Link with students to expand education about the consequences of nuclear war and the planetary health imperative to eradicate nuclear weapons as part of initial and continuing health professional education Urge health journals to correct their widespread failure to publish on and address nuclear weapons on an ongoing basis
Build wide civil society collaboration and coalitions	The founding of the International Campaign to Abolish Nuclear Weapons (ICAN) by IPPNW—see Case Study	Expanding and deepening civil society collaboration, e.g., with Red Cross/Red Crescent movement; other scientific, humanitarian, development, faith, human rights, trade union, service, environmental, social justice, and other partners
Encourage, support, and collaborate with governments joining the Treaty on the Prohibition of Nuclear Weapons and otherwise working to stigmatize, prohibit, and eliminate nuclear weapons	IPPNW contributions to the 2013–2014 international conferences on the humanitarian impacts of nuclear weapons, the 2016 UN Working Group on nuclear disarmament, and the 2017 UN conference to negotiate the nuclear weapons ban treaty	Join with the Red Cross and Red Crescent movement (Council of Delegates, 2017), IPPNW, ICN, WMA, WFPHA, and others in calling on all states to promptly sign, ratify, or accede to, and faithfully implement the Treaty on the Prohibition of Nuclear Weapons

Table 21.1 Continued

Encourage divestment of public and private institutions from companies which produce nuclear weapons	Public health evidence and advocacy for divestment from landmines and cluster munitions producers, tobacco, and fossil fuels	Use positive examples, such as those outlined by Don't Bank on The Bomb (Snyder, 2022), Quit Nukes (Australia) and Don't Bank on the Bomb Scotland to promote government funds, banks, pension funds, and other private financial institutions to divest from companies producing nuclear weapons

ICN—International Council of Nurses

IPPNW—International Physicians for the Prevention of Nuclear War

Red Cross and Red Crescent movement comprises the International Committee of the Red Cross, International Federation of Red Cross Red Crescent Societies, and 190 Red Cross Red Crescent National Societies

WMA—World Medical Association

WFPHA—World Federation of Public Health Associations

References

Council of Delegates of the International Red Cross and Red Crescent Movement. (2017). *Working towards the elimination of nuclear weapons: 2018–2021 action plan*. Resolution CD/17/R4.

Coupe, J., Bardeen, C. G., Robock, A., Toon, O. B. (2019). Nuclear winter responses to nuclear war between the United States and Russia in the Whole Atmosphere Community Climate Model Version 4 and the Goddard Institute for Space Studies ModelE. *Journal of Geophysical Research: Atmospheres, 124,* 8522–8543.

Europe Integration and Foreign Affairs Federal Ministry, Republic of Austria. (2014a). Vienna Conference on the Humanitarian Impact of Nuclear Weapons 8 to 9 December 2014 Report and Summary of Findings of the Conference, Dec 9, 2014.

Europe Integration and Foreign Affairs Federal Ministry, Republic of Austria. (2014b). "Humanitarian Pledge". Vienna Conference on the Humanitarian Impacts of Nuclear Weapons, Dec 9, 2014.

Food and Agriculture Organization of the United Nations (FAO), IFAD, UNICEF, WFP and WHO (2021). *The state of food security and nutrition in the world 2021*. Rome: Food and Agriculture Organization.

Forrow, L., Ruff, T., & Thurlow, S. (2018). The 2017 Nobel Peace Prize and the Doomsday Clock—The end of nuclear weapons or the end of us? *New England Journal of Medicine, 378,* 2258–2261.

Helfand, I. (2013). *Nuclear famine: Two billion people at risk*. Boston, MA: International Physicians for the Prevention of Nuclear War.

Helfand, I., Haines, A., Ruff, T., Kristensen, H., Lewis, P., & Mian, Z., (2016). The growing threat of nuclear war and the role of the health community. *World Medical Journal, 62*(3), 86–94.

International Panel on Fissile Materials (IPFM). (2021). *Fissile material stocks, September 4, 2021*. Retrieved from http://fissilematerials.org.

Kristensen, H. M., & Korda, M. (2021). *Status of world nuclear forces*. Federation of American Scientists. Retrieved from http://fas.org/issues/nuclear-weapons/status-world-nuclear-forces/.

Lewis, P., Unal, B., & Aghlani, S. (2017). *Nuclear disarmament. The Missing link in multilateralism*. Research Paper, updated April 2017. London: Chatham House.

Mills, M., Toon, O., Lee-Taylor, J., & Robock, A. (2015). Multi-decadal global cooling and unprecedented ozone loss following a regional nuclear conflict. *Earth's Future*, *2*, 161–176.

The Norwegian Nobel Committee. (2017). *The Nobel Peace Prize for 2017*. Oslo: The Norwegian Nobel Committee.

Ruff, T. A. (2013). The health consequences of nuclear explosions. In B. Fihn (Ed.), Unspeakable suffering—the humanitarian impact of nuclear weapons (14–27). Geneva: Reaching Critical Will, Women's International League for Peace and Freedom.

Ruff, T. A. (2017). Health implications of ionising radiation. In P. van Ness & M. Gurtov (Eds.), *Learning from Fukushima. Nuclear power in East Asia* (pp. 221–260). Acton: ANU Press.

Ruff, T. A. (2018a). The Treaty on the Prohibition of Nuclear Weapons: A planetary health good of the highest order. *Journal of Public Health Policy, 39*, 382–387.

Ruff, T. A. (2018b). Negotiating the UN Treaty on the Prohibition of Nuclear Weapons and the role of ICAN. *Global Change, Peace and Security*, *30*(2), 233–241.

Science and Security Board, Bulletin of the Atomic Scientists. (2020, January 23). It is 100 seconds to midnight. 2020 Doomsday Clock Statement, edited by John Mecklin. Chicago, IL: Bulletin of the Atomic Scientists. https://thebulletin.org/doomsday-clock/current-time/.

Snyder, S. (2022). Rejecting risk. Utrecht: PAX, ICAN. Retrieved from https://www.dontbankonthebomb.com/wp-content/uploads/2022/01/RejectingRisk-web.pdf.

Toon, O. B., Bardeen, C. G., Robock, A., Xia, L., Kristensen, H., McKinzie, M., ... Turco R. P. (2019). Rapidly expanding nuclear arsenals in Pakistan and India portend regional and global catastrophe. *Science Advances, 5*(10), eaay5478.

Toon, O. B., Robock, A., Mills, M., & Xia, L. (2017). Asia treads the nuclear path, unaware that self-assured destruction would result from nuclear war. *The Journal of Asian Studies*, *76*(2), 437–56.

Toon, O. B., Turco, R. P., Robock, A., Bardeen, C., Oman, L., Stenchikov, G. L. Atmospheric effects and societal consequences of regional scale nuclear conflicts and acts of individual nuclear terrorism. *Atmospheric Chemistry and Physics*, 2007;7,1973–2002.

United Nations General Assembly. (2016). *The health and humanitarian case for banning and eliminating nuclear weapons. Working paper A/AC.286/NGO/18, 4 May 2016*. New York, NY United Nations General Assembly.

United Nations General Assembly. (2017). Treaty on the Prohibition of Nuclear Weapons. A/CONF.229/2017/8. New York, NY United Nations General Assembly.

United Nations and World Bank. (2018). *Pathways for peace: inclusive approaches to preventing violent conflict*. Washington, DC, World Bank. 18. https://www.worldbank.org/en/topic/fragilityconflictviolence/publication/pathways-for-peace-inclusive-approaches-to-preventing-violent-conflict.

World Health Assembly. (1983). *The role of physicians and other health workers in the preservation of peace as the most significant factor for the attainment of health for all. WHA 36.28*. Geneva: World Health Organization.

World Health Organization. (1987). *Effects of nuclear war on health and health services* (2nd ed.). Geneva: World Health Organization.

22

Learning from Case Studies in Global Health

Joseph Rhatigan

What is a Case Study?

The term "case study" refers to a form of qualitative and descriptive research that examines a particular event, a specific problem, or an organization's behavior over a defined time period. Usually, a case study is written as a descriptive narrative that seeks to provide a comprehensive and objective view of the events that occurred. Methods employed for collecting data vary but often involve interviews with informants who participated in the events being examined or who have particular knowledge about them. These methods can range from open-ended discussions to structured interviews. In addition, data can also be collected through focus groups or surveys, or by examination of documents (such as emails, memos, reports, news stories) that are relevant to the case. In his seminal book on case study research, Yin defines a case study as "an empirical inquiry that investigates a contemporary phenomenon within its real world context" (Yin, 2003:13).

The author of the case study uses the data to construct a narrative that describes the events as completely as possible. Usually, the exposition of the case is separated from the analysis. For analysis, the author can offer an interpretation of the case in several ways: (i) by making claims of cause and effect within the events described, (ii) by comparing the case with other similar cases and making claims across cases, or (iii) by applying an accepted framework to the case and interpreting the case's events through this explanatory model.

Case studies are subject to all the biases that affect qualitative research. The strength of the results is dependent on how well the case author is able to establish a comprehensive and "objective" narrative description of the events in the case that avoids being unduly influenced by a particular informant's or group of informants' viewpoints or interests. If a particular event, organization, or person's behavior is interesting enough to warrant a case study, then it is likely to elicit emotions in informants that can influence their objective reporting of events. To limit this inherent bias, case authors must incorporate a range of different informants' viewpoints into their narrative and use documentation to arrive at a narrative that is consistent, plausible, and agreed upon by most observers.

While the strength of evidence generated by case studies is generally considered lower than other methods, case studies are able to examine phenomenon that elude other research methods. Case studies are useful in examining complex social phenomenon that involve multiple actors, have multiple causes, and that are context-specific. Case studies are best suited to asking questions about how and why events occurred

Joseph Rhatigan, *Learning from Case Studies in Global Health* In: *Systems Thinking for Global Health.* Edited by: Fiona Larkan, Frédérique Vallières, Hasheem Mannan, and Naonori Kodate, Oxford University Press.
DOI: 10.1093/oso/9780198799498.003.0022

and to generate hypotheses that can be tested using other methods. In addition, they promote systems thinking by integrating multiple perspectives and examining problems that are best viewed through a multidisciplinary lens.

Application to Global Health

Case studies are particularly useful tools for examining global health phenomena because of the complex, heterogeneous, and context-dependent nature of many of these phenomena. Case studies employ a systems-thinking approach to global health because they require input from multiple respondents across a variety of disciplines and positions and seek to examine the interrelationship between various causative forces. In addition, case-study writing involves examining multiple forms of evidence, including sources diverse as community members' testimony, policy documents, and technical reports. Unlike more traditional forms of inquiry in global health, such as epidemiological studies or clinical trials that seek to examine narrow questions with high reliability, case studies seek to integrate local context within larger health and social systems to examine multifactorial causation and context-dependent effects. Because of this, systems thinking is critical in accurately interpreting and analyzing case studies.

In particular, (i) policy formation and process in global health, (ii) understanding global health outbreaks and the response to them, and (iii) implementation of global health programs both internationally and within nations are domains where case studies can generate useful information.

(i) Policy formation and process in global health

How policy is crafted and implemented are questions that are commonly examined through case studies, and case studies are often the preferred way to examine these questions Policy formation involves multiple actors with competing agendas that negotiate to achieve an agreement. Case studies are able to describe these different actors, their agendas, and the strategies they employ to achieve a resolution. They are effective ways of unpacking complex health policy systems where context, content and process matter, and various actors in the middle interact and influence each other (Walt & Gilson, 1994). A well-crafted case study will demonstrate how multiple outcomes were possible give the circumstances, and it will examine how various factors contributed to result in the outcome that occurred. Policy cases are often analyzed through application of particular frameworks or models that can help elucidate behaviors of particular actors or organizations in the domains of advocacy, negotiation, and the political process of policy formation.

(ii) Disease outbreak and response

While epidemiological methods are commonly employed to investigate disease outbreaks in real time, case studies can provide useful additional data retrospectively. Epidemics are inherently social phenomenon and often are influenced by policy- and decision-making that epidemiological methods are ill-suited to capture. Outbreak response is subject to all the politics and competing agendas that policy formation comprises, and case studies can provide helpful analysis in dissecting the factors that lead to a particular response. Rarely are disease outbreak responses successful solely on the basis of technical intervention, but rather success usually hinges on mobilization of resources, political will, and community mobilization. These are all issues that case studies are able to document and explore. Case studies also provide important documentation of events that can be referenced in future disease outbreaks and responses.

(iii) Program design and implementation

Case studies are useful in understanding how global health programs are designed and implemented. Global health program implementation involves elements of strategy, design, community engagement, financing, and management that interact in complex ways. Programs are also dependent on local and national contexts which case studies can capture through their description and exposition. In understanding program implementation, case studies are able to examine complex questions. For example, a case study that sought to examine the design and implementation of a national disease control program—for example a program run by a national government to reduce the incidence of malaria—might try to answer some set of the following questions:

- What is the program trying to deliver? What are its mission and goals?
- What exactly is its value proposition (i.e., how does it explain why its activities will benefit the community/population it is serving)?
- What do the program's designers consider to be the factors that influence the burden and determinants of the disease in the population it is serving? How did they arrive at this interpretation?
- Is the program designers' interpretation of these factors accurate?
- What is the programs strategy for influencing and/or accounting for these factors? What activities does it pursue and why?
- How does the program manage these activities and measure their performance?
- How operationally effective is the program regarding key administrative functions such as finance, human resources, information management, infrastructure, and supply chain management?
- How does the program seek to improve its performance? How well does it adapt and learn?
- How does the program's leaders understand its role in relation to the healthcare system? How does the program's designers and managers view the program's ability to sustain its activities and increase its scale?

These questions show the breadth of concerns that can be addressed by case studies and how case studies can foster systems-thinking approaches to global health. In our example above, the very context-specific questions (e.g., how the program manages key activities) cannot be truly understood unless one also enquires about larger-scale issues within a biosocial framework of health and disease. To come to a comprehensive understanding of a particular health program, it is not enough simply to measure a few outputs, but rather one must also use systems thinking to investigate how the program is positioned within the larger social and healthcare system to appreciate the interrelationships between these. This will allow one to appreciate the effects of the program on the system and the effects of the system on the program.

These three types of application can all highlight complexity and how systems-level forces influence events, processes of program design, implementation strategies, and program effectiveness in global health.

Teaching Cases

Case studies, as we have discussed, are a research method used to examine some social phenomenon within the context in which it occurred. Teaching cases are similar texts but are written to be discussed in a classroom with particular learning objectives in mind. The "case method" of instruction involves the active participation of the class in analyzing a case and articulating key lessons learned. Teaching cases are designed to present experiences in a value-neutral voice so that students can draw their own conclusions about the experience; however, they are specifically framed to inspire productive classroom discussion of important issues. Everything that is presented in the cases is true; however, the cases might omit other events if they are not relevant to the educational objectives of the case. This educational method is often called "virtual-experiential learning" or "participant-centered learning," reflecting both the method's process and goals. Teaching cases are written to allow students to experience the challenges facing the featured organizations and programs through the eyes of those involved in the actual events. The goal is to encourage students to "walk in the shoes" of the protagonist. Instead of the instructor presenting information and analysis to the class that they need to learn, the students generate the "lessons" through their participation in facilitated classroom discussion. Teaching cases are effective tools to aid students in learning systems thinking in global health as they describe complex phenomenon that are not easily understood through simple notions of cause and effect. Teaching cases capture the multifactorial aspect of social phenomenon and help elucidate how outcomes are often contingent and context-dependent. They can help students learn to view causality as an ongoing process that is constantly reshaped by results that then feedback to influence other causes of different effects.

Examples of Case Studies in Global Health

One of the easiest ways to appreciate the usefulness of case studies in global health is to read one. Following are four examples of case collections that examine global health issues.

(iv) Millions saved

Millions Saved is a collection of "success stories in global health" written by the Center for Global Development that describes the impacts of eighteen different global health programs. These include Eliminating Meningitis Across Africa's Meningitis Belt; Botswana's Mass Antiretroviral Therapy Program; South Africa's Child Support Grant; Vietnam's Comprehensive Helmet Law; Indonesia's Total Sanitation and Sanitation Marketing Program; Thailand's Universal Coverage Scheme; Thailand's Campaign for Tobacco Control; Argentina's Plan Nacer; Eliminating Polio in Haiti; and Kenya's Social Cash Transfer Program. Most of the cases are detailed descriptions of how a particular program was designed and implemented with a focus on how it was able to achieve its goals.

The *Millions Saved* cases are used extensively as teaching cases as well and have been gathered into a textbook (Glassman & Temin, 2016). For further information see http://millionssaved.cgdev.org/.

Many of the cases illustrate important concepts in systems thinking. For example, the case, "Kenya's School-Based Deworming Program" traces the development of Kenya's mass deworming project from the early evidence, generated in 2001, that deworming children had positive effects not only on health but also on improved school attendance and children's growth. The case then traces how these findings were taken up by policy-makers to secure international funding to scale up the program in Kenya. A few years into the program, evidence of poor financial management led to funding of the program by international donors being withdrawn. A non-governmental organization, Deworm the World, stepped up to help improve financial management of the program and re-engage funders. The results were that the program was successfully able to scale up coverage to the entire nation. Results from an evaluation of the program showed an over 50% decrease in the number of children with worm infestations, improved school attendance for all children, and taller overall stature in children (Baird, Hicks, Kremer, & Miguel, 2016).

There are several important systems-thinking insights that the case highlights. One is the important interplay between scientific research (in discovering the effects of deworming), policy formation (in creating a plan for translating these findings into action), and political will (in securing funding and popular support for the program). Another is the collaborative successes that can be achieved when government works with the private sector and civil society organizations to scale up and manage large-scale public health programs. A third is the important intersectoral synergies that can arise between the often siloed domains of education, economic development, and health when programs work across these sectors to achieve multiple goals (improved health, better school attendance, and more vigorous human capital).

(v) Case studies-attaining SDGs

The UN Sustainable Development Goals Fund wrote a series of sixty-three case studies examining how different countries have implemented programs to attain the Sustainable Development Goals (SDGs). These cases provide well-documented examples of systems-thinking in global health as they detail large-scale, strategic programs that are designed to provide enduring progress across all the domains of the SDGs. Each case study provides a concise background of the situation, the approach taken, results of program, and a discussion of the challenges and lessons learned. Although many of the case studies do not deal with health SDGs directly, they all are written from a systems-thinking framework that tries to account for historical, political, economic, environmental, and cultural issues that programs need to navigate to be successful. These cases highlight the importance of systems thinking not only in global health but also in global development and global environmental sustainability. To access the cases, visit https://www.sdgfund.org/case-studies.

(vi) Maximizing positive synergies

From 2008 to 2009, the World Health Organization (WHO) convened the Maximizing Positive Synergies Collaborative Group made up of global health academics and civil society groups to examine the effects of global health initiatives on national health systems. The group conducted a number of case studies to investigate this question using a systems-thinking approach. The studies looked at how disease-focused initiatives, such as the US President's Emergency Program for AIDS Relief (PEPFAR), influenced the overall health system in both positive and negative ways. A paper summarizing the results was published in 2009 (World Health Organization Maximizing Positive Synergies Collaborative Group, 2009). For instance, while outcomes for target populations improved greatly, there was some evidence suggesting that other portions of the health system were weakened, such as maternal and child health programs, most likely by the loss of human capital that was redeployed to the targeted disease-control programs. The case studies that form the basis of these results can be found at http://www.who.int/healthsystems/publications/MPS_academic_case_studies_Book_01.pdf?ua=1 and at http://www.who.int/healthsystems/publications/MPS_civil_society_case_studies.pdf

(vii) Global health delivery case collection

The Global Health Delivery Case Collection is a set of forty-one teaching cases written by faculty members at Harvard University. The cases are designed to be used as educational tools to teach fundamental principles about healthcare delivery especially in low- and middle-income countries (LMICs). Written through a systems-thinking lens, these cases allow students to carefully consider the question of how epidemiology, pathophysiology, culture, economics, and politics inform the design and performance of global health programs. They are written with the goal of helping students to (i) learn the ability to analyze the design, operations, and outcomes of global healthcare programs in low-resource settings; (ii) appreciate the role of local context-specific factors such as culture, history, and politics in the design and implementation of global health programs; (iii) understand the role of strategic analysis in solving global health problems and the use of frameworks such as care delivery value chain analysis. Each case seeks to contextualize the specific program being examined within the larger historical, political, and economic forces that influence the structure and function of the health system with a focus on the interrelationship between these forces. The cases cover a large spectrum of issues in global health using country-specific examples such as improving healthcare delivery for specific conditions including HIV, tuberculosis, malaria, malnutrition, and several neglected tropical diseases; ensuring universal health coverage and access on a national scale; improving maternal and child health; increasing the effectiveness of international vaccination programs; healthcare policy development; and use of community health workers in integrated healthcare delivery systems. The entire library is available via open access at http://www.globalhealthdelivery.org/case-collection

Many of the pressing issues in global health are difficult to fully understand without adopting a systems-thinking perspective. For instance, many would agree that the issue of universal health coverage (UHC) is a leading global health issue in LMICs. This issue is often framed in narrow terms as fundamentally an economic or a political problem. However, from a systems-thinking perspective, the problem clearly extends beyond these domains. Attaining UHC will not only involve solving the political and economic issues, but will also require development of human capital, expansion and spread of healthcare facilities, creation of better information and knowledge management systems, community engagement and empowerment to demand higher-quality health services, mitigation of environmental impacts, and improved physical infrastructure such as electrification and roads. A systems-thinking approach to UHC, which is sorely lacking in many contemporary discussions of this issue, would acknowledge that all these domains need to be addressed and the interrelationships between them understood before UHC becomes more than a series of empty commitments that lacks a robust health system to deliver on those promises.

Case studies are particularly helpful in applying a systems-thinking approach to UHC as they allow detailed comparisons between the path to UHC that different nations have embarked on. They can elucidate the different strategies these countries have adopted and describe the differences between the strategic frameworks that each country has used. As more nations make commitments to UHC, case studies will help illuminate best practices from successful countries that can be disseminated to help struggling countries improve.

Conclusion: Case Studies as Systems Thinking

This chapter explored how case studies are helpful in applying systems thinking to global health research and education. It examined how case studies are created and what kind of questions they seek to elucidate. It discussed how case studies can bring a systems-thinking approach to issues in global health such as global health policy formation, disease outbreak and response, and program design and implementation. It also described the use of teaching cases that can help foster systems thinking in examining myriad issues in global health. The chapter concluded with some examples of teaching case series that educators can freely access and adopt for use in various educational programs.

References

Baird, S., Hicks, J. H., Kremer, M., & Miguel, E. (2016). Worms at work: Long-run impacts of a child health investment, *The Quarterly Journal of Economics, 131*(4), 1637–1680. Retrieved from https://doi.org/10.1093/qje/qjw022.

Glassman, A., & Temin, M. (2016). *Millions saved: new cases of proven success in global health.* Washington, DC: Center for Global Development.

Walt G. I., & Gilson, L. (1994). Reforming the health sector in developing countries: the central role of policy analysis. *Health Policy & Planning, Dec;9*(4), 353–370.

World Health Organization Maximizing Positive Synergies Collaborative Group. (2009). An assessment of interactions between global health initiatives and country health systems. *The Lancet, 373,* 2137–2169.

Yin, R. K. (2003). *Case study research: Design and methods* (3rd ed.). London: Sage. Pg13.

23

Statelessness, the Right to Health, Policy, and Case Law

The Potential Role of Feminist Development Education and the Campaign for Universal Birth Registration

Patricia Erasmus

Healthcare and Exclusion

The right to healthcare is a vital component of human dignity and a human right which should transcend considerations of documentation or legal status. A person who is unable to access healthcare because of their legal status in a country faces a form of discrimination which not only places their lives in direct risk if they are denied medical assistance but also increases the spaces in which non-nationals are made to feel unwelcome and unworthy. Kingston, Cohen, and Morley (2010) describe this type of exclusion as being denied "medical citizenship." When policies and laws draw lines in the sand between who is worthy of medical treatment and who is not, this is the quintessential "othering" of the group being denied their rights.

A stateless person is someone who is not a national of any country (Hanley, 2014), who has no identity in the legal sense. They are a "legal ghost," unable to prove who they are and unable to call on any country to protect their rights as a citizen. They belong to nobody, and no country belongs to them. Their very existence is fraught with unimaginable difficulty and uncertainty. Legal status or nationality is the key to accessing rights such as education, health, housing, and welfare (Fullerton, 2015). Even travelling, finding employment, and getting married is impossible without an identity (De Chickera and Whiteman, 2014). One only has to consider how many activities in our daily lives ask us to prove who we are before we can access a particular service to understand the obstacles stateless people confront when they cannot fulfil this condition in any country in the world, for any activity. Wherever they do manage to settle, they will always be outsiders and legal nobodies. One imagines a stowaway on a ship, yet the ship in this analogy may be the person's country of residence, connection, and affiliation.

Statelessness may be persecutory and deliberate. One thinks of the millions of people in India having their nationality revoked suddenly by a "citizenship list" or the Rohingya people in Myanmar being deliberately denied nationality rights as part of mass-targeted human rights atrocities and alienation (Balazo, 2015). Statelessness may also be arbitrary (where laws are simply inadequate to deal with anomalous situations and leave people without remedy) or it may be caused by laws which discriminate

Patricia Erasmus, *Statelessness, the Right to Health, Policy, and Case Law* In: *Systems Thinking for Global Health.* Edited by: Fiona Larkan, Frédérique Vallières, Hasheem Mannan, and Naonori Kodate, Oxford University Press.
DOI: 10.1093/oso/9780198799498.003.0023

along gender lines (e.g., by preventing a mother from passing her nationality to her child) or by historic divisions rooted in colonial policies of cultural division. In this chapter, we will focus on statelessness which is caused by a very specific cause: a lack of access to (or a lack of awareness about) birth registration.

Birth registration is hugely important, especially in the context of healthcare, and this chapter will discuss how increasing access to birth registration has the potential not only to improve the quality and availability of healthcare to registered people but also to go some way toward reducing the number of people who are stateless and are therefore denied all their rights in addition to healthcare. Birth registration is therefore a mechanism which serves multiple purposes. The symbiosis between increasing access to healthcare services (such as better documented vaccination schedules, tracking of milestones, and development and other benefits) and statelessness eradication in a specific but surprisingly large group of affected people is an exciting opportunity to alleviate human suffering.

Stateless people are an extremely marginalized group (Baluarte, 2015) whose vulnerability is often exacerbated by policies which make it impossible to regularize their documentation and condemns them to a life of living in the shadows, never legally settled, never legally entitled to the most basic elements of human existence—including, devastatingly, healthcare. The impact of becoming stateless also permeates down generations. If a mother has no nationality to pass onto her child, or if discriminatory laws prevent the maternal passing of nationality to a child, whole families will become stateless and the tragic denial of rights and dignity continues (Edwards & Van Waas, 2014).

Against that background, this chapter will consider that development education has a powerful role to play in furthering global equality and fostering a sense of global citizenship. It has vast potential to explore and amplify feminist and gender empowerment themes in meaningful ways to achieve global solidarity and awareness of gender-based inequalities which impact on health and human rights negatively. Statelessness in Africa, when it is caused by inadequate access to (or knowledge about) birth registration mechanisms, is an issue linked to the feminization of poverty, the cycle of poverty, and inequality. Crucial in overcoming this type of statelessness is education, both of a frontline community and grassroots nature in Africa, and also, it will be suggested, in the context of feminist development education in the Global North. A feminist pedagogy in education is a necessary approach to further achieve global equality and it is an approach which in essence resists hierarchical structures, uses experiences as a valuable resource, and opens the possibility for transformative learning (Lawrence, 2016). Issues of identity and difference can be authentically approached through a feminist approach to learning (Macdonald and Sánchez-Casal, 2002). The inclusion of men in the conversation is a vital part of the success of feminist pedagogy (Flood, 2011) as well as creating room for learning which is safe and embraces all views and experiences (Kishimoto & Mwangi, 2009).

Feminist development education has the potential to be an innovative tool for furthering our understanding of the interconnected nature of rights, policies, and practices that result cumulatively in the exclusion of people generally (Lawrence, 2016) and in this context, specifically stateless people from healthcare. This approach will allow for a systems-thinking approach toward enabling birth registration as a dual-pronged mechanism for the alleviation of some forms of statelessness and an increase in access to (among other rights) healthcare.

Before dealing with the rather niche scenario of statelessness when it is caused by a lack of birth registration, it might be helpful to paint in broad strokes the environment in which migrants attempt to access healthcare in general terms. Using South Africa as a case study, a couple of points are pertinent. First, xenophobic attacks have been a devastating part of the lived realities of non-nationals in South Africa and have in many cases been fueled by the words and conduct of politicians and influential leaders who adopt a rhetoric of "othering" and scapegoating. Non-nationals are blamed for all manner of societal ills (see generally Piper & Charman, 2016), including "stealing" jobs and healthcare resources from locals. This unfortunately translates into non-nationals being treated differently and often being excluded from healthcare services, either by the attitudes of frontline staff or by policy decisions (Crush & Tawodzera, 2013).

Three cases I have dealt with at Lawyers for Human Rights (a non-governmental legal organization working to protect the rights of vulnerable communities) stick out to demonstrate the exclusion which non-nationals face on a daily basis in South Africa. The first concerns a young Somali child who was denied access to life-saving heart surgery on the basis that her asylum application was not yet processed (she had collapsed immediately upon arriving in the country) and she was therefore undocumented. It took approaching the High Court to force the Department of Health to treat her and save her life, despite doctors being willing to perform the procedure but being curtailed from doing so by hospital policy (Dadi Patel, 2014).

The second case deals with widespread maternal and child healthcare abuses. In our consultations around the country with numerous migrant women, we were told stories of mothers in labor being denied access to hospital to give birth, babies being born in toilets, or even outside in the road, and xenophobic language being used during birth. One specific example struck me: when a young mother was in the height of labor pain and let out a cry, she was slapped and pinched by nurses and told to go back home and stop having so many babies here. Similar experiences are well documented by Human Rights Watch (2011) in their damning report entitled *Stop making excuses: Accountability for maternal health care in South Africa*, which highlights not only systemic human rights abuses in maternal health but an additional layer of suffering for migrant women.

The third case deals with a man who died outside our refugee legal advice clinic because he was refused kidney dialysis in circumstances where he would have survived if he had received it. The reason for his refusal was that the policy in place stated that kidney dialysis was only available to people who were eligible for transplants (Erasmus, 2015). The transplant policy stated that refugees and asylum seekers were ineligible for transplants and the knock-on effect was his undignified death in a van outside my office. I have also had to sit before a dying Ethiopian woman, with her sister sitting next to me offering to donate her kidney and explain to her that even in the presence of a willing donor, her sister (as an asylum seeker) would be ineligible for a transplant and would die because of her documentation status.

It is a harsh and brutal landscape where policy and law collide to divide and exclude humans from healthcare that would save their life. This is the sobering reality we must bear in mind when discussing stateless people whose lack of documentation may quite literally be a death sentence. There are many causes of statelessness which will not be addressed by the approach suggested in this chapter, for example laws which discriminate against women passing their nationality down to their children, or policies of citizenship discrimination such as those occurring in India and Myanmar. Those causes of statelessness must be addressed through diplomatic pressure for policy change and, where appropriate, litigation. In this chapter, we will focus on birth registration, aware of its limitations as a strategy but also fully embracing the idea that even one life saved is a noble aim.

Statelessness—Definitions, Causes, Prevalence, and Impact

Individual cases of statelessness demonstrate the stark realities of exclusion from legal recognition and identity. A child denied access to life-saving healthcare appears to be an act of unimaginable cruelty. Investigating the cause of an act which appears so impossibly callous often reveals that these individual accounts of human suffering occur because of broader policies and laws which exclude groups of people in an exercise of "othering." Systems thinking is a valuable way to approach understanding statelessness and its impact on healthcare because although the suffering is individual, the causes are systemic. According to the Convention Relating to the Status of Stateless Persons (1954), a stateless person is "a person who is not considered as a national by any State under the operation of its law." It is well recognized that a person may either be born stateless or they may become stateless by some other act (United Nations High Commissioner for Refugees, 2019). The consequence is the same: a stateless person may not call him/herself a national of any country and is therefore unable to avail him/herself of the ordinary benefits which stem from nationality, such as access to basic services and socio-economic rights (Manly & Persaud, 2009).

It is also interesting to note that when determining whether a person is stateless or not, the investigation must not focus exclusively on the law. Indeed, the inquiry needs to be informed by both law and fact. For example, in the case where a person meets the requirements for nationality under a particular legal system but is in fact not regarded/treated as a national by a certain state, that person is nonetheless stateless (United Nations High Commissioner for Refugees, 2019). This means that a distinction may be drawn between what is known as *de jure* statelessness and *de facto* statelessness (Milbrandt, 2014).

A useful definition of a "national" was included in the judgement of *Liechtenstein v. Guatemala [1955] ICJ 1* where the International Court of Justice described nationality thus:

> [a]ccording to the practice of States, to arbitral and judicial decisions and to the opinion of writers, nationality is a legal bond having as its basis a social fact of attachment, a genuine connection of existence, interest and sentiments, together with the existence of reciprocal rights and duties.

While the exact number of stateless individuals is not known, the UNHCR estimates there to be, conservatively, at least 10 million people. Some of the consequences of statelessness are identified in the "IBelong" campaign and include barriers to access to basic rights including freedom of movement, education, healthcare, work, banking, access to property, and the ability to even get married (United Nations High Commissioner for Refugees, 2019).

Mutegi (2016) notes that the lack of access to legal identification has the worst impact on rural populations, the vulnerable (such as women) and children. Problems such as accessing property rights and accessing financial services are identified. Mutegi also highlights the specific struggles that lack of identification may have for children—namely exclusion from healthcare, vaccination schemes, and education. These obstacles will be exacerbated in the already marginalized and vulnerable population group of children in Africa and so even a perfunctory consideration of the impact of statelessness provides robust justification for the investigation of the most effective way to formulate a response to statelessness eradication. In fact, the Citizenship Rights Initiative in Africa (CRAI) describes the impact of statelessness on access to basic rights as "devastating" (CRAI, 2019). Manby (2016) also notes the vulnerability of stateless persons in Africa in her comprehensive overview of citizenship in Africa. The link between the denial of socio-economic rights such as healthcare and education and the continuation of the cycle of poverty is well documented (Swanepoel & De Beer, 2006), providing further underpinning justification for the relevance of intervention strategies. Once again, the fact that "othering" occurs through the exclusion of certain groups is compelling reason to employ systems thinking and try to get to the bottom of what systems are in place which continue the cycle of "othering" and what systems-based approaches might be effective in breaking into the cycle and bringing relief and dignity to those marginalized groups whose very existence is under threat due to their non-recognition.

Hussein (2009: 20) has suggested that "stateless people become less than fully human and are reduced to mere targets of humanitarian assistance." More sinister consequences of statelessness are also identified by Manby (2016) when she highlights that stateless persons are more likely to be victims of human rights abuses and that statelessness contributes to intercommunity, ethnic, and racial tensions. This, in a continent already ravaged along arbitrary geographic, ethnic, religious, and cultural lines established by the legacy of colonialism, should be of particular concern (see Mamdani, 1996; Lefebvre, 2011).

(i) Causes of statelessness

The global causes of statelessness vary from region to region and indeed from state to state within those regions. This has been sharply demonstrated by the jurisprudence emerging from regional human rights tribunals/bodies in different regions. Bialosky (2015) notes, for example, that the Inter-American system has focused largely on the deprivation of nationality whereas European jurisprudence has focused largely on the right to access nationality and Africa has often dealt with nationality in the situation of expulsion. Regardless of differing approaches and opinions, Bialosky notes that nationality is recognized as a fundamental right. Statelessness obviously places this fundamental right in serious jeopardy (Blitz & Lynch, 2011).

The African Commission for Human and Peoples' Rights (2015: 3) notes with regret that:

> the right to nationality, described as a "fundamental human right", is not really protected in Africa, for reasons including the arbitrary denial or deprivation of the nationality of persons on grounds of race, ethnicity, language, religion, gender discrimination, non-compliance with the rules on the prevention of statelessness pursuant to transfers of territory between States, and the failure of many African States to ensure that all children are systematically registered at birth.

The United Nations High Commissioner for Refugees (2019) identifies some of the broader categories of the causes of statelessness as gaps in nationality laws, intercountry movement, establishment of new states or movement of borders, and loss/deprivation of nationality (including for persecutory goals).

The African situation bears unique scrutiny and causes of statelessness in the African context do not always mirror those which present themselves globally. The African Commission on Human and Peoples' Rights (2015) captures some of the causes of statelessness in Africa as *inter alia* the legacy of colonialism, migration of populations, a lack of state borders, discrimination along gender/ethnic/racial lines, nomadic lifestyles, barriers to movement, persecutory withdrawal or denial of nationality, and a lack of adequate laws within states to deal with stateless persons.

It also bears mentioning at the outset that the causes and impact of statelessness will naturally differ from country to country and Africa cannot be treated with a level of generality that would prevent the individual circumstances of each country from being addressed. The benefits of addressing the situation continentally though will be evident in the discussion around universal birth registration.

(ii) The special rights of children

Although there may be room for academic and political debate about the precise status of broad nationality rights in international law generally, there is compelling reason to treat the specific rights of children to nationality differently for a number of reasons. In the first instance, Article 7 of the 1989 Convention on the Rights of the Child provides that a child "shall be registered immediately after birth and shall have the right from birth to a name, the right to acquire a nationality and as far as possible, the right to know and be cared for by his or her parents" and states are also obliged, in terms of Article 7, to "ensure the implementation of these rights in accordance with their national law and their obligations under the relevant international instruments in this field, in particular where the child would otherwise be stateless."

African children's "double disadvantage" is also an important contextual factor: first, they are disadvantaged by virtue of their status as children and secondly, they are disadvantaged by living on a continent where human rights abuses are more likely to happen to them (Assefa, 2014). It is crucially important to be mindful of the special place children's rights have in the international legal order (Sloth-Nielsen, 2016). Much reliance should be placed on the special positioning children have in international law (such as the UN Convention on the Rights of the Child, 1989 and the African Charter on the Rights and Welfare of the Child, 1990) when formulating responses to the scourge of statelessness in African children. Indeed the "best interests of the child" principle has been recognized as a "general/cross-cutting" principle on the continent (Fokala & Chenwi, 2014). The Open Society Justice Initiative (2016) has noted the particular importance of the Convention on the Rights of the Child since all but two states have ratified it. The African Charter on the Rights and Welfare of the African Child confirms the specific right to a nationality for children.

Birth Registration and Advocacy

Recognizing the value of systems thinking in approaching statelessness eradication as a method of increasing access to healthcare for those who are excluded due to their lack of legal identity, what strategies might form a vital role in changing existing systems to be more inclusive? We will now consider both advocacy movements and development education as means of increasing awareness about and access to birth registration.

The United Nations Children's Fund (UNICEF) (2016) estimates that approximately 230 million children (under five) have not had their births officially registered and approximately 290 million are without birth certificates. UNICEF (2016) explains its strategies for birth registration include legal reform, state policy reform, registration strategy assistance, building of capacity, raising of awareness/advocacy, integration of birth registration (e.g., into health or education services), community registration campaigns, and technology and innovation as tools (e.g., online systems/SMS).

It is evident that there is some overlap and consistency in the approaches. Plan International (2016) reports that its campaign to promote birth registration has resulted in the registration of approximately 40 million children since 2005 and has contributed to law reform in ten countries.

In addition, numerous grassroots projects advocate for awareness around birth registration and the vindication of stateless persons' rights. Litigation has been used successfully on the continent in a number of cases to secure access to nationality rights for stateless persons. This public interest litigation is a form of advocacy in itself, given the generation of interest surrounding it. This chapter suggests in summary that the body of literature points to a very clear picture: advocacy and awareness is not the holy grail but are vital tools to be used in the eradication of statelessness caused by a lack of birth registration awareness or mechanisms. The literature also suggests that the expansion of advocacy projects which seek to enlighten communities, governments, and policymakers about the importance of birth registration must be encouraged.

Development Education and Feminism

On the face of it, it may appear that statelessness (especially when caused by inadequate birth registration in Africa) is an issue too far away, too remote, and too unconnected to the European experience to warrant inclusion in Global North development education initiatives. Indeed, it will be seen from the discussion which follows that statelessness, although disturbingly common globally, is caused by very different factors in different regions. For example, in Europe, inadequate access to birth registration is not as large a contributing factor to statelessness as it is in Africa. Why then is it important to include this apparently remote issue on the development education agenda in Europe?

First, it will be seen that systems thinking and highlighting issues of inequality, human rights, and injustice fit within the goals and purposes of development education generally. And secondly, it will be seen that development education aims to foster responsible global citizenship and solidarity and to spark change globally by recognizing inequality and injustice where it occurs and working toward sustainability (IDEA, 2019).

Statelessness is a major (and possibly lesser known) cause of inequality and injustice and the fostering of global solidarity and awareness about this fits within the goals and potential of development education initiatives. Thirdly, it will be seen that statelessness is linked to ideas about the feminization of poverty, especially when it is linked to the mostly mother-initiated task of birth registration. This provides compelling justification for its inclusion in feminist education, especially feminist development education.

Daly, Regan, & Regan (2017: 12) adopt a helpful working definition of development education: "Development education is directly concerned with the educational policies, strategies and processes around issues of human development, human rights and sustainability (and immediately related areas)."

The Irish Development Education Association (IDEA, 2019) captures the very character of development education in saying on its website:

> Development Education works to tackle the root causes of injustice and inequality, globally and locally. The world we live in is unequal, rapidly changing and often unjust. Our everyday lives are affected by global forces. Development Education is about understanding those forces and how to change them to create a more just and sustainable future for everyone.

Statelessness in Africa is a highly appropriate topic to incorporate into development education initiatives precisely because statelessness in Africa is a massive cause of inequality and injustice. Statelessness causes suffering on a major scale within some of the most vulnerable populations in the world. It also has a direct impact on gender disempowerment in Africa and for those reasons it is an important issue of global justice and inequality.

IDEA (2019) divides the goals of development education into values, knowledge, skills, and actions. More specifically about values, it notes that development education "aims to bring about positive change, informed by values of equality, diversity, sustainability and human rights and responsibilities." Regarding knowledge, they note that "it explores cultural, environmental, economic, political and social relationships and challenges local and global power inequalities caused by patterns of production, distribution and consumption." Relating to skills, they say "it equips people to explore multiple perspectives and critically engage with local and global issues, using participative and creative approaches." And finally, in relation to actions, it notes that "it enables people to make connections between their own lives and global justice issues, and empowers them to make a positive difference in the world." These themes and goals resonate with discussions about statelessness and the resultant hardship it creates, and the inequality which causes it and also is perpetuated by it. The very dignity and survival of a stateless person is at stake and there can be no greater call to action for global justice and empowerment than that.

The importance of solidarity in feminist movements is well established (Sweetman, 2013) and recognizing the innate power of every global citizen to advocate for and create change is a crucial aspect of the systems thinking needed to deconstruct inequality wherever it arises.

Birth registration is primarily a mother-initiated exercise and steps taken to improve access to birth registration mechanisms are vital to meaningful gender empowerment. Therefore, advocacy and awareness campaigns in Africa and complementary discussions and advocacy in the Global North have huge potential to spark change globally.

Statelessness creates a situation where rights cannot be vindicated and this occurs (in the present discussion) where birth registration cannot occur, either due to a lack of availability of adequate birth registration mechanisms or due to lack of awareness of the importance of birth registration. In either situation, the risk of the continuation of the cycle of poverty is increased. Theories about the feminization of poverty are helpful ways of understanding why this matters so much from a gender perspective. Regan (2012) notes that "feminization of poverty" is generally used to mean three distinct things: "That women have a higher incidence of poverty than men", "that their poverty is more severe than that of men" and "that there is a trend toward a greater poverty among women, particularly associated with rising rates of female headed households."

Regan (2012) also notes that the feminization of poverty means that "women face more barriers to lifting themselves out of poverty," "female-headed households are considered to be the poorest of the poor," and "women are prone to suffering more persistent or longer-term poverty than men." This captures intuitively what we already know. Women are more likely to be poor and more likely to be unable to extricate themselves from the poverty cycle. When the poverty cycle is being perpetuated by statelessness and this is being caused frequently by the failure to register births (which is primarily a mother-initiated task), it is an inevitable conclusion that gender empowerment in the arena of birth registration is of crucial importance from a human rights and feminist perspective.

This chapter is therefore suggesting that in addition to justifying the role out of advocacy and educational campaigns (among vulnerable communities, policy-makers, and the donor/philanthropic community) in Africa, all of these issues also contain the potential to be rich springboards for robust feminist discussions in the context of development education in the Global North.

There is a growing trend of activism in favor of universal birth registration and the idea finds support across sectors. It is not only role players in the field of statelessness who find the concept appealing, but medical professionals too (Comandini et al., 2016; Abouzahr & de Savigny, 2015).

There can be no illusion that this idea would be the magical and singular solution to statelessness. At best, this idea could be part of multifaceted approach which is needed to address statelessness (Achmad, 2015). It is against this background that this chapter now turns to the birth registration inquiry and what role, if any, should a strategy of universal or regional birth registration play in statelessness eradication? While it may seem obvious that birth registration will assist to eradicate statelessness, especially since it has been recognized as such a large contributing factor to the prevalence of statelessness in African children (Baquele, 2005), some points warrant further reflection.

Heap and Cody (2009) advocate for universal birth registration with the following cogent justifications: that birth registration is essential to prove legal identity; birth registration is essential for protection of rights and reducing the possibility of child abuse and exploitation, especially in the case of separated children; the UN Convention on the Rights of the Child recognizes children's right to a nationality and compel states to register children immediately after birth. The UN Convention on the Rights of the Child also compels states to give a child born in that state citizenship if they are not recognized as a citizen of another country; and that despite international law imperatives, an estimated 51 million children are not registered at birth per year.

When analyzing why this shockingly high number of children are not registered at birth every year, the authors proffer the following reasons: a lack of awareness among parents; cost and time involved in registration processes; the availability of/distance to a registration facility; doubt about whether a child will survive or not; political unrest; legal barriers; social barriers; cultural barriers; and fear of persecution by authorities.

The authors also point to the very harsh reality that in countries and families besieged by HIV/AIDS and poverty, birth registration is not high on the list of priorities. The fact that children often die young is also a tragic fact which impacts on the number of children who will ultimately be registered (since parents may not see the point).

The potential value of increasing awareness within communities, governmental bodies and policy makers in Africa cannot be overstated. Similarly, recognizing the urgency of gender empowerment initiatives when the consequences of a lack of birth registration are so dire provides strong justification for the incorporation of this cross-cutting feminist issue onto the global agenda and specifically into discussions happening in development education settings.

Conclusion

Policies, laws, and practices which exclude people from accessing healthcare based on the status of their documentation are egregious threats to human dignity. Using systems thinking to tackle the question of how policies and laws view some people as worthy and some as unworthy exposes the very rhetoric which we need to counter in the strongest terms. Statelessness is a human rights issue, obviously not specific to women since any person may find themselves stateless. This chapter has suggested that there is practical sense in approaching statelessness specifically caused by a lack of birth registration as an issue of feminist importance, given the primarily mother-initiated process of registration of births. It has been suggested that there is strong justification for including this topic on the feminist discussion agenda in the Global North, especially in the context of development education initiatives. What may appear to be a remote and fringe issue is in fact an issue of global gender empowerment and solidarity, something which resonates with the broad goals of development education and movements for the sparking of change. Of particular interest is the movement advocating for universal birth registration as a mechanism to break down the perpetual cycle of poverty and the feminization of poverty.

References

Abouzahr, C., & de Savigny, D. (2015). Towards universal civil registration and vital statistics systems: The time is now. *The Lancet, 386*(10001), 1407–1418.

Achmad, C. (2015). Combating statelessness. *New Zealand International Review, 40*(1), 22–26.

Adam Hussein, A. (2009). Kenyan Nubians: Standing up to statelessness. *Forced Migration Review, 32*, 19–20.

African Charter on Human and People's Rights, 1981.

African Charter on the Rights and Welfare of the Child, 1990.

African Commission on Human and Peoples' Rights. (2015) The Right to Nationality in Africa (ACHPR)

Assefa, A. (2014). Advancing children's rights in Africa: The role of the African Children's Charter and Its Monitoring Body. *Mekelle University Law Journal, 2*(1), 66–101.

Balazo, P. (2015). Truth & rights: Statelessness, human rights, and the Rohingya. *Undercurrent, 11*(1), 6–15.

Baluarte, D. (2015). Life after Limbo: Stateless persons in the United States and the role of international protection in achieving a legal solution. *Georgetown Immigration Law Journal, 29*(3), 351–390.

Baquele, A. (2005). Universal birth registration: The challenge in Africa. *The African Child Policy Forum, 1*(1), 1–25.

Bialosky, J. (2015). Regional protection of the right to a nationality. *Cardozo Journal of International & Comparative Law, 24*(1), 153–192.

Blitz, B., & Lynch, M. (2011). *Statelessness and citizenship: A comparative study on the benefits of nationality*. London: Edward Elgar.

Citizenship Rights Africa. (2019). *Statelessness: Citizenship rights in Africa initiative*. Retrieved from http://citizenshiprightsafrica.org/theme/statelessness.

Comandini, O., Cabras, S., & Marini, E. (2016). Birth registration and child undernutrition in sub-Saharan Africa. *Public Health Nutrition, 19*(10), 1757–1767.

Convention Relating to the Status of Stateless Persons, 1954.

Crush, J., & Tawodzera, G. (2013). Medical xenophobia and Zimbabwean migrant access to public health services in South Africa. *Journal of Ethnic and Migration Studies, 40*(4), 655–670.

Dadi Patel, A. (2014). *Court orders treatment for gravely ill Somali girl*. The Daily Vox. Retrieved from https://www.thedailyvox.co.za/update-court-orders-treatment-for-gravely-ill-somali-girl/.

Daly, T., Regan, C., & Regan, C. (2019). *Developmenteducation.ie*. Retrieved from https://developmenteducation.ie/app/uploads/2017/11/Learning-to-Change-the-World-DE-Resources-Audit-2017-web.pdf.

De Chickera, A., & Whiteman, J. (2014). Discrimination and the human security of stateless people. *Forced Migration Review, 46*, 56–59. Refugee Studies Centre, University of Oxford.

Edwards, A., & Van Waas, L. (2014) *Nationality and statelessness under international law*. Cambridge: Cambridge University Press.

Erasmus, P. (2015). *Dying for a transplant*. Thoughtleader.co.za. Retrieved from https://thoughtleader.co.za/dying-for-a-transplant/

Flood, M. (2011) Men as students and teachers of feminist scholarship. *Men and Masculinities, 14*(2), 135–154.

Fokala, E., & Chenwi, L. (2014) Statelessness and rights: Protecting the rights of Nubian children in Kenya through the African Children's Committee. *African Journal of Legal Studies, 2*(2), 357–374.

Fullerton, M. (2015). Comparative perspectives on statelessness and persecution. *Kansas Law Review, 16*(4), 863–902.

Hanley, W. (2014). Statelessness: An invisible theme in the history of international law. *European Journal of International Law, 25*(1), 321–327.

Heap, S., & Cody, C. (2009). The universal birth registration campaign. *Forced Migration Review, 4*(32), 20–23.

Human Rights Watch. (2011). *Stop making excuses: Accountability for maternal health care in South Africa*. Human Rights Watch. Retrieved from https://reliefweb.int/sites/reliefweb.int/files/resources/Full_Report_2004.pdf.

The Irish Development Education Association. (2019). *Development education the Irish Development Education Association (IDEA)*. Retrieved from https://www.ideaonline.ie/development-education.

Kingston, L. N., Cohen, E. F., & Morley, C. P. (2010). Debate: Limitations on universality: the" right to health" and the necessity of legal nationality. *BMC International Health and Human Rights, 10*(1), 11. https://doi.org/10.1186/1472-698X-10-11

Kishimoto, K., & Mwangi, M. (2009) Critiquing the rhetoric of "safety" in feminist pedagogy: Women of color offering an account of ourselves. *Feminist Teacher, 19*, 2, 87–102.

Lawrence, E. (2016). *Feminist pedagogy*. Genderandeducation.com. Retrieved from http://www.genderandeducation.com/issues/feminist-pedagogy/.

Lefebvre, C. (2011). We have tailored Africa: French colonialism and the "artificiality" of Africa's borders in the interwar period. *French Geography, Cartography and Colonialism, 37*(2), 191–202.

Liechtenstein v. Guatemala [1955] ICJ 1

Macdonald, A. A., & Sánchez-Casal, S. (2002). *Twenty-first-century feminist classrooms: Pedagogies of identity and difference*. New York, NY: Palgrave Macmillan.

Mamdani, M. (1996). *Citizen and subject: contemporary Africa and the legacy of late colonialism*. Princeton, NJ: Princeton University Press.

Manby, B. (2016). *Citizenship law in Africa: A comparative study*. Cape Town: African Minds. Retrieved from https://www.refworld.org/docid/56a77ffe4.html.

Manly, M., & Persaud, S. (2009). UNHCR and responses to statelessness. *Forced Migration Review, 32*, 7–10.

Milbrandt, J. (2014). Adopting the stateless. *Brooklyn Journal of International Law, 39*(2), 694–793.

Mutegi, L. (2016). *Africa: Mobile technology could be the answer to unlocking digital identity for Africa*. All Africa. Retrieved from https://allafrica.com/stories/201608011383.html.

Open Society Justice Initiative. (2016). *Open Society Justice Initiative: Children's Right to a Nationality*. Geneva: Office of the United Nations High Commissioner for Human Rights. Retrieved from http://www.ohchr.org/Documents/Issues/Women/WRGS/RelatedMatters/OtherEntities/OSJIChildrenNationalityFactsheet.pdf.

Piper, L., & Charman, A. (2016). Xenophobia, price competition and violence in the spaza sector in South Africa. *African Human Mobility Review, 2*(1), 332–362.

PLAN. (2016). *Birth registration.* Plan International. Retrieved from https://plan-international.org/birth-registration#.

Regan, C. (2012). *Women & development—DevelopmentEducation.ie.* Retrieved from https://developmenteducation.ie/feature/women-development/.

Sloth-Nielsen, J. (2016). *Children's rights in Africa: A legal perspective.* London: Routledge.

Swanepoel, H., & De Beer, F. (2006). *Community development: Breaking the cycle of poverty* (4th ed.) South Africa, Cape Town: Juta and Co.

Sweetman, C. (2013). Introduction, feminist solidarity and collective action. *Gender & Development, 21*(2), 217–229.

United Nations. (1961). UN Convention on the Reduction of Statelessness, 1961. New York, NY: United Nations.

United Nations. (1989). UN Convention on the Rights of the Child, 1989. New York, NY: United Nations.

United Nations Children's Fund. (2016). *Child protection from violence, exploitation and abuse: Birth registration.* New York, NY: United Nations Children's Fund. Retrieved from http://www.unicef.org/protection/57929_58010.html.

United Nations High Commissioner for Refugees. (2019). *Ending statelessness.* Geneva: United Nations High Commissioner for Refugees. Retrieved from https://www.unhcr.org/en-ie/ending-statelessness.html.

(1948). Universal Declaration on Human Rights, 1948.

24
Systems Thinking to Combat Malaria
A Literature Review of Building Blocks

Savyasachee Jha and Anjula Gurtoo

Introduction

Malaria is one of the best known and most widely understood mosquito-borne illnesses. Africa bears a disproportionate burden of malarial patients as well as deaths, with nearly 212 million cases of Malaria occurring in 2018 causing around 380,000 deaths (World Health Organization, 2015). Malaria gets linked with the burden of poverty as well, with an estimated loss of around $12 billion in Africa due to lost tourism, productivity, and additional health expenditure (Greenwood, Bojang, Whitty, & Targett, 2005; Worrall, Basu, & Hanson, 2005). The World Health Organization (WHO) has taken cognizance of the fact and undertaken to create consistent, constantly updating strategies for combating malaria (World Health Organization, 2015). However, despite numerous attempts at control and elimination, the disease remains a threat in developing nations.

The WHO systems-thinking framework (detailed in Chapter 1) forms the basis for evaluating most of these interventions. The framework goes beyond the doctor–patient paradigm and defines a health system as encompassing "all organizations, people and actions whose primary intent is to promote, restore or maintain health." The framework consists of six building blocks, namely service delivery, workforce, information systems, medical technologies (including access to medicines and vaccines, henceforth referred to as access to medical technologies), financing, and leadership and governance. Using a systems-thinking approach, the framework aims for a deep understanding of linkages and interactions between the various parts of a health system (de Savigny, Adam, Alliance for Health Policy and Systems Research, & World Health Organization, 2009).

Many disease control and elimination programs have traditionally been described as "vertical" programs, labeled as such due to their independence from other programs for health provisions (henceforth referred to as health systems). For example, India's National AIDS Control Programme is a typical "vertical" program. On the other hand, the Revised National Tuberculosis Control and the National Vector Borne Disease Control Programmes are well-integrated into India's national health services. These are referred as "diagonal" programs because while they have their own funding and leadership/governance structures, the programs share management and resources with other disease eradication programs (Rao, Ramani, Hazarika, & George, 2014).

Savyasachee Jha and Anjula Gurtoo, *Systems Thinking to Combat Malaria* In: *Systems Thinking for Global Health.* Edited by: Fiona Larkan, Frédérique Vallières, Hasheem Mannan, and Naonori Kodate, Oxford University Press.
DOI: 10.1093/oso/9780198799498.003.0024

In this chapter, we review literature on malaria interventions and categorize them using the six building blocks of the WHO framework. We also review some frameworks deviating from the standard set by the WHO which have incorporated systems thinking in their approach. Previously published literature reviews (Atkinson, Vallely, A., Fitzgerald, Whittaker, & Tanner, 2011; Rao, Schellenberg, & Ghani, 2013; Ray & Tilak, 2017) have not given weightage to the systems awareness of programs or interventions. Throughout this chapter, we attempt to highlight gaps and oversights in existing anti-malarial interventions and their effects on health systems.

Methodology

A qualitative review of literature mentioning systems thinking in the context of malaria intervention was conducted. Systems thinking refers to an approach of targeting parts of a health system while being aware of the effect of this intervention on other parts. This definition is similar to the one used by the WHO (de Savigny et al., 2009). However, no effort was made to restrict the search to studies explicitly using the WHO systems-thinking framework in order to find alternate concepts and frameworks. The PubMed, Scopus, and Web of Science databases were searched. A search strategy using key words (Box 24.1) was developed for PubMed and then applied to other databases. The search identified 3,826 studies which were sorted as given in Figure 24.1.

The review focused on original research. Thus, reviews and expert opinions were excluded from the analysis, and workshop and conference studies were included. The search was restricted to articles written in English and was not restricted to any geographical area. Cross-country case studies were included. There were no further filters for study design. The studies were then subjected to a title and keyword analysis and further shortlisted by abstract screening. Finally, full-text screening was performed to identify studies relevant for the chapter. Figure 24.2 illustrates the selection plan. The study had to satisfy one of the following criteria for inclusion in the review:

1. Discuss the effect of an anti-malarial intervention on one or more health subsystem as defined by the WHO with respect to strengthening the local or national health system.
2. Explore the relationship between two or more different building blocks of the health system as defined by the WHO framework in the context of malaria intervention.
3. Propose, use, or evaluate an anti-malaria intervention using a framework that utilizes systems thinking, but defined a health system and its parts differently from the WHO.

Box 24.1 Keywords used for review

((Systems Thinking) OR (Health Systems)) AND ((Mosquitoes) OR (Malaria)) NOT (Dengue) NOT (Chikungunya)

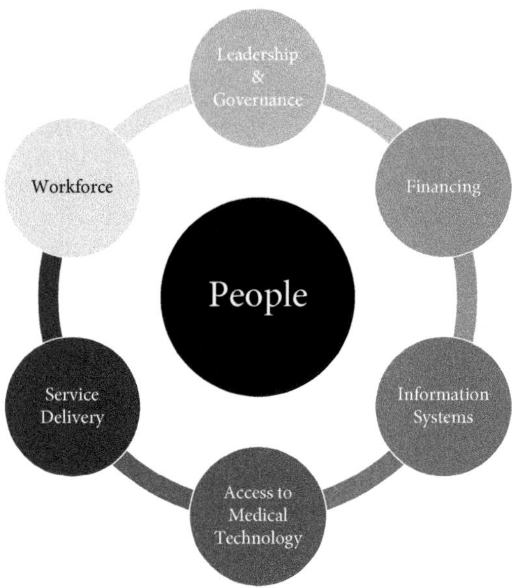

Figure 24.1 The WHO's health system building blocks

Adapted with permission from de Savigny, D., Adam, T., Alliance for Health Policy and Systems Research, & World Health Organization (Eds.). (2009). *Systems thinking for health systems strengthening. Alliance for Health Policy and Systems Research.* Geneva: World Health Organization.

Table 24.1 presents the final list of papers reviewed. Thirty-nine papers fall within the building blocks specified by WHO. Five papers describe systems-thinking frameworks which differ from the WHO framework.

Review of Building Blocks: An Evaluation Focus

This section explores the effects of anti-malaria interventions upon the six building blocks of healthcare systems as identified by the WHO with an emphasis on

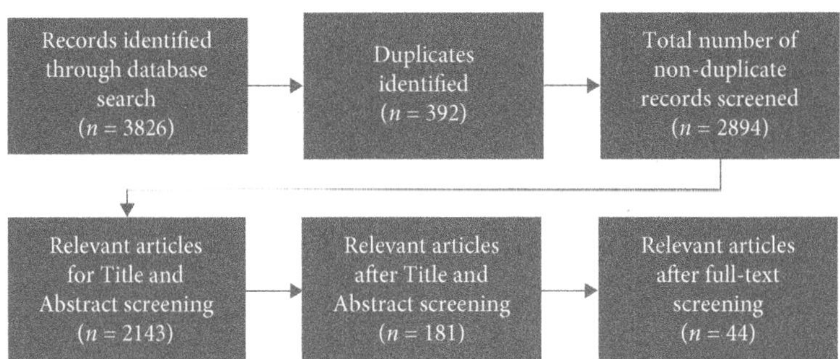

Figure 24.2 Process of identifying relevant studies

Table 24.1 Reviewed papers working with WHO framework building blocks

Paper	Countries/Regions	Building Blocks considered
Abdelgader et al. (2012)	Sudan	Access to Medical Technologies
Asale et al. (2019)	Ethiopia	Access to Medical Technologies
Beisel et al. (2016)	Uganda, Tanzania, Sierra Leone	Access to Medical Technologies
Berthe et al. (2019)	Malawi	Access to Medical Technologies
Boyce et al. (2015)	Uganda	Access to Medical Technologies
Chandler et al. (2010)	Ghana	Workforce
de Savigny et al. (2012)	Ghana, Tanzania	Access to Medical Technologies, Financing
Evans et al. (1997)	Gambia	Service Delivery, Financing
Fan et al. (2017)	Worldwide (111 countries)	Financing (Global Fund health system investments)
Febir et al. (2015)	Ghana	Access to Medical Technologies, Workforce
Guyant et al. (2015)	The African continent, The Greater Mekong subregion, India	Governance and Leadership
Hanvoravongchai et al. (2010)	Thailand	Financing
Heerdegen et al. (2020)	Ghana	Governance and Leadership
Hetzel et al. (2014)	Papua New Guinea	Workforce, Information Systems, Governance and Leadership
Kivumbi et al. (2004)	Uganda	Financing, Leadership and Community Response
Koenker et al. (2013)	Tanzania	Access to Medical Technologies
Kroeger et al. (2002)	Colombia	Workforce, Financing, Governance and Leadership
Lal et al. (2015)	Uganda	Workforce
Macharia et al. (2017)	Kenya	Access to Medical Technologies
McLean et al. (2018)	Myanmar	Workforce
Minja et al. (2001)	Tanzania	Access to Medical Technologies, Financing
Mukonka et al. (2015)	Zambia	Access to Medical Technologies, Information Systems, Workforce
Murhandarwati et al. (2015)	Indonesia	Access to Medical Technologies, Financing
Mwendera et al. (2019)	Malawi	Governance and Leadership
Nabyonga Orem et al. (2013)	Uganda	Workforce
Okell et al. (2012)	The African Continent	Access to Medical Technologies
Pradhan et al. (2019)	India	Service Delivery, Workforce, Information Systems, Governance and Leadership

(continued)

Table 24.1 Continued

Paper	Countries/Regions	Building Blocks considered
Rao et al. (2013b)	Tanzania	Service Delivery
Rao et al. (2014)	India	Service Delivery, Governance and Leadership
Roman et al. (2014)	Malawi, Senegal, Zambia	Workforce, Information Systems, Financing, Governance and Leadership
Rosewell et al. (2017)	Papua New Guinea	Financing
Rowe et al. (2007)	Kenya	Workforce
Sahu et al. (2020)	Worldwide (105 countries)	Service Delivery, Information Systems, Governance and Leadership
Salje et al. (2016)	Bangladesh	Information Systems
Sarriot et al. (2015)	Rwanda	Workforce, Governance and Leadership
Semwanga et al. (2016)	Uganda	Governance and Leadership
Umlauf and Park (2018)	Uganda	Access to Medical Technologies
Warren et al. (2013)	N/A	Financing (Global Fund health system investments)
Webster et al. (2018)	Indonesia	Service Delivery, Workforce, Governance and Leadership

understanding the effects of increased diagonalization, that is integration with existing health systems.

(i) Service delivery

Literature on service delivery tends to look at hard-to-reach areas (de Savigny et al., 2012; Koenker et al., 2013; Webster et al., 2018) These areas present distinct challenges which precipitate a cycle of limited access to malaria services, which leads to areas becoming hotspots and therefore requiring resource-intensive care and services (Pradhan et al., 2019). Improving access, thus, is a point highlighted by several studies.

In addressing this, national governments (e.g., Tanzania, Ghana, Indonesia) have implemented various strategies such as utilizing existing vaccine distribution channels, government subsidy for distribution through other channels, social marketing, and cost-sharing with private players (Evans, Azene, & Kirigia, 1997). In 2012, Indonesia introduced a single screening system for pregnant women which included malaria testing during the first antenatal visit to a clinic (Webster et al., 2018). These strategies demonstrate the importance of increased integration between disease-specific programs and the wider health system.

Working with onsite doctors and nurses, instead of hiring new ones, has also been positively correlated with success in malaria control (Rao et al., 2014), allowing for optimal resource utilization without creating parallel leadership structures. Sahu, Tediosi, Noor, Aponte, and Fink (2020) modelled data between 2000 and 2016 from 105 countries and found a positive correlation between anti-malaria coverage and measles immunization, tuberculosis treatment success, insecticide-treated bed net coverage, cases of children with fever, and malaria surveillance, demonstrating the need for anti-malaria interventions to become diagonal.

(ii) Workforce

Community health workers are the backbone of a successful health strategy, especially in areas with unreliable public healthcare services (Sarriot et al., 2015). The positive role of appropriately trained community health workers in treating childhood respiratory tract and diarrheal infections has been demonstrated previously by Rowe et al. (2007). Lal et al. (2015) highlight the same for endemic malaria as well. The case in point can be found in a study performed in Myanmar, where the remit of community health workers was expanded beyond malaria testing and treatment to general healthcare service delivery, leading to higher uptake of their services (McLean et al., 2018).

Literature demonstrates that targeted training of health workers leads to several benefits. When trained healthcare workers are directed toward distributing anti-malaria drugs for children, quick access to healthcare can be achieved (Nabyonga Orem, Mugisha, Okui, Musango, & Kirigia, 2013). Furthermore, the formation and use of trained community health worker groups may produce better results in terms of awareness and education (Roman et al., 2014). Chandler, Whitty, and Ansah (2010) found existing conceptualizations of malaria risk and diagnosis worked as impediments to introducing new rapid diagnostic testing (RDT) kits due to the inadequate knowledge and awareness of health workers. Formal mechanisms for learning, for example classes, lectures, and group discussions, were emphasized by the authors. Evidence shows that while horizontal integration of the workforce within the health system ought to be a goal, the need for training healthcare workers in a targeted manner, typical of a vertical program, is still required.

Unfortunately, structural issues linked to the relationship between health workers and financial incentives tend to hinder workforce effectiveness (Kroeger, Ordoñez-Gonzalez, & Aviña, 2002; McLean et al., 2018). Results-based financing can produce perverse effects including gaming of the system and introduction of unwanted dependencies. At the same time, conditional cash transfers can yield positive outcomes such as an increase in the uptake of certain services (Oxman & Fretheim, 2009). These relationships ought to be analyzed more deeply on a case-by-case basis.

(iii) Information systems

Provision of effective healthcare requires the availability of relevant and reliable data (Sahu et al., 2020). Early diagnosis through surveillance reduces the duration of sickness and prevents its escalation to a more severe stage (Pradhan et al., 2019), thereby reducing the burden on other subsystems. However, this requires highly trained staff who are willing to go out into the field and supervise field workers (Hetzel et al., 2014), which implies greater investment in training. Furthermore, the literature highlights the lack of a proper health management system which leads to deficiencies in surveillance. Limited integration of disease-specific surveillance systems with an existing health information system tends to reduce the effectiveness of local and national policy formulation (Pradhan et al., 2019).

Population data is gathered through programs of mass screening as well. Mass screening data has immediate actionability as reliable raw data (Pradhan et al., 2019). For example, Salje et al. (2016) demonstrate viral spread being driven by transmissions between neighboring households in Bangladesh. The transmission remains largely unaffected by the use of mosquito coils and occurs during summers. These data can be used by information systems for maintaining stocks and preparedness. However, lack of integration among various data collection programs into a formal information management system limits potential impact.

(iv) Access to medical technologies

The availability of artemisinin combined therapy (ACT), RDTs, and insecticide-treated nets (ITNs) have significantly enhanced the effectiveness of a country's anti-malaria response (Umlauf & Park, 2018). However, access to medicine and support infrastructure impacts effectiveness. For example, Abdelgader et al. (2012), in their discussion on the National Malaria Strategic Plan (2007–2012) of Sudan, highlight that replacing chloroquine monotherapy with ACT led to suboptimal availability of second-level treatments.

Introduction of RDTs in Uganda led to improvements in clinical measures and outcomes as well as a significant reduction in antibiotic prescription levels (Boyce et al., 2015). Unfortunately, RDTs require robust infrastructure and systems-level support for effective functioning (Beisel, Umlauf, Hutchinson, & Chandler, 2016). Furthermore, frequent stockouts impact effective implementation (Febir et al., 2015; Mukonka et al., 2015).

ITNs, the most well-known population-facing therapy, have been deployed in countries like Tanzania, Ghana (Minja et al., 2001; de Savigny et al., 2012; Febir et al., 2015), Malawi (Berthe et al., 2019), Kenya (Macharia, Odera, Snow, & Noor, 2017), and Indonesia (Murhandarwati et al., 2015). Tanzania provides a sterling example of achieving 100% coverage with ITNs and has built on its success through a continuous distribution system (Koenker et al., 2013). Other countries have been less successful. Berthe et al. (2019) describe the difficulties faced by poverty-stricken families and the sale of ITNs for food and their use in fishing. Asale, Kussa, Girma, Mbogo, and Mutero (2019) point out the reluctance to spend money on repairs to damaged ITNs. Modelling various ITN delivery strategies shows that targeted antenatal care is an effective way of reducing malaria deaths (Okell, Paintain, Webster, Hanson, & Lines, 2012) in poverty-stricken areas, highlighting the need for diagonal integration.

(v) Financing

Financial incentives like vouchers and discount coupons are a popular means of influencing public sentiment toward malaria prevention over cure. Tanzania and Ghana, for example, have integrated vouchers with ITNs. Tanzania took an integrated approach by working with both private and public players, thereby creating a diagonal program. The same scheme did not work as effectively in Ghana because of improper stakeholder management, half-hearted implementation of the voucher strategy, and a lack of integration into the wider public health system (de Savigny et al., 2012).

Governments have tried various decentralized financing mechanisms such as public–private partnerships and subsidies (Evans et al., 1997). Unfortunately, financial decentralization led to long and cumbersome bureaucratic processes in Uganda and increased corruption (Kivumbi, Nangendo, & Ndyabahika, 2004). Columbia's experience also showed that replacing centralized systems with decentralized ones can lead to slower service delivery (Kroeger et al., 2002).

A number of governments depend upon donor support (Roman et al., 2014). A prominent donor is the Global Fund to Fight AIDS, Tuberculosis and Malaria (Fan et al., 2017; Roman et al., 2014). Fan et al. (2017) found TB-related strengthening as the greatest benefactor of the fund, followed by HIV and malaria. Regardless, the authors suggest further tweaking of the Global Fund because countries often improve on variables which can be easily reported, ignoring other significant variables. For example, many indicators used by the Global Fund measure number of health workers hired or their training, not their distribution or retention (Fan et al., 2017).

Warren, Wyss, Shakarishvili, Atun, and de Savigny (2013) found mixed impact of the Global Fund on the health system in Thailand. While the fund led to expansion of the health system to previously uncovered populations, organizational conflicts and motivational problems limited the impact (Hanvoravongchai, Warakamin, & Coker, 2010). Furthermore, parallel health information systems set up in Cambodia, Uganda, and Cameroon by the Global Fund undermined existing information systems and increased transaction costs (Rosewell et al., 2017; Warren et al., 2013), further highlighting inefficiencies in vertically designed programs.

(vi) Governance and leadership

Lack of governmental commitment tends to result in uneven and patchy implementations of policy (Mwendera et al., 2019). Pradhan et al. (2019) found that political support from the health secretary, good leadership at the state level, and support from national-level vector control programs resulted in a decline in the malaria burden of the Indian state of Odisha between 2013 and 2018. Government commitment also plays a large role in quality control (Roman et al., 2014; Sarriot et al., 2015).

The Population Movement Framework in Cambodia is an example of malaria elimination through community involvement (Guyant et al., 2015). However, community responses require effective leadership and the implementation manager forms an essential component of the exercise (Roman et al., 2014). The implementation manager's skill in communication, organization, and teamwork had a positive effect on the performance of a region (Heerdegen, Aikins, Amon, Agyemang, & Wyss, 2020).

Reliable transport (air, sea, and land) and a stable law and order situation are important requirements as well (Hetzel et al., 2014). Political interference and nepotism, though not specific to health systems, can cause mismanagement (Kroeger et al., 2002). The involvement of civil society and journalists has been proposed as a counterbalance to this (Mwendera et al., 2019). Creating targeted programs may also increase patient confidence and perception of good governance (Rao et al., 2014), with the downside of creating purely vertical interventions. The formation of worker cooperatives in Rwanda is a unique example of solving this issue. These cooperatives generate their own income and also receive donor funds, making them resistent to political pressure (Sarriot et al., 2015).

Alternative Frameworks for Malaria Intervention

In this section we evaluate three anti-malaria frameworks which differ from the WHO systems-thinking framework.

(i) The roll back malaria framework

This framework is tailored specifically toward malaria management and built around variables for measuring malarial load, while the WHO framework was devised for designing and evaluating a wider variety of interventions. In contrast, this framework has wider scope within the context of malaria and incorporates a broader range of contextual factors such as environment, climate, poverty levels, and various macroeconomic factors in addition to the building blocks of the WHO model (Rowe et al., 2007; Yé et al., 2017; Ashton, Prosnitz, Andrada, Herrera, & Yé, 2020).

The Roll Back Malaria Monitoring and Evaluation Reference Group is a global platform comprising various community health worker groups and malaria researchers. The group created a series of recommendations predating the WHO's latest report on systems thinking by a couple of years in the context of the Millennium Development Goals 2005. The framework may be summarized thus: "If intervention coverage increases, anaemia prevalence decreases, and malaria-associated mortality decreases, then malaria control efforts would reduce malaria-associated mortality" (Rowe et al., 2007).

Yé et al. (2017) expanded the framework using past experiences in designing the evaluation criteria for malaria control. The authors introduce systems thinking by including causal inferences and listing fifteen indicators for assessing malaria control scale-up, ranging from the prevalence of insecticide-treated nets in households to the proportion of households with children receiving treatment using first-line anti-malarial drugs.

Other papers making use of this system emphasizes the need for high-quality surveillance data for evaluation. Ashton et al. (2020) modified the framework to separate evaluation into process and impact. The authors suggest the use of process evaluation in a low transmission setting first, which can then be used to assess the requirement for a detailed impact assessment.

(ii) Loop analysis for evaluation of malaria control initiatives

The Loop Analysis framework by Yasuoka, Jimba, and Levins (2014) does not have equivalents of all six WHO subsystems. Instead, it starts with the assumption of current malaria control relying heavily on a one-size-fits-all approach rather than tailor-made interventions taking local contexts into account. The framework defines seven loop diagrams namely, source reduction, insecticide/larvicide use, biological control, treatment with antimalarials, ITNs, non-chemical personal protection measures, and educational intervention. These loops have some differences from the WHO framework as this framework considers an unwanted side effect of any chemical intervention. For example, the biological control loop includes the introduction of larvivorous fish for reducing mosquito larvae population, and the insecticide and larvicide loop takes predator–prey relationships into account so as to not disturb the natural balance of an ecosystem.

This framework utilizes malaria-specific variables such as biting rate, predators for mosquito larvae, predators for mosquito adults, etc., which supports easier understanding of the relationship between medical technologies and their outcomes. For example, it points out that both ITNs and larvicides/insecticides show similar effects for managing the spread of insecticide resistance, yet many studies advocate using both together (Kleinschmidt et al., 2009; Okumu & Moore, 2011; Fullman, Burstein, Lim, Medlin, & Gakidou, 2013;). However, financing, governance, and service delivery are not part of this framework, and therefore are not considered (Yasuoka et al., 2014).

(iii) Integrated risk and vulnerability assessment framework for climate change and malaria transmission

Onyango, Sahin, Awiti, Chu, and Mackey (2016) have created an integrated framework to examine the role of systemic factors that can cause stress to an area or community. It stands in contrast to the WHO framework as it discusses the interrelation between systems at similar levels, namely the health system and climate, and thus defines variables differently. For example, risk of malaria infection can be identified as a climate-related hazard, influenced by climate variability and land-use change. Further, infection vulnerability is determined by genetic susceptibility, biological susceptibility, and community and individual preparedness as well. The integration of factors outside of the typical health system allows for comprehensive assessment of impacts on a community and their preparedness to cope.

Thirty-six variables (twenty-one biophysical and fifteen socio-economic) are identified and a causal loop diagram created between them. The framework divides them into influential, relay, dependent, and autonomous variables. Twenty-five of them are used to create the main diagram, out of which four variables, namely agriculture, air temperature, average rainfall, and El Niño were found to be influential variables and three of them (vector biting, vector abundance, and vector infection rate) were classified as dependent variables. The rest were all found to be autonomous (Onyango et al., 2016).

Discussion

The WHO's systems-thinking model highlights the codification of years of study into health systems. Infectious disease programs for vector-borne diseases such as malaria are gradually incorporating systems thinking and thus influencing health systems in turn. Our review indicates that the transition from a purely vertical intervention to a diagonal one requires concerted effort and a deliberate desire to enhance integration for which the WHO framework is a major step forward. However, some major gaps and oversights remain.

1. Digitization has the potential to increase transparency and visibility of fund utilization and management for funding agencies. It also has the potential to ease resource management and reduce stockouts of essential medicines and supplies. More research is required in this area.
2. Lack of trained healthcare personnel and educated supervisors remains a concern. The presence of community health workers as first-line staff moderates the lack of adequate doctors and nurses. While team-building exercises and extending the scientific knowledge of health workers has begun to be explored, the effect of local superstitions and religious beliefs on the effectiveness of community health workers and consequently their effect on service delivery needs to be investigated.
3. Managing finance emerges as a critical part of governance. Efforts at decentralization of finance have not always led to favorable outcomes. Are long and bureaucratic procedures in decentralized financial systems justifiable, considering time-sensitive programs such as malaria control? Are stringent financial regulations, where donors decide on the characteristics of the funding, practical? These questions need to be addressed through further research and discussion.

Other frameworks exist for evaluation of systems-level interventions. There are some overlaps with the WHO's but the alternative frameworks naturally place a greater focus on malarial interventions, and therefore have malaria-specific variables.

The long-term merit of all these frameworks remains open for debate. Some points of concern are highlighted here.

1. The WHO framework should incorporate other variables such as population movement, climate change-led health changes, and cultural practices. The intersection between socio-economic factors, environmental factors, and biological factors has been aptly demonstrated by many studies. Some examples include drug misuse, inadequate knowledge of disease control, myths and superstitions at the household level, female education, and population density (Wandiga et al., 2010; Dickin & Schuster-Wallace, 2014; Lyth & Holbrook, 2015).

2. Vertical programs need to evolve into diagonal ones. The use of systems thinking to battle malaria can yield many synergistic gains in a diagonally integrated health system. There are two key advantages. First, failure of the program will not compromise the fight against a disease because the requisite expertise still exists in the system. Second, the integration of vertical programs into health systems has demonstrated increased performance, better resource utilization, and more efficient leadership.
3. Most frameworks are designed for output evaluation. A forward-looking framework should incorporate process, outcome, and impact evaluation.

Conclusion

The use of systems thinking in designing malaria interventions has gained widespread acceptance by the WHO as well as national governments. The data suggest that strengthening service delivery, medical workforce training, information systems, access to medical technologies, financing, and governance can lead to synergetic effects across a health system. Malarial interventions have historically started off as "vertical" interventions which were deliberately removed from the health systems of the countries at which they were targeted and are now being reintegrated into these systems, becoming "diagonal" programs.

While the WHO framework is the most commonly used paradigm for health system evaluation, other frameworks also exist. Regardless of the framework used for evaluation, health systems with efficient and integrated building blocks are positively correlated with a successful malaria strategy. Utilizing systems thinking to evaluate the effect of an intervention on a health system has the potential to understand them more analytically, and thus provide the ability to better design them in the future. The importance of strengthening health systems holistically cannot be emphasized enough.

References

Abdelgader, T. M., Ibrahim, A. M., Elmardi, K. A., Githinji, S., Zurovac, D., Snow, R. W., & Noor, A. M. (2012). Progress towards implementation of ACT malaria case-management in public health facilities in the Republic of Sudan: A cluster-sample survey. *BMC Public Health, 12*, 11. Retrieved from https://doi.org/10.1186/1471-2458-12-11

Asale, A., Kussa, D., Girma, M., Mbogo, C., & Mutero, C. M. (2019). Community based integrated vector management for malaria control: Lessons from three years' experience (2016–2018) in Botor-Tolay district, southwestern Ethiopia. *BMC Public Health, 19*, 1318. Retrieved from https://doi.org/10.1186/s12889-019-7606-3

Ashton, R.A., Prosnitz, D., Andrada, A., Herrera, S., & Yé, Y. (2020). Evaluating malaria programmes in moderate- and low-transmission settings: Practical ways to generate robust evidence. *Malaria Journal, 19*, 75. Retrieved from https://doi.org/10.1186/s12936-020-03158-z

Atkinson, J.-A., Vallely, A., Fitzgerald, L., Whittaker, M., & Tanner, M. (2011). The architecture and effect of participation: A systematic review of community participation for communicable disease control and elimination. Implications for malaria elimination. *Malaria Journal, 10,* 225. Retrieved from https://doi.org/10.1186/1475-2875-10-225

Beisel, U., Umlauf, R., Hutchinson, E., & Chandler, C. I. R. (2016). The complexities of simple technologies: Re-imagining the role of rapid diagnostic tests in malaria control efforts. *Malaria Journal, 15,* 64. Retrieved from https://doi.org/10.1186/s12936-016-1083-2

Berthe, S., Harvey, S. A., Lynch, M., Koenker, H., Jumbe, V., Kaunda-Khangamwa, B., & Mathanga, D. P. (2019). Poverty and food security: Drivers of insecticide-treated mosquito net misuse in Malawi. *Malaria Journal, 18,* 320. Retrieved from https://doi.org/10.1186/s12936-019-2952-2

Boyce, R. M., Muiru, A., Reyes, R., Ntaro, M., Mulogo, E., Matte, M., & Siedner, M. J. (2015). Impact of rapid diagnostic tests for the diagnosis and treatment of malaria at a peripheral health facility in Western Uganda: An interrupted time series analysis. *Malaria Journal, 14,* 203. Retrieved from https://doi.org/10.1186/s12936-015-0725-0

Chandler, C. I. R., Whitty, C. J. M., & Ansah, E. K. (2010). How can malaria rapid diagnostic tests achieve their potential? A qualitative study of a trial at health facilities in Ghana. *Malaria Journal, 9,* 95. Retrieved from https://doi.org/10.1186/1475-2875-9-95

de Savigny, D., Adam, T., Alliance for Health Policy and Systems Research, & World Health Organization (Eds.). (2009). *Systems thinking for health systems strengthening. Alliance for Health Policy and Systems Research.* Geneva: World Health Organization.

de Savigny, D., Webster, J., Agyepong, I. A., Mwita, A., Bart-Plange, C., Baffoe-Wilmot, A., ... Lengeler, C. (2012). Introducing vouchers for malaria prevention in Ghana and Tanzania: Context and adoption of innovation in health systems. *Health Policy Planning, 27*(Suppl 4), iv32–43. Retrieved from https://doi.org/10.1093/heapol/czs087

Dickin, S. K., & Schuster-Wallace, C. J. (2014). Assessing changing vulnerability to dengue in northeastern Brazil using a water-associated disease index approach. *Global Environmental Change, 29,* 155–164. Retrieved from https://doi.org/10.1016/j.gloenvcha.2014.09.007

Evans, D. B., Azene, G., & Kirigia, J. (1997). Should governments subsidize the use of insecticide-impregnated mosquito nets in Africa? Implications of a cost-effectiveness analysis. *Health Policy Planning, 12,* 107–114. Retrieved from https://doi.org/10.1093/heapol/12.2.107

Fan, V. Y., Tsai, F.-J. J., Shroff, Z. C., Nakahara, B., Vargha, N., & Weathers, S. (2017). Dedicated health systems strengthening of the Global Fund to Fight AIDS, Tuberculosis, and Malaria: An analysis of grants. *International Health, 9,* 50–57. Retrieved from https://doi.org/10.1093/inthealth/ihw055

Febir, L. G., Baiden, F. E., Agula, J., Delimini, R. K., Akpalu, B., Tivura, M., ... Webster, J. (2015). Implementation of the integrated management of childhood illness with parasitological diagnosis of malaria in rural Ghana: Health worker perceptions. *Malaria Journal, 14,* 174. Retrieved from https://doi.org/10.1186/s12936-015-0699-y

Fullman, N., Burstein, R., Lim, S. S., Medlin, C., & Gakidou, E. (2013). Nets, spray or both? The effectiveness of insecticide-treated nets and indoor residual spraying in reducing malaria morbidity and child mortality in sub-Saharan Africa. *Malaria Journal, 12,* 62. Retrieved from https://doi.org/10.1186/1475-2875-12-62

Greenwood, B. M., Bojang, K., Whitty, C. J., & Targett, G. A. (2005). Malaria. *The Lancet 365,* 1487–1498. Retrieved from https://doi.org/10.1016/S0140-6736(05)66420-3

Guyant, P., Corbel, V., Guérin, P. J., Lautissier, A., Nosten, F., Boyer, S., ... White, N. (2015). Past and new challenges for malaria control and elimination: The role of operational research for innovation in designing interventions. *Malaria Journal, 14,* 279. Retrieved from https://doi.org/10.1186/s12936-015-0802-4

Hanvoravongchai, P., Warakamin, B., & Coker, R. (2010). Critical interactions between Global Fund-supported programmes and health systems: A case study in Thailand. *Health Policy Planning 25*, i53–i57. Retrieved from https://doi.org/10.1093/heapol/czq059

Heerdegen, A. C. S., Aikins, M., Amon, S., Agyemang, S. A., & Wyss, K. (2020). Managerial capacity among district health managers and its association with district performance: A comparative descriptive study of six districts in the Eastern Region of Ghana. *PloS One, 15*, e0227974. Retrieved from https://doi.org/10.1371/journal.pone.0227974

Hetzel, M. W., Pulford, J., Maraga, S., Barnadas, C., Reimer, L. J., Tavul, L., ... Mueller, I. (2014). Evaluation of the Global Fund-supported National Malaria Control Program in Papua New Guinea, 2009–2014. *Papua New Guinea Medical Journal, 57*, 7–29.

Kivumbi, G. W., Nangendo, F., & Ndyabahika, B. R. (2004). Financial management systems under decentralization and their effect on malaria control in Uganda. *International Journal of Health Planning and Management, 19*, S117–S131. Retrieved from https://doi.org/10.1002/hpm.773

Kleinschmidt, I., Schwabe, C., Shiva, M., Segura, J. L., Sima, V., Mabunda, S. J. A., & Coleman, M. (2009). Combining indoor residual spraying and insecticide-treated net interventions. *American Journal of Tropical Medicine and Hygiene, 81*, 519–524.

Koenker, H. M., Yukich, J. O., Mkindi, A., Mandike, R., Brown, N., Kilian, A., & Lengeler, C. (2013). Analysing and recommending options for maintaining universal coverage with long-lasting insecticidal nets: The case of Tanzania in 2011. *Malaria Journal, 12*, 150. Retrieved from https://doi.org/10.1186/1475-2875-12-150

Kroeger, A., Ordoñez-Gonzalez, J., & Aviña, A.I. (2002). Malaria control reinvented: Health sector reform and strategy development in Colombia. *Tropical Medicine and International Health, 7*, 450–458. Retrieved from https://doi.org/10.1046/j.1365-3156.2002.00876.x

Lal, S., Ndyomugenyi, R., Alexander, N. D., Lagarde, M., Paintain, L., Magnussen, P., ... Clarke, S. E. (2015). Health facility utilisation changes during the introduction of community case management of malaria in South Western Uganda: An interrupted time series approach. *PloS One, 10*, e0137448. Retrieved from https://doi.org/10.1371/journal.pone.0137448

Lyth, A., & Holbrook, N. J. (2015). Assessing an indirect health implication of a changing climate: Ross River Virus in a temperate island state. *Climate Risk Management, 10*, 77–94. Retrieved from https://doi.org/10.1016/j.crm.2015.06.004

Macharia, P. M., Odera, P. A., Snow, R. W., & Noor, A. M. (2017). Spatial models for the rational allocation of routinely distributed bed nets to public health facilities in Western Kenya. *Malaria Journal, 16*, 367. Retrieved from https://doi.org/10.1186/s12936-017-2009-3

McLean, A. R. D., Wai, H. P., Thu, A. M., Khant, Z. S., Indrasuta, C., Ashley, E. A., ... Smithuis, F. M. (2018). Malaria elimination in remote communities requires integration of malaria control activities into general health care: An observational study and interrupted time series analysis in Myanmar. *BMC Medicine, 16*, 183. Retrieved from https://doi.org/10.1186/s12916-018-1172-x

Minja, H., Schellenberg, J. A., Mukasa, O., Nathan, R., Abdulla, S., Mponda, H., Tanner, M., Lengeler, C., & Obrist, B. (2001). Introducing insecticide-treated nets in the Kilombero Valley, Tanzania: The relevance of local knowledge and practice for an Information, Education and Communication (IEC) campaign. *Tropical Medicine & International Health, 6*(8), 614–623.

Mukonka, V. M., Chanda, E., Kamuliwo, M., Elbadry, M. A., Wamulume, P. K., Mwanza-Ingwe, M., ... Haque, U. (2015). Diagnostic approaches to malaria in Zambia, 2009–2014. *Geospatial Health, 10*, 63–68. Retrieved from https://doi.org/10.4081/gh.2015.330

Murhandarwati, E. E. H., Fuad, A., Wijayanti, M. A., Bia, M. B., Widartono, B. S., Lobo, N. F., & Hawley, W. A. (2015). Change of strategy is required for malaria elimination: A case study in Purworejo District, Central Java Province, Indonesia. *Malaria Journal, 14*, 318. Retrieved from https://doi.org/10.1186/s12936-015-0828-7

Mwendera, C. A., de Jager, C., Longwe, H., Kumwenda, S., Hongoro, C., Phiri, K., & Mutero, C. M. (2019). Challenges to the implementation of malaria policies in Malawi. *BMC Health Services Research, 19,* 194. Retrieved from https://doi.org/10.1186/s12913-019-4032-2

Nabyonga Orem, J., Mugisha, F., Okui, A.P., Musango, L., & Kirigia, J. M. (2013). Health care seeking patterns and determinants of out-of-pocket expenditure for malaria for the children under-five in Uganda. *Malaria Journal, 12,* 175. Retrieved from https://doi.org/10.1186/1475-2875-12-175

Okell, L. C., Paintain, L. S., Webster, J., Hanson, K., & Lines, J. (2012). From intervention to impact: modelling the potential mortality impact achievable by different long-lasting, insecticide-treated net delivery strategies. *Malaria Journal, 11,* 327. Retrieved from https://doi.org/10.1186/1475-2875-11-327

Okumu, F. O., & Moore, S. J. (2011). Combining indoor residual spraying and insecticide-treated nets for malaria control in Africa: A review of possible outcomes and an outline of suggestions for the future. *Malaria Journal, 10,* 208. Retrieved from https://doi.org/10.1186/1475-2875-10-208

Onyango, E. A., Sahin, O., Awiti, A., Chu, C., & Mackey, B. (2016). An integrated risk and vulnerability assessment framework for climate change and malaria transmission in East Africa. *Malaria Journal, 15,* 551. Retrieved from https://doi.org/10.1186/s12936-016-1600-3

Oxman, A. D., & Fretheim, A. (2009). Can paying for results help to achieve the Millennium Development Goals? Overview of the effectiveness of results-based financing. *Journal of Evidence-Based Medicine, 2,* 70–83. Retrieved from https://doi.org/10.1111/j.1756-5391.2009.01020.x

Pradhan, M. M., Anvikar, A. R., Daumerie, P. G., Pradhan, S., Dutta, A., Shah, N. K., … Valecha, N. (2019). Comprehensive case management of malaria: Operational research informing policy. *Journal of Vector Borne Diseases, 56,* 56–59. Retrieved from https://doi.org/10.4103/0972-9062.257776

Rao, V. B., Schellenberg, D., & Ghani, A. C. (2013). Overcoming health systems barriers to successful malaria treatment. *Trends in Parasitology, 29,* 164–180. Retrieved from https://doi.org/10.1016/j.pt.2013.01.005

Rao, K. D., Ramani, S., Hazarika, I., & George, S. (2014). When do vertical programmes strengthen health systems? A comparative assessment of disease-specific interventions in India. *Health Policy and Planning, 29,* 495–505. Retrieved from https://doi.org/10.1093/heapol/czt035

Ray, S., & Tilak, R. (2017). Systems thinking approach in Malaria control: A qualitative health system strengthening interventions. *International Journal of Current Advanced Research, 6,* 6497–6499. Retrieved from https://doi.org/10.24327/ijcar.2017

Roman, E., Wallon, M., Brieger, W., Dickerson, A., Rawlins, B., & Agarwal, K. (2014). Moving malaria in pregnancy programs from neglect to priority: Experience from Malawi, Senegal, and Zambia. *Global Health: Science and Practice, 2,* 55–71. Retrieved from https://doi.org/10.9745/GHSP-D-13-00136

Rosewell, A., Makita, L., Muscatello, D., John, L. N., Bieb, S., Hutton, R., … Shearman, P.,(2017). Health information system strengthening and malaria elimination in Papua New Guinea. *Malaria Journal, 16,* 278. Retrieved from https://doi.org/10.1186/s12936-017-1910-0

Rowe, S. Y., Kelly, J. M., Olewe, M. A., Kleinbaum, D. G., McGowan, J. E., McFarland, D. A., … Deming, M. S. (2007). Effect of multiple interventions on community health workers' adherence to clinical guidelines in Siaya district, Kenya. *Transactions of the Royal Society of Tropical Medicine and Hygiene, 101,* 188–202. Retrieved from https://doi.org/10.1016/j.trstmh.2006.02.023

Sahu, M., Tediosi, F., Noor, A. M., Aponte, J. J., & Fink, G. (2020). Health systems and global progress towards malaria elimination, 2000–2016. *Malaria Journal, 19*, 141. Retrieved from https://doi.org/10.1186/s12936-020-03208-6

Salje, H., Lessler, J., Paul, K. K., Azman, A. S., Rahman, M. W., Rahman, M., … Cauchemez, S. (2016). How social structures, space, and behaviors shape the spread of infectious diseases using Chikungunya as a case study. *Proceedings of the National Academy of Sciences of the United States of America, 113*, 13420–13425. Retrieved from https://doi.org/10.1073/pnas.1611391113

Sarriot, E., Morrow, M., Langston, A., Weiss, J., Landegger, J., & Tsuma, L. (2015). A causal loop analysis of the sustainability of integrated community case management in Rwanda. *Social Science and Medicine, 131*, 147–155. Retrieved from https://doi.org/10.1016/j.socscimed.2015.03.014

Umlauf, R., & Park, S.-J. (2018). Stock-outs! Improvisations and processes of infrastructuring in Uganda's HIV/Aids and malaria programmes. *Global Public Health, 13*, 325–338. Retrieved from https://doi.org/10.1080/17441692.2017.1414287

Wandiga, S. O., Opondo, M., Olago, D., Githeko, A., Githui, F., Marshall, M., … Achola, P. (2010). Vulnerability to epidemic malaria in the highlands of Lake Victoria basin: the role of climate change/variability, hydrology and socio-economic factors. *Climate Change, 99*, 473–497. Retrieved from https://doi.org/10.1007/s10584-009-9670-7

Warren, A. E., Wyss, K., Shakarishvili, G., Atun, R., & de Savigny, D. (2013). Global health initiative investments and health systems strengthening: A content analysis of global fund investments. *Global Health, 9*, 30. Retrieved from https://doi.org/10.1186/1744-8603-9-30

Webster, J., Burdam, F. H., Landuwulang, C. U. R., Bruce, J., Poespoprodjo, J. R., Syafruddin, D., Ahmed, R., & Hill, J. (2018). Evaluation of the implementation of single screening and treatment for the control of malaria in pregnancy in Eastern Indonesia: A systems effectiveness analysis. *Malaria Journal, 17*, 310. Retrieved from https://doi.org/10.1186/s12936-018-2448-5

World Health Organization. (2015). *Global technical strategy for malaria, 2016–2030*. Geneva: World Health Organization.

Worrall, E., Basu, S., & Hanson, K. (2005). Is malaria a disease of poverty? A review of the literature. *Tropical Medicine and International Health, 10*, 1047–1059. Retrieved from https://doi.org/10.1111/j.1365-3156.2005.01476.x

Yasuoka, J., Jimba, M., & Levins, R. (2014). Application of loop analysis for evaluation of malaria control interventions. *Malaria Journal, 13*, 140. Retrieved from https://doi.org/10.1186/1475-2875-13-140

Yé, Y., Eisele, T. P., Eckert, E., Korenromp, E., Shah, J. A., Hershey, C. L., … Bhattarai, A. (2017). Framework for evaluating the health impact of the scale-up of malaria control interventions on all-cause child mortality in Sub-Saharan Africa. *American Journal of Tropical Medicine and Hygiene, 97*, 9–19. Retrieved from https://doi.org/10.4269/ajtmh.15-0363

25

The Utility of Systems Thinking in the Context of Infectious Disease Surveillance in India

Rosemary James, Anish Jammu, Annabel Taks, Tapashi Adhikary, Hasmik Nazaryan, Sreya Abraham, Upasna Gaba, Zeenath Roohi, Alexandra Humpert, and Isabel Foster

Background

From the twentieth to the twenty-first century, India has evolved from once being one of the poorest nations in the world into the fifth largest economy (World Bank, 2011). However, developments in health remain only moderate by international standards, partly due to chronic underfunding (Davies, 2012) and unequal health coverage (Reddy, 2018). Consequently, India has one of the highest private, out-of-pocket healthcare expenditures globally (Patel, Kumar, Paul, Rao, & Reddy, 2011). Resulting health disparities allow both non-communicable and infectious diseases to flourish, the latter contributing to 30% of the national disease burden (John, Dandona, Sharma, & Kakkar, 2011). This gap in high-quality universal care can be narrowed by the successful implementation of both infectious disease surveillance and vaccine coverage (Andre et al., 2008; Krieger, Waterman, Chen, Soobader, & Subramanian, 2016).

Sensitive, integrated systems of surveillance are essential for disease control (Davies, 2012). This point has been well-articulated by the director-general of the World Health Organization (WHO), Tedros Adhanom Ghebreyesus, during the COVID-19 pandemic: "You cannot fight a fire blindfolded. And we cannot stop this pandemic if we don't know who is infected" (World Health Organization, 2020a). This analogy has long held true for the containment of both emerging and resurgent infectious diseases (Zaidi, Awasthi, & deSilva, 2004).

The Indian Ministry of Health and Family Welfare (MoHFW) collects infectious disease (ID) surveillance data via two main avenues. The first means is deeply rooted in the WHO's Integrated Disease Surveillance and Response (IDSR) of 1998 and the International Health Regulations (IHR) of 2005 (Kumar, Goel, Jain, & Khanna, 2014). The IDSR is an evidence-based strategy that aims to strengthen national public health surveillance at the community, health facility, district, and national levels (Fall et al., 2019). The effect of the IDSR was tested during the 2003 SARS outbreak. In the aftermath, global health authorities recognized that they must maintain an equilibrium whereby states held principal authority over the containment (through implementation of the IDSR) of outbreaks within borders, while simultaneously ensuring that clusters

Rosemary James, Anish Jammu, Annabel Taks, Tapashi Adhikary, Hasmik Nazaryan, Sreya Abraham, Upasna Gaba, Zeenath Roohi, Alexandra Humpert, and Isabel Foster, *The Utility of Systems Thinking in the Context of Infectious Disease Surveillance in India* In: *Systems Thinking for Global Health.* Edited by: Fiona Larkan, Frédérique Vallières, Hasheem Mannan, and Naonori Kodate, Oxford University Press. © Oxford University Press 2023. DOI: 10.1093/oso/9780198799498.003.0025

of cases do not develop into epidemics that spread into neighboring countries and beyond (Davies, 2012; Honigsbaum, 2017). As a result, the IHR were developed in 2005, a legal instrument requiring all 194 member states to operate and manage real-time health event monitoring and strengthening of existing disease surveillance systems (Mandyata, Olowski, & Mutale, 2017). Significant efforts have been made in India to operationalize these two global health surveillance regulations through its Integrated Disease Surveillance Programme (IDSP), established in 2004 (Pilot, Rao, Jena, & Krafft, 2014).

The IDSP is a decentralized, state- and case-based surveillance system intended to detect early warning signs of potential outbreaks (Kumar et al., 2014). It has been praised as one of the most advanced national-level implementations of the IDSR in the WHO-South East Asia Region (SEAR) (Phalkey, Yamamoto, Awate, & Marx, 2015). The system captures syndromic, presumptive, and laboratory-confirmed cases of acute infections. The IDSP also predicts disease trends, allowing for preventative action (Yasobant, Patel, & Saxena, 2019).

During the 1990s, many low- and middle-income countries developed vertical disease surveillance and response strategies for priority IDs (Mandyata et al., 2017). These programs are heavily funded and relatively autonomous with central, state, and district officers working solely toward surveillance of a single disease (John et al., 2011). While they have proven to be very successful in India's eradication of leprosy and smallpox and containment of HIV/AIDS, empirical evidence has demonstrated that it is not feasible, nor preferred, for this to be replicated for all IDs, given India's limited resources and vast geography (John et al., 2011; Yasobant et al., 2019).

This chapter explores the complex system of ID surveillance in India using systems thinking, specifically general systems theory (explained in Chapter 1 and Table 1.1 of this book). Focus is placed on measles and TB surveillance, covered by the IDSP and vertical disease program, respectively, to demonstrate these two avenues of data flow, and because both infections are highly prevalent in India.

From using the WHO's Health System Strengthening (HSS) building blocks as a lens, a review of literature and policy, coupled with key informant interviews, system maps and a causal loop diagram (CLD) were created to understand which variables are essential in India's complex, contemporary ID surveillance system.

Using Systems Thinking to Strengthen Health Systems

The WHO has defined a "Framework for Action" on health systems which identifies six Health System Building Blocks as essential components for a complete system. These blocks include *service delivery* which provides quality, access, safety, and coverage; *health workforce* equipped with human resources management, skills, and policies; *health information* facilitating the production, analysis, and efficient use of information; *medical technologies and products* with supply programs to ensure equitable access and quality; *health financing* with adequate funds and appropriately allocated resources; as well as *leadership and governance* that implement strategic policy frameworks to ensure accountability, incentives, and effective coalition building.

Beyond these building blocks, a health system consists of many interconnected parts that must unite in function to be effective as explained in Chapter 1 of this book.

A health system's ID surveillance is likewise multicomponent and includes many actors, both in the field and at the policy level. Each has its unique function such that any study of one in isolation limits understanding of the system as a whole (de Savigny & Adam, 2009; Xia, Zhou, & Liu, 2017).

As discussed in Chapter 1, systems thinking is a useful approach to analysis as it provides a holistic understanding of complex interrelationships between various actors in a system, permitting more insightful interpretations. The HSS building block framework demonstrates how the health system is indeed shaped by multiple and complex interactions; therefore, employing a systems-thinking lens can ensure that relationships among the blocks are captured in the systems analysis. Systems thinking is derived from various theories including complexity theory, which explains the increasing interest in employing a systems-thinking lens in the practical context of examining the health system.

Within systems thinking, general systems theory best suits a health system as it allows for the development of a general conceptual framework to represent a theory or problem whereby the essential features are maintained. Systems dynamics modelling is a systems-thinking method that involves using a set of tools, which commonly include causal loop or stocks and flows diagrams, to understand the behavior of complex systems over time. This method allows for variables to be changed over small periods of time while feedback, interactions, and delays occur simultaneously, thereby facilitating the analysis of systems involving mutual causation. CLDs, in particular, are a system dynamics tool that can be used to produce models illustrating causality and feedback loops, highlighting their role within a system. It is important to acknowledge that there is continued debate surrounding the widespread adoption of systems thinking in health systems practice (Peters, 2014), as there are limitations that caution one's ability to fully understand a system in-depth, from all perspectives (Kast & Rosenzweig, 1972; Mutale, Balabanova, Chintu, Mwanamwenge, & Ayles, 2016).

Overview of ID Surveillance System in India

Prior to exploring India's ID system as a whole, it is important to understand its existing components. Using the framework of the six WHO HSS building blocks this section provides a general overview of key elements of the surveillance system.

(i) Policies, leadership and governance, and financing

In the 1990s, ID surveillance was increasingly recognized as an area warranting greater attention on the Indian national agenda. In response, the Government of India (GoI) developed a National Apical Advisory Committee for National Disease Surveillance and Response System in 1998 and launched the National Surveillance Programme for Communicable Diseases (NSPCD) between 1997 and 1998 across 101 districts (Raut & Bhola, 2014). The NSPCD was implemented on the premise of two key objectives: (i) capacity building (early warning systems, laboratory strengthening, network development) to allow for early identification of ID outbreaks and (ii) appropriate and timely response to prevent and control communicable disease outbreaks. Vertical single disease control programs typically incorporate vertical case-based surveillance as one element of the program objectives (Phalkey et al., 2013). Following the institution of the NSPCD, case-based reporting remained low and did not yield a representative image of the state of ID burden within India (Raut & Bhola, 2014). The global lack of success with vertical single disease control programs, despite significant economic investment and the rise in other health challenges, motivated the WHO to establish the IDSR.

As such, the GoI decided to discontinue the NSPCD by 2002 and implemented the IDSP in 2004, based on the provisions set forth by the WHO IDSR Strategy and the US-based Center for Disease Control & Prevention to address "unresolved issues in the surveillance efforts in low-and middle-income countries" (Phalkey et al., 2015: 132). On a national level, the MoHFW governs surveillance as per the National Health Policy (Ministry of Health and Family Welfare, 2017b). The National Health Policy (2017) includes specific provisions for disease surveillance including Article 4.5 (Communicable Diseases) which addresses the link between communicable disease control programs and the public health strengthening in the context of IDSP and Article 13.9 (Disease Surveillance) which addresses collaboration and engagement with the non-government sector and private sector to strengthen disease surveillance particularly through data pooling and sharing (Ministry of Health and Family Welfare, 2017b). The National Centre for Disease Control (NCDC), which cooperates with the Central Surveillance Unit (CSU), manages the IDSP which reports on infectious diseases with outbreak potential. The IDSP involves "a combination of active and passive systems that use a single infrastructure to gather information about multiple diseases" (Raut & Bhola, 2014; Phalkey et al., 2015: 132). Initially, the World Bank provided financing to support the IDSP but this funding ceased in 2012 and currently the GoI funds the IDSP with state budgets allocated annually (Phalkey et al., 2013), ultimately contributing to the achievement of Universal Health Coverage (UHC) (Balasubramaniam & Hira, 2014; Kieny et al., 2017; Reddy et al., 2011).

(ii) Service delivery: health workforce, information flow, and technologies

Data collection

The WHO broadly defines three types of ID surveillance: passive, active, and sentinel (Pilot, Murthy, & Nittas, 2020; World Health Organization, 2000). India's surveillance infrastructure is composed of three major levels—district (DSU), state (SSU), and central (CSU). The main actors are appointed surveillance officers and public health specialists (Raut & Bhola, 2014).

Active surveillance involves labor-intensive searching, testing, and responding to a disease for either elimination purposes, or to respond to an outbreak (Iskander & M'ikanatha, 2015). A Media Scanning and Verification Cell (MSVC) and 24×7 toll-free call center, part of the NCDC in Delhi, have teams of analysts responding to informal media reports and calls to aid in outbreak surveillance (Davies, 2012). These additional surveillance methods are used as an early warning system and have been found to support and fill gaps within the main formal surveillance system in detecting disease threats effectively (Kant & Krishnan, 2010; Davies, 2012; Raut & Bhola, 2014). Sentinel surveillance involves recruiting several health facilities known to be outbreak-prone or in an endemic-area instead of the overall population, to actively identify and notify on certain diseases (Iskander & M'ikanatha, 2015). Passive surveillance is the most commonly applied type of ID surveillance (Iskander & M'ikanatha, 2015). Surveillance units rely on local actors to report at the district level weekly, through hardcopy registers and forms. Primary passive surveillance is undertaken at all reporting units by an appointed medical officer. For example, pyrexia is kept under regular passive surveillance by reporting units both in the public and private sectors of rural and urban areas of the district.

Reporting

Hard-copy data collected at the local level is digitalized via electronic reporting portals, at the DSU (Kant & Krishnan, 2010; Pilot et al., 2017). As mentioned earlier, the principle aim of implementing the IDSP was to strengthen the Indian disease surveillance system by decentralizing disease (outbreak) detection, reporting, and response (Kumar et al., 2014; Pilot et al., 2017). Within the IDSP, surveillance is formally conducted through data collection of both suspected and confirmed infectious disease cases at the community level through reports completed by both public and private healthcare workers in each DSU (Raut & Bhola, 2014; Pilot et al., 2017). These forms are available in an electronic format from the primary health center (PHC) level upwards (Raut & Bhola, 2014). The reports consist of three distinct forms known as "S," "P," and "L" forms which are developed weekly and relayed to the designated DSUs (Raut & Bhola, 2014). The "S" form is the reporting format for *syndromic (symptom-based) surveillance*, the primary source of active surveillance performed by the IDSP. This is filled mainly by community health workers (CHWs), who also carry out contact tracing and are responsible for reaching all members of the population in their assigned local area. More specifically, to enable contact tracing, at-risk individuals get their assigned personal identification number (Aadhaar number) and location based on landmarks recorded. The "P" form, the reporting format for *presumptive surveillance*, contains a list of provisional diagnoses and is filled by medical officers in primary care settings. Finally, the "L" forms are the reporting format for *laboratory surveillance*. The "L" form includes the number of samples tested and their respective outcomes (e.g., positive/negative). Diagnostic services and facilities for the collection of laboratory samples are to be provided at community health centers (CHCs) and PHCs and are sent to public and private microscopy centers as appropriate. Next to reporting cases and outbreaks, *nil-reporting* in the instance of no cases is mandatory (Raut & Bhola, 2014; Integrated Disease Surveillance Programme, 2017).

Analysis

The IDSP portal provides the opportunity to analyze and communicate ID surveillance data from the DSUs upwards (Kant & Krishnan, 2010; Raut & Bhola, 2014). Therefore, the focal point of integrated disease surveillance is located at the DSU level where the data collection ("P," "S," and "L") forms are collated on a weekly basis (Raut & Bhola 2014; Pilot et al., 2017). This happens often still by manual digitization, with which the ID data are analyzed for the first time (Raut & Bhola, 2014) by trained data managers, data entry operators, microbiologists, and epidemiologists (Kant & Krishnan, 2010). Via the portal, the data flows to the respective SSU or Union Territory where disease outbreak reports are developed (Integrated Disease Surveillance Programme, 2017).

The CSU receives all outbreak reports from each of the twenty-six SSUs and UTs to generate a weekly national outbreak report and annual national epidemiological situation report (Suresh, 2008; Integrated Disease Surveillance Programme, 2017).

Appropriate data analysis, at the different surveillance levels, is important to ensure a swift containment of clusters of cases to prevent outbreaks, and to predict disease trends (e.g., seasonality) and disease burden (Kant & Krishnan, 2010; Davies, 2012). With ID surveillance data analysis, the progression of the current national disease control programs can be monitored, which in turn can direct necessary resource allocation (Kumar et al., 2014). This highlights the importance of comprehensive surveillance in disease control, which some underfunded regions and disease programs lack to begin with. The IDSP web portal provides epidemiological analysis software to analyze ID surveillance data (Kant & Krishnan, 2010), however, access is limited at district level, and requires specialized skills to be used effectively (Phalkey et al., 2013; Raut & Bhola, 2014). Alongside the main IDSP surveillance system, the web portal also includes information regarding disease outbreak alerts and unusual media reporting regarding outbreaks, acquired via the call center and MSVC (Kant & Krishnan, 2010; Raut & Bhola, 2014).

Response

Based on this retrieved ID surveillance data and analysis, concerned officials at the respective organizational level are contacted who direct rapid response teams (RRTs) to handle further investigation and verification (Kant & Krishnan, 2010; Integrated Disease Surveillance Programme, 2017). Each disease requires a unique response, with different actors, policies, and infrastructure at play. Unusual cases or outbreaks are investigated by the corresponding district RRT (Kant & Krishnan, 2010). An RRT is composed of various experts depending on the disease, trained in outbreak surveillance, investigation, vector control, and containment (Kadri, Rehana, Benetou, Ahmad, & Abdullah, 2018). Their primary role is validating the initial report of the outbreak (National Disaster Management Authority (NDMA) 2008). This is essential, particularly given that many of the gaps in public collecting are filled by the informal reports from the media and the hotline but also to prevent the possibility of instigating undue panic if the outbreak claim is invalid (Davies, 2012).

RRTs sent from the district level are responsible for directing and mobilizing essential components needed for initial containment. The RRTs from the state level are reserved for crisis situations (National Disaster Management Authority, 2008). There are also RRTs at the national level deployed for large-scale outbreaks (Raut & Bhola, 2014). As discussed, veterinary and animal husbandry officers are included in the RRT when the outbreak is zoonotic in nature (Kadri et al., 2018).

The next sections will place particular focus on the surveillance of two IDs: measles and tuberculosis.

Measles Surveillance

Measles, a highly contagious viral disease, is one of the leading causes of childhood mortality in India and can lead to severe complications among vulnerable populations (Wong et al., 2019). To control the severe consequences of measles, India has committed to the WHO-SEAR goal of eliminating measles by 2023 (World Health

Organization, 2019a). India is leveraging the WHO National Polio Surveillance Program (WHO-NPSP) model for measles and rubella (fever and rash) surveillance alongside acute flaccid paralysis surveillance under one integrated system (World Health Organization, 2017). Besides the WHO-NPSP, the measles surveillance system involves several other actors, vertical national programs, and institutions that provide early warning signs of an outbreak. Each of these elements comprising the surveillance system operating within a hierarchy. Figure 25.1 depicts the interactions of each element at various levels.

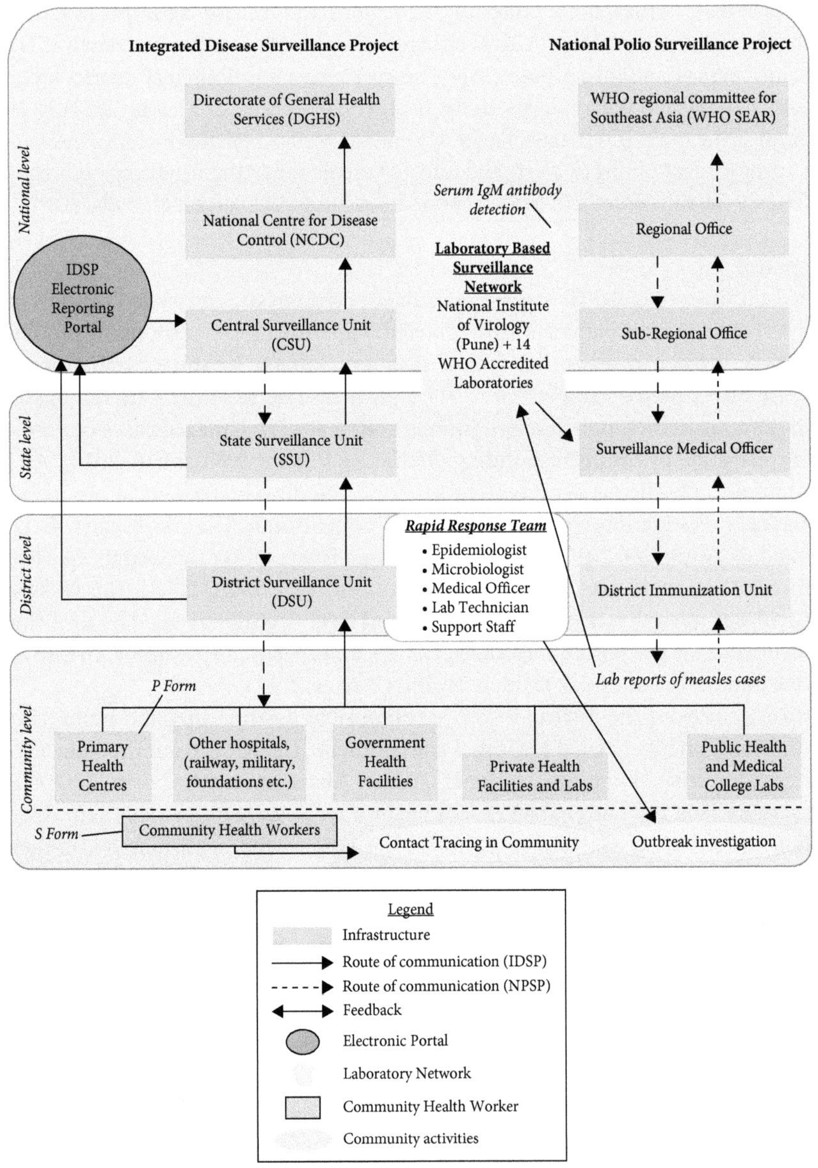

Figure 25.1 System map of measles surveillance in India

Data collection, compilation, and reporting are done at PHCs, where web-enabled technology connects PHCs with DSUs (Raut & Bhola, 2014). Health facilities with physicians (PHCs, CHCs, and sub-district hospitals) report on measles by syndromic surveillance using the "P" forms. These reports are analyzed at the district and sub-district levels before their dissemination in the IDSP portal. Separate reports on outbreaks that are occurring more than their expected patterns are filed by the districts. Following the reporting of an outbreak, DSUs assess the situation before deploying specialized RRTs for further investigation of the outbreak. On the field, blood samples are collected and sent for serum IgM antibody detection to designated laboratories that are identified under the IDSP program. Feedback response is generally initiated at the DSUs and flows upwards toward the SSU and CSU (Raut & Bhola, 2014). To improve the reporting of surveillance data, IDSP has requested all private practitioners to comply with voluntary reporting of measles cases (National Centre for Disease Control, Government of India, 2013).

All surveillance-based activities are primarily guided by the IDSP while the WHO-NPSP provides technical support and capacity building workshops for accelerated measles control and immunization across the country (World Health Organization, 2020b). India has fourteen WHO-accredited laboratories that conduct lab-based surveillance for measles, and five among these perform genetic characterization of the virus (Ministry of Health and Family Welfare, 2017b). Lab-confirmed samples are referred for further investigation to the National Institute of Virology, Pune (Raut & Bhola 2014). The transition from outbreak-based surveillance to case-based surveillance is currently being rolled out with the support of NPSP (World Health Organization, 2017).

Tuberculosis Surveillance

India has the highest prevalence of tuberculosis (TB) cases worldwide (World Health Organization, 2019b). The active pulmonary TB surveillance system in India is complex, with a hierarchy of many actors and institutions working toward the ambitious goals set by WHO's End TB Strategy, which aims to reduce the incidence of TB cases by 90% by 2035 (World Health Organization, 2015a). Surveillance data on TB have a fourfold importance: to monitor trends, plan for programming, evaluate policy effectiveness, and provide information for education and awareness (Iskander & M'ikanatha, 2015). Using an HSS approach is crucial for TB control (Atun, Weil, Eang, & Mwakyusa, 2010), as outlined in the WHO's Checklist for TB Surveillance (World Health Organization, 2014). System mapping is applied in this section to visualize the key actors and infrastructure involved in India's TB surveillance reporting system, from community level upwards (Figure 25.2).

The surveillance system is driven by the National Tuberculosis Elimination Program (NTEP) 2017–2025 HSS strategy (Ministry of Health and Family Welfare, 2017a). There is little focus and no national policy for latent TB screening or surveillance (Saha et al., 2020). An online portal, Nikshay, was implemented in 2014 by the Central TB unit, by which all medical professionals and laboratories are mandated by

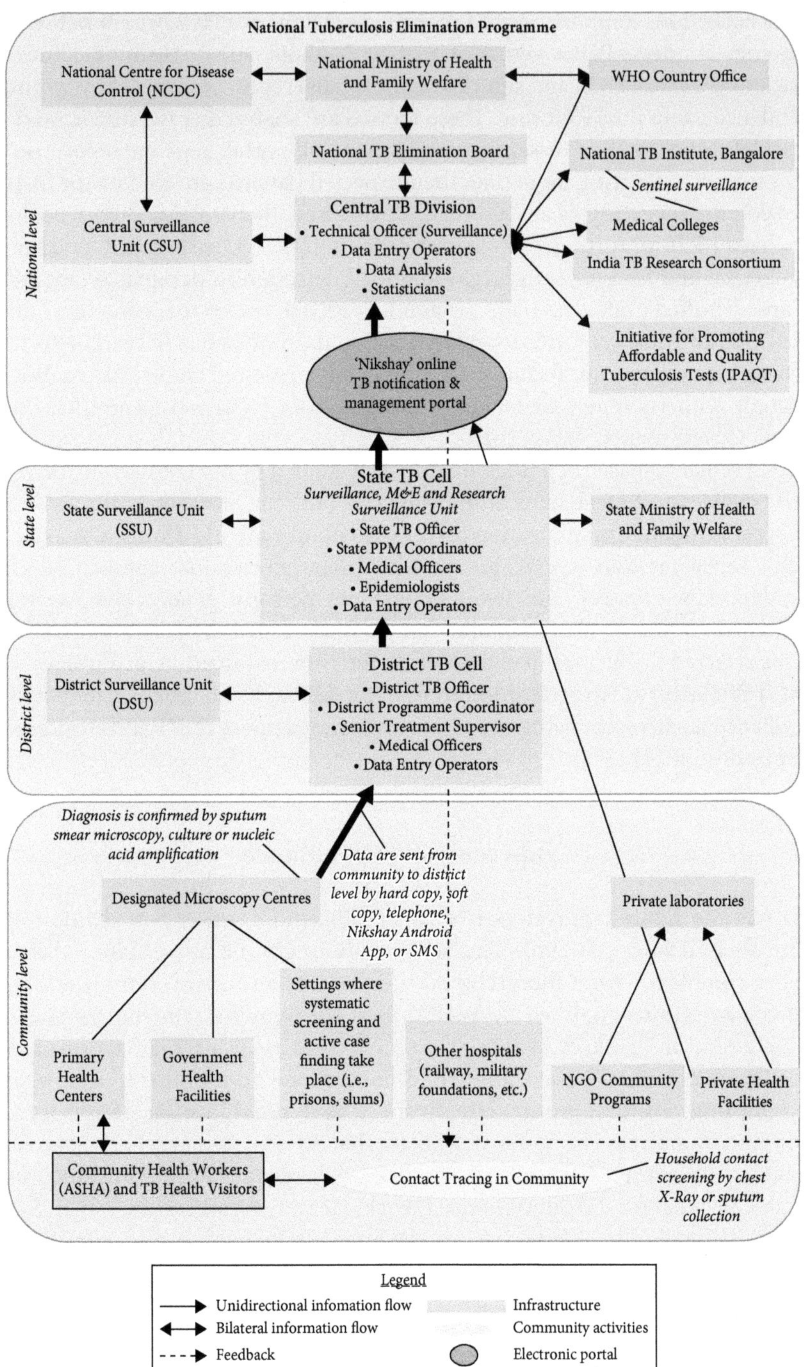

Figure 25.2 System map of tuberculosis surveillance in India

law to report any active TB diagnoses (Yadav, Atif, & Rawal, 2018; Dey, Rao, Kumar, & Narayanan, 2020). Much of the sentinel surveillance and staff training for TB is provided by the National TB Institute.

Active TB symptom-based surveillance is conducted by CHWs, who refer suspected cases to PHCs. It is required that all household contacts are screened, which can pose social and mental issues due to stigma (Shamanewadi, 2020). Medical practitioners in PHCs and government hospitals assess individuals and refer sputum samples to a district-level designated microscopy center (DMCs). Once a case is lab-confirmed, hard-copy TB registers in government health facilities require staff to document and report to the Nikshay portal weekly. Individual's demographic, clinical, socio-economic, geographic, and spatial variables are documented to enable data stratification and contact tracing (Prathiksha, Daniel, & Natrajan, 2019). Data are then sent from community to district level by hard copy, soft copy, telephone, Android Nikshay App, or SMS. Newer diagnostic machines in DMCs can transmit data directly to the Nikshay portal, and tablets for real-time field data entry are also being rolled out (Ministry of Health and Family Welfare, 2017a).

India continues to use the globally adopted strategy of Directly Observed Treatment Short Course (DOTS), which aims to ensure treatment adherence. In the community, PHCs function as DOTS centers to deliver free treatment through DOTS providers, the majority being community health workers. Certified TB "Health Visitors" are also trained to visit patients to ensure compliance and nutritional support. At each district TB unit, monthly meetings are held with key actors, and a quarterly report on new and retreatment cases is compiled. Analysis of TB surveillance data is then conducted at the state and national level, by several institutions and actors including epidemiologists and the WHO to inform program prioritization and subsequent response (Nishikioria & Morishitaa, 2013).

It is estimated that up to 80% of people with TB attend private health services at first contact in India, and half continue to seek treatment privately (Satyanarayana et al., 2011; Salve, Harris, Sheikh, & Porter, 2018). This often leads to underreporting as well as diagnostic and treatment delays (Khan et al., 2012; Sreeramareddy, Qin, Satyanarayana, Subbaraman, & Pai, 2014). A public–private mix (PPM), backed by the WHO, was first adopted in 2013 to improve the integration of the private sector in surveillance functions (Chauhan, 2007; Wells, Uplekar, & Pai, 2015), allowing DOTS facilities to scale up reporting in collaboration with private facilities and medical colleges (Khan et al., 2012). Further, the India TB Research Consortium was established in 2016 to support PPM in improving diagnostic capabilities (Pai, 2018). Diagnostic tools are being made more affordable through a non-profit PPM, the Initiative for Promoting Affordable and Quality Tuberculosis Tests, which also ensures affiliated labs report all cases to the Nikshay portal (Dabas et al., 2019). Financial incentives and access to TB diagnostics for private practitioners, who report to the Nikshay portal, are now offered (Yadav et al., 2018; Dey et al., 2020). Since the introduction of the NTEP, reporting seems to be improving, with notifications of new cases rising by 60% between 2013 and 2018 (World Health Organization, 2019b).

Exploring Interrelationships within the System

Causal loop diagrams are a system dynamics tool that aid in conceptualizing a system by focusing on causality and feedback loops (Peters, 2014). A typical CLD is composed of feedback loops (balancing or reinforcing), polarities, causalities, delays, clockwise, and counterclockwise symbols. Loops are considered as reinforcing if the variables influence each other in the same direction, they are said to be balancing if they influence each other in the opposite direction. CLDs are of great value when it comes to exploring complex interplays between different factors acting in a surveillance system (Littlejohns, Baum, Lawless, & Freeman, 2018). Stakeholder engagement is an important aspect of designing a CLD as it makes a mental model appear more concrete, rational, and easier for readers to comprehend. Thus, a participatory approach was used to gain insight into the design of the CLD. Key informants with expertise in surveillance and systems thinking were interviewed. Frontline health workers (CHWs and a medical officer) were also interviewed for more grassroots level insights.

The CLD (Figure 25.3) demonstrates various causal relationships within the Indian ID surveillance system. The model focuses mainly on two HSS building blocks; service delivery and information, which are represented in the model as data quality and reporting of cases, respectively. The reinforcing loop at the top left of Figure 25.3 represents a virtuous cycle that shows how an increase in resource allocation can enhance the data quality of surveillance. The model also identifies a complex notification system that can affect health workers' performance as they often fail to comprehend such systems. This may produce a vicious cycle that affects data quality. The model also highlights contentious events such as civil unrest that may lead to a lack of trust in the system, and this can be exacerbated by existing political factors and data privacy concerns. These events indirectly compromise the data quality and volume of cases that are being reported. Data quality can also be compromised due to lack of laboratory capacity, inadequate regulatory norms, and lack of reporting from private sectors. Balancing loops, such as the one at the lower right corner of the model, shows the rising disease burden leading to disease intervention. Increasing disease burden may also lead to the implementation of multiple programs which results in a fragmented system of reporting. In such cases, mandatory reporting of surveillance data of all programs under one integrated system can help in managing surveillance more effectively.

This CLD was developed based on interviews with key informants, data from the IDSP website, and relevant contemporary literature, to gain an in-depth understanding of the factors that affect quality and reporting systems of ID surveillance in India. The derived conclusions are context specific and can be ambiguous. The model can be utilized to identify leverage points for robust surveillance.

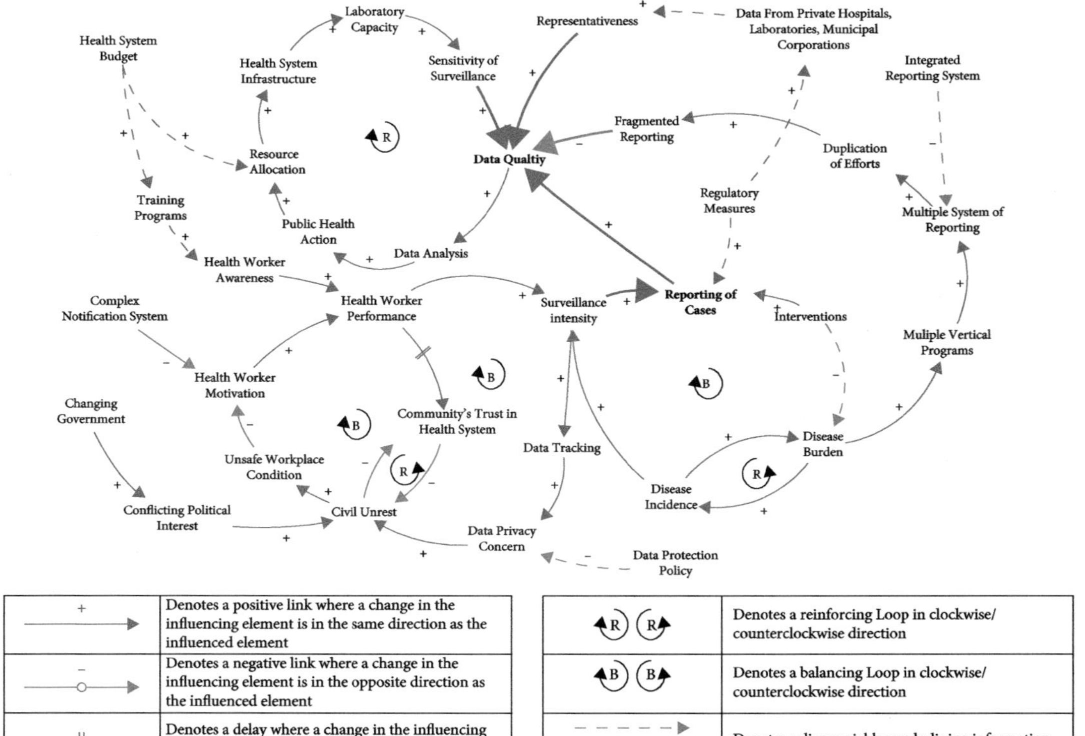

+	Denotes a positive link where a change in the influencing element is in the same direction as the influenced element
–	Denotes a negative link where a change in the influencing element is in the opposite direction as the influenced element
	Denotes a delay where a change in the influencing element produces a change in the influenced element only after a delay

R R	Denotes a reinforcing Loop in clockwise/ counterclockwise direction
B B	Denotes a balancing Loop in clockwise/ counterclockwise direction
	Denotes ruling variables underlining information and service delivery

Figure 25.3 Causal loop diagram exploring the intricacies of India's infectious disease surveillance system

Challenges and Opportunities

In global health, depicting and thereby understanding complex systems is challenging (Greenhalgh & Papoutsi, 2018). Simple blueprint approaches show limited success. A holistic approach enables practitioners of global health to see the broader contextual pattern, helps identify gaps and weaknesses, and allows for the discovery of out-of-the-box solutions (Peters, 2014). Analyzing the Indian surveillance system through a systems-thinking lens, mapping the TB and measles surveillance data flow, and creating a CLD disclosed several gaps and weaknesses as well as opportunities for improvement.

Key activities for public health surveillance include case detection, registration, laboratory confirmation, reporting, analysis, and feedback (McNabb et al., 2002). Shortcomings in these steps reduce the reliability and validity of the collected health information. India's surveillance system has undergone large improvements since its IDSP introduction in 2004. However, there are spatial differences of surveillance coverage and captured data quality which can distort the display of India's ID disease burdens. The system is complex, highly thematic, and administratively fragmented and subdivided into multiple vertical (disease-specific) programs. This makes the linkage of information from several separately operating health systems, and bridging knowledge and information gaps among programs and stakeholders challenging (Pilot et al., 2020). Further, lack of (designated) human and financial resources (Dehal, Krishan, Kanchan, Unnikrishnan, & Singh, 2015; Pilot et al., 2020) and an uneven distribution of these resources negatively impacts reporting practices (John et al., 2011).

At the community level, healthcare workers are not sufficiently acquainted with different vertical health programs in place and are found to have incomplete knowledge about their role in the surveillance system (Kumar et al., 2014). This knowledge gap can lead to insufficient case detection and registration practices. A further systemic gap that hampers this is the system's public–private division. Many cases are not being captured as the majority of the Indian population seeks healthcare in the private sector (Rajagopalan & Choutagunta, 2020), and this sector has little regulation and obligation to report, although there are recent efforts to address this (Shinde, Kembhavi, Kuwatada, & Khandednath, 2012; Raut & Bhola, 2014, Pilot et al., 2019).

Further, there are quality differences between laboratories. In the private sector, laboratories are often well equipped and regulated, providing timely and sensitive results. However, this is not consistent in the public sector (Sheikh et al., 2005). Delayed diagnosis is common, as repair of equipment and the purchase of reagents are delayed, rapid tests are too expensive, and a high turnover of laboratory technicians costs time and funding in a system with a high health workforce shortage (Labonté & Ruckert, 2019). Further, in public health facilities, many ID samples are sent outside to the required reference laboratories only when patients have the financial means to fund the service (Engel et al., 2015). To establish a high-functioning laboratory network with increased capacity and reach, more high-quality laboratories should be included in the surveillance system, and well supported (John et al., 2011). India also suffers from a chronic systematic underreporting of some IDs and reduced data quality due not only to a lack of trained staff and resources, but from fear of blame, stigmatization, and political consequences, as demonstrated by the CLD (Figure 25.3). Further, monitoring water quality, food safety, and security, or zoonotic sanitation are important preventive measures for ID prevention, however environmental risk factor surveillance is not yet a fundamental component of the IDSP (Chatterjee, Kakkar, & Chaturvedi, 2016; Yasobant et al., 2019).

(iii) Measles surveillance

Despite considerable efforts to strengthen surveillance via the IDSP, measles surveillance, in particular, the timely detection and early warning of outbreaks, remains challenging. Absence of formalization of community reporting, lack of ownership, and knowledge among health workers regarding the surveillance system are some of the key obstacles toward the goal of eliminating measles (Suresh, 2008). In 2018, seventy-two districts in India did not report a single suspected case, indicating a need for increased sensitization for reporting (Shastri, 2019). Serosurveillance of immunization coverage also needs to be scaled up by expanding the measles laboratory network, while also engaging professional societies to strengthen routine immunization surveillance programs (Bavdekar & Karande, 2017).

(iv) Tuberculosis surveillance

From mapping the flow of information through the key actors and infrastructure in place from the community to national level, challenges facing the TB surveillance system were identified. Political commitment is of utmost importance (Dias, Pai, & Raviglione, 2018; Nadda, 2019). To attain the NTEP and WHO's End TB strategy, TB surveillance need not only focus on passive diagnosis reporting. Continuous surveillance of drug-resistance (Pai, Bhaumik, & Bhuyan, 2017; Zignol et al., 2016), and treatment outcomes (Ministry of Health and Family Welfare, 2017a), and latent TB case reporting should also be integrated into the system. Systematic active case finding (ACF) should be expanded to reach all vulnerable groups (World Health Organization, 2015b; Bhatnager, Ralte, Ralte, Sundaramoorthy, & Chhakchhuak, 2019; Prathiksha et al., 2019). However, ACF can be effective only by scaling up diagnostic facilities and promoting positive health-seeking behavior of the vulnerable population (Gupta, Saibannavar, & Kumar, 2016; Shamanewadi et al., 2020). There is also a need for accessible, point-of-care tests, to reduce the often complex diagnostic journey (Engel et al., 2015; Yellapa et al., 2017). Further, investments in staff training and infrastructure should be made when new reporting systems, such as novel diagnostic tools, or information systems are introduced (Engel et al., 2015; Shamanewadi et al., 2020). Finally, it is of utmost importance to end the stigma surrounding TB through community engagement (Pai et al., 2017; Chakrabartty, Basu, Ali, Sarkar, & Ghosh, 2018). Systemically connecting the interlinkages between these gaps in the surveillance system will in turn help to strengthen the entire health system and health outcomes (Atun et al., 2010).

Way Forward

The COVID-19 pandemic, which has disrupted ID testing and tracing to a magnitude like never before, could mark a turning point in the reform of ID surveillance systems worldwide. For the system to function coherently, and to address the aforementioned gaps and weaknesses, strong political support and leadership are required (Amrith, 2007; Shiffman & Smith, 2007; Nadda, 2019). This is challenging as health system responsibilities are shared among central and state governments, and oftentimes, these exhibit divergent or competing political and developmental agendas (Pilot et al., 2020). The right political prioritization needs to be given to ascertain that there are adequate actors and institutions, in quantity and quality within the system, working in timely collaboration. The largest opportunity to be harnessed is improved inclusion of the private sector (Pilot et al., 2014). Going forward, to strengthen health systems holistically, multisectoral and interdisciplinary action should be taken to adopt the latest evidence and proven innovations adapted to the local context. It is also important to apply systems thinking when introducing innovations, such as diagnostics or IT systems, to ensure they align with the existing system. Implementation requires a ground-up approach, to reduce rural-urban inequities. Geographic Information Systems (GIS) are promising tools that can enable visualization of clustered cases while retaining data security and protection as a key priority (Apte et al., 2019). The Integrated Health Information Platform (IHIP), established in 2018, offers real-time GIS case-based surveillance, and could greatly improve the system, provided that adequate training, resources, and infrastructure is available. The IHIP will also be a tool for tracking antimicrobial resistance (World Health Organization, 2019c). Medical colleges were also identified as key actors in India's surveillance system. Their resources and expertise could be harnessed further, by commissioning more systems-thinking research, both quantitative and qualitative. Further, using available electronic health and emergency medical service data from the private sector could enable rapid outbreak detection while conserving limited resources (Pilot et al., 2014, 2017). A One Health approach, where animals and ecosystems are considered as a whole, to disease outbreaks could be improved by enhancing communication between the IDSP and the National Animal Disease Reporting System (Chatterjee et al., 2016; Yasobant et al., 2019). Looking ahead, as NCDs are estimated to account for 63% of the total deaths in India (World Health Organization, 2018), lessons learnt from the successes of the IDSP could also be translated to NCD surveillance. These opportunities must be harnessed if India is to succeed in its ambitious goals of attaining measles elimination, the End TB Strategy, and UHC. An interdisciplinary approach to surveillance, with political engagement at all levels, is essential.

Conclusion

Through systems mapping using general systems theory, it is possible to analyze the Indian infectious disease surveillance system in depth and holistically, to a certain extent. Applying the HSS building blocks as the basis for an ideal system for India, the mapping process provided insights into what actors and institutions are involved, what interactions and communication take place, the weaknesses and gaps, and ultimately, opportunities for improvement.

Acknowledgments

We would like to extend our thanks to our key informants and reviewers who provided valuable insight: Professor Carjin Beumer, Eva Pilot, Ricky Janssen (Maastricht University), Professor Shah Hossain (Manipal Academy of Higher Education), and Professor Ashish Joshi (City University of New York).

References

Amrith, S. (2007). Political culture of health in India: A historical perspective. *Economic and Political Weekly, 42*(2), 114–121.

Andre, F. E., Booy, R., Bock, H. L., Clemens, J., Datta, S. K., John, T. J., . . . Santosham, M. (2008). Vaccination greatly reduces disease, disability, death and inequity worldwide. *Bulletin of the World Health Organization, 86*, 140–146.

Apte, A., Ingole, V., Lele, P., Marsh, A., Bhattacharjee, T., Hirve, S., . . . Juvekar, S. (2019). Ethical considerations in the use of GPS-based movement tracking in health research–lessons from a care-seeking study in rural west India. *Journal of Global Health, 9*(1), 1–7.

Atun, R., Weil, D. E., Eang, M. T., & Mwakyusa, D. (2010). Health-system strengthening and tuberculosis control. *The Lancet, 375*(9732), 2169–2178.

Balasubramaniam, P., & Hira, S. (2014). Operational pathways for integrating national disease control programmes for universal health coverage. *SSRN Electronic Journal*, 1–128. https://papers.ssrn.com/sol3/papers.cfm?abstract_id=2821364

Bavdekar, S. B., & Karande, S. (2017). Elimination of measles from India: Challenges ahead and the way forward. *Journal of Postgraduate Medicine, 63*(2), 75.

Bhatnagar, T., Ralte, M., Ralte, L., Sundaramoorthy, L., & Chhakchhuak, L. (2019). Intensified tuberculosis and HIV surveillance in a prison in Northeast India: Implementation research. *PloS One, 14*(7), e0219988.

Chatterjee, P., Kakkar, M., & Chaturvedi, S. (2016). Integrating one health in national health policies of developing countries: India's lost opportunities. *Infectious Diseases of Poverty, 5*(1), 1–5.

Chakrabartty, A., Basu, P., Ali, K. M., Sarkar, A. K., & Ghosh, D. (2018). Tuberculosis related stigma and its effect on the delay for sputum examination under the Revised National Tuberculosis Control Program in India. *Indian Journal of Tuberculosis, 65*(2), 145–151.

Chauhan, L. S. (2007). Public–private mix DOTS in India. *Bulletin of the World Health Organization, 85*(5), 399.

Dabas, H., Deo, S., Sabharwal, M., Pal, A., Salim, S., Nair, L., . . . Chitalia, M. (2019). Initiative for Promoting Affordable and Quality Tuberculosis Tests (IPAQT): A market-shaping intervention in India. *BMJ Global Health, 4*(6), e001539.

Davies, S. E. (2012). The challenge to know and control: Disease outbreak surveillance and alerts in China and India. *Global Public Health, 7*(7), 695–716.

Dehal, N., Krishan, K., Kanchan, T., Unnikrishnan, B., & Singh, J. (2015). Integrated disease surveillance in India—Progress and pitfalls. *Perspectives in Public Health, 135*(6), 290.

de Savigny, D., & Adam, T. (Eds.). (2009). *Systems thinking for health systems strengthening.* Geneva: World Health Organization.

Dey, S., Rao, A. P., Kumar, A., & Narayanan, P. (2020). Awareness & utilization of NIKSHAY and perceived barriers for tuberculosis case notification among the private practitioners in Udupi district, Karnataka. *Indian Journal of Tuberculosis, 67*(1), 15–19.

Dias, H. M. Y., Pai, M., & Raviglione, M. C. (2018). Ending tuberculosis in India: A political challenge & an opportunity. *The Indian Journal of Medical Research, 147*(3), 217.

Engel, N., Ganesh, G., Patil, M., Yellappa, V., Pai, N. P., Vadnais, C., & Pai, M. (2015). Barriers to point-of-care testing in India: Results from qualitative research across different settings, users and major diseases. *PLoS One, 10*(8), e0135112.

Fall, I. S., Rajatonirina, S., Yahaya, A. A., Zabulon, Y., Nsubuga, P., Nanyunja, M., ... Kasolo, F. C. (2019). Integrated Disease Surveillance and Response (IDSR) strategy: Current status, challenges and perspectives for the future in Africa. *BMJ Global Health, 4*(4), e001427.

Greenhalgh, T., & Papoutsi, C. (2018). Studying complexity in health services research: Desperately seeking an overdue paradigm shift. *BMC Medicine, 16*(1), 95.

Gupta, M., Saibannavar, A. A., & Kumar, V. (2016). Household symptomatic contact screening of newly diagnosed sputum smears positive tuberculosis patients—An effective case detection tool. *Lung India, 33*(2), 159.

Honigsbaum, M. (2017). Between securitisation and neglect: Managing Ebola at the borders of global health. *Medical History, 61*(2), 270–294.

Integrated Disease Surveillance Programme. (2017). *IDSP Annual Report 2017*. Retrieved from https://www.idsp.nic.in/WriteReadData/l892s/36105768501527248161.pdf

Iskander, J. K., & M'ikanatha, N. M. (2015). *Concepts and methods in infectious disease surveillance*. Chichester: Wiley-Blackwell.

John, T. J., Dandona, L., Sharma, V. P., & Kakkar, M. (2011). Continuing challenge of infectious diseases in India. *The Lancet, 377*(9761), 252–269.

Kadri, S. M., Rehana, K., Benetou, D. R., Ahmad, D. F., & Abdullah, A. (2018). Ten years of disease surveillance in Kashmir, India under Integrated Disease Surveillance Programme (IDSP) During 2006–2016. *Annals of Medical and Health Sciences Research, 8*(1), 19–23.

Kant, L., & Krishnan, S. K. (2010). Information and communication technology in disease surveillance, India: A case study. *BMC Public Health, 10*(1), S11, 1–4.

Kast, F. E., & Rosenzweig, J. E. (1972). General systems theory: Applications for organization and management. *Academy of Management Journal, 15*(4), 447–465.

Khan, A. J., Khowaja, S., Khan, F. S., Qazi, F., Lotia, I., Habib, A., ... Becerra, M. C. (2012). Engaging the private sector to increase tuberculosis case detection: An impact evaluation study. *The Lancet Infectious Diseases, 12*(8), 608–616.

Kieny, M. P., Bekedam, H., Dovlo, D., Fitzgerald, J., Habicht, J., Harrison, G., ... Siddiqi, S. (2017). Strengthening health systems for universal health coverage and sustainable development. *Bulletin of the World Health Organization, 95*(7), 537.

Krieger, N., Waterman, P. D., Chen, J. T., Soobader, M. J., & Subramanian, S. V. (2016). Monitoring socioeconomic inequalities in sexually transmitted infections, tuberculosis, and violence: Geocoding and choice of area-based socioeconomic measures—the public health disparities geocoding project (US). *Public Health Reports*.

Kumar, A., Goel, M. K., Jain, R. B., & Khanna, P. (2014). Tracking the implementation to identify gaps in integrated disease surveillance program in a block of district Jhajjar (Haryana). *Journal of Family Medicine and Primary Care, 118*(3), 240–260.

Labonté, R., & Ruckert, A. (2019). Global flows: Health workers and patients on the move. In *Health Equity in a Globalizing Era: Past Challenges, Future Prospects* (pp. 192–219). Oxford: Oxford University Press.

Littlejohns, L. B., Baum, F., Lawless, A., & Freeman, T. (2018). The value of a causal loop diagram in exploring the complex interplay of factors that influence health promotion in a multisectoral health system in Australia. *Health Research Policy and Systems, 16*(1), 1–12.

Mandyata, C. B., Olowski, L. K., & Mutale, W. (2017). Challenges of implementing the integrated disease surveillance and response strategy in Zambia: A health worker perspective. *BMC Public Health, 17*(1), 1–12.

McNabb, S. J., Chungong, S., Ryan, M., Wuhib, T., Nsubuga, P., Alemu, W., ... Rodier, G. (2002). Conceptual framework of public health surveillance and action and its application in health sector reform. *BMC Public Health, 2*(1), 1–9.

Ministry of Health and Family Welfare. (2017a). *National strategic plan for tuberculosis elimination 2017–2025. Revised national tuberculosis control programme*. Central TB Division, 109. New Delhi: Government of India.

Ministry of Health and Family Welfare. (2017b). *Measles-Rubella (MR) vaccine introduction plan*. New Delhi: Government of India. Retrieved from https://www.gavi.org/sites/default/files/temp/gavi_1570473800/India-MR-2017/MR%20Introduction%20Plan%20-%20India.pdf.

Mutale, W., Balabanova, D., Chintu, N., Mwanamwenge, M. T., & Ayles, H. (2016. Application of system thinking concepts in health system strengthening in low-income settings: A proposed conceptual framework for the evaluation of a complex health system intervention: The case of the BHOMA intervention in Zambia. *Journal of Evaluation in Clinical Practice, 22*(1), 112–121.

National Centre for Disease Control, Government of India. (2013). Delhi. https://idsp.nic.in/WriteReadData/OldSite/pediatrics.pdf.

National Disaster Management Authority. (2008). *National Disaster Management Guidelines—Management of Biological Disasters*. New Delhi: Government of India.

Nadda, J. P. (2019). India's leadership to end tuberculosis. *The Lancet, 393*(10178), 1270–1272.

Nishikiori, N., & Morishita, F. (2013). Using tuberculosis surveillance data for informed programmatic decision-making. *Western Pacific Surveillance and Response Journal, 4*(1), 1.

Pai, M. (2018). Time for high-burden countries to lead the tuberculosis research agenda. *PLoS Medicine, 15*(3), e1002544.

Pai, M., Bhaumik, S., & Bhuyan, S. S. (2017). India's plan to eliminate tuberculosis by 2025: Converting rhetoric into reality. *BMJ Global Health, 2*(2), e000326.

Patel, V., Kumar, A. S., Paul, V. K., Rao, K. D., & Reddy, K. S. (2011). Universal health care in India: The time is right. *The Lancet, 377*(9764), 448.

Peters, D. H. (2014). The application of systems thinking in health: Why use systems thinking?. *Health Research Policy and Systems, 12*(1), 1–6.

Phalkey, R. K., Shukla, S., Shardul, S., Ashtekar, N., Valsa, S., Awate, P., & Marx, M. (2013). Assessment of the core and support functions of the Integrated Disease Surveillance system in Maharashtra, India. *BMC Public Health, 13*(1), 1–15.

Phalkey, R. K., Yamamoto, S., Awate, P., & Marx, M. (2015). Challenges with the implementation of an Integrated Disease Surveillance and Response (IDSR) system: A systematic review of the lessons learned. *Health Policy and Planning, 30*(1), 131–143.

Pilot, E., Murthy G. V. S., & Nittas, V. (2020). Understanding India's urban dengue surveillance: A qualitative policy analysis of Hyderabad district. *Global Public Health, 15*(11), 1702–1717.

Pilot, E., Nittas, V., & Murthy, G. V. S. (2019). The organization, implementation, and functioning of dengue surveillance in India—A systematic scoping review. *International Journal of Environmental Research and Public Health, 16*(4), 661.

Pilot, E., Rao, R., Jena, B., & Krafft, T. (2014). Emergency Medical Service (EMS) data for syndromic surveillance in Andhra Pradesh, India. In W. Wang, T. Krafft, M. Rosenberg, E. Pilot (Eds.), *Environment and Health in Urban Areas*; Part V International Perspectives on Disease Surveillance. Chapter 18. China Environmental Press: Beijing, China.

Pilot, E., Roa, R., Jena, B., Kauhl, B., Krafft, T., & Murthy, G. V. S. (2017). Towards sustainable public health surveillance in India: Using routinely collected electronic emergency medical service data for early warning of infectious diseases. *Sustainability, 9*(4), 604.

Prathiksha, G., Daniel, B. D., & Natrajan, M. (2019). Active case-finding for tuberculosis in India. *The National Medical Journal of India, 32*(2), 90.

Rajagopalan, S., & Choutagunta, A. (2020). *Assessing healthcare capacity in India.* Mercatus Center at George Mason University, Arlington, VA.

Reddy, K. S. (2018). Health care reforms in India. *JAMA, 319*(24), 2477–2478.

Reddy, K. S., Patel, V., Jha, P., Paul, V. K., Kumar, A. S., Dandona, L., & Lancet India Group for Universal Healthcare. (2011). Towards achievement of universal health care in India by 2020: A call to action. *The Lancet, 377*(9767), 760–768.

Raut, D. K., & Bhola, A. K. (2014). Integrated disease surveillance in India: Way forward. *Global Journal of Medicine and Public Health, 3*(4), 1–10.

Saha, S., Kumar, A., Saurabh, K., Shankar, S. H., Kashyap, A., ... Wig, N. (2020). Current status of treatment of latent tuberculosis infection in India. *Indian Journal of Medical Sciences, 71*(2), 54–59.

Salve, S., Harris, K., Sheikh, K., & Porter, J. D. (2018). Understanding the complex relationships among actors involved in the implementation of public-private mix (PPM) for TB control in India, using social theory. *International Journal for Equity in Health, 17*(1), 1–15.

Satyanarayana, S., Nair, S. A., Chadha, S. S., Shivashankar, R., Sharma, G., Yadav, S., ... Dewan, P. K. (2011). From where are tuberculosis patients accessing treatment in India? Results from a cross-sectional community based survey of 30 districts. *PLoS One, 6*, e24160.

Shamanewadi, A. N., Naik, P. R., Thekkur, P., Madhukumar, S., Nirgude, A. S., Pavithra, M. B., ... Shakila, N. (2020). Enablers and challenges in the implementation of active case findings in a selected district of Karnataka, South India: A qualitative study. *Tuberculosis Research and Treatment, 2020*, 9746329.

Shastri, D. (2019). Measles and rubella surveillance. *Indian Pediatrics, 56*(9), 723.

Sheikh, K., Rangan, S., Kielmann, K., Deshpande, S., Datye, V., & Porter, J. (2005). Private providers and HIV testing in Pune, India: Challenges and opportunities. *AIDS Care, 17*, 757–766.

Shiffman, J., & Smith, S. (2007). Generation of political priority for global health initiatives: A framework and case study of maternal mortality. *The Lancet, 370*(9595), 1370–1379.

Shinde, R. R., Kembhavi, R. S., Kuwatada, J. S., & Khandednath, T. S. (2012). To develop a public private partnership model of disease notification as a part of integrated disease surveillance project (IDSP) for private medical practitioners in Mumbai City, India. *Global Journal of Medicine and Public Health, 1*(6), 1–11.

Sreeramareddy, C. T., Qin, Z. Z., Satyanarayana, S., Subbaraman, R., & Pai, M. (2014). Delays in diagnosis and treatment of pulmonary tuberculosis in India: A systematic review. *The International Journal of Tuberculosis and Lung Disease, 18*(3), 255–266.

Suresh, K. (2008). Integrated Diseases Surveillance Project (IDSP) through a consultant's lens. *Indian Journal of Public Health, 52*(3), 136–43.

Wells, W. A., Uplekar, M., & Pai, M. (2015). Achieving systemic and scalable private sector engagement in tuberculosis care and prevention in Asia. *PLoS Medicine, 12*(6), e1001842.

Wong, B. K., Fadel, S. A., Awasthi, S., Khera, A., Kumar, R., Menon, G., & Jha, P. (2019). The impact of measles immunization campaigns in India using a nationally representative sample of 27,000 child deaths. *Elife, 8*, e43290. https://elifesciences.org/articles/43290.pdf

World Bank. (2011). *World development report 2011: Conflict, security, and development.* Washington, DC: World Bank.

World Health Organization. (2000). *Report on global surveillance of epidemic-prone infectious diseases. (No. WHO/CDS/CSR/ISR/2000.1).* Geneva: Department of Communicable Disease Surveillance and Response, World Health Organization.

World Health Organization.(2005). *International health regulations.* Geneva: World Health Organization.

World Health Organization. (2014). *Standards and benchmarks for tuberculosis surveillance and vital registration systems: Checklist and user guide (No. WHO/HTM/TB/2014.02).* Geneva: World Health Organization.

World Health Organization. (2015a). *Implementing the end TB strategy: The essentials (No. WHO/HTM/TB/2015.31).* Geneva: World Health Organization.

World Health Organization. (2015b). *Systematic screening for active tuberculosis: An operational guide (No. WHO/HTM/TB/2015.16).* Geneva: World Health Organization.

World Health Organization. (2017). *Introduction of measles-rubella vaccine. National Operational Guidelines.* Geneva: World Health Organization.

World Health Organization. (2018). *Noncommunicable diseases country profiles 2018.* Geneva: World Health Organization.

World Health Organization. (2019a). *WHO South-East Asia regional high-level consultation on adopting the revised goal of measles and rubella elimination, New Delhi, India, March 14–15, 2019 (No. SEA-Immun-131).* World Health Organization. Regional Office for South-East Asia.

World Health Organization. (2019b). *Global tuberculosis report 2019.* Geneva: World Health Organization.

World Health Organization. (2019c). *The WHO India country cooperation strategy 2019–2023: A time of transition.* Geneva: World Health Organization.

World Health Organization. (2020a). *Director-General's opening remarks at the media briefing on COVID-19.* Retrieved from https://www.who.int/dg/speeches/detail/who-director-general-s-opening-remarks-at-the-media-briefing-on-covid-19---16-march-2020.

World Health Organization. (2020b). *WHO South-East Asia Regional Meeting on Strengthening Capacity of National Immunization Technical Advisory Groups (NITAGs) (No. SEA-Immun-134).* World Health Organization. Regional Office for South-East Asia. Licence: CC BY-NC-SA 3.0 IGO. New Delhi, India.

Yadav, S., Atif, M., & Rawal, G. (2018). Nikshay Poshan Yojana—Another step to eliminate TB from India. *IP Indian Journal of Immunology and Respiratory Medicine*, *3*(2), 28–29.

Yasobant, S., Patel, K., & Saxena, D. (2019). Hastening One health collaboration in Gujarat, India: A SWOT analysis. *Journal of Public Health Policy*, *3*(2).

Yellapa, V., Devadasan, N., Krumeich, A., Pant Pai, N., Vadnais, C., Pai, M., & Engel, N. (2017). How patients navigate the diagnostic ecosystem in a fragmented health system: A qualitative study from India. *Global Health Action*, *10*(1).

Zaidi, A. K., Awasthi, S., & deSilva, H. J. (2004). Burden of infectious diseases in South Asia. *British Medical Journal*, *328*(7443), 811–815.

Zignol, M., Dean, A. S., Falzon, D., van Gemert, W., Wright, A., van Deun, A., ... Bloom, A. (2016). Twenty years of global surveillance of antituberculosis-drug resistance. *New England Journal of Medicine*, *375*(11).

Xia, S., Zhou, X. N., & Liu, J. (2017). Systems thinking in combating infectious diseases. *Infectious Diseases of Poverty*, *6*(1), 1–7.

26

Human Rights and Social Inclusion in Health Policies

HIV/AIDS, Tuberculosis, and Malaria Policies across Namibia, Malawi, South Africa, and Sudan

Mutamad Amin, Malcolm MacLachlan, Hasheem Mannan, Durria M. Elhussein, Leslie Swartz, Alister Munthali, Gert Van Rooy, and Joanne McVeigh

Introduction

Trochim, Cabrera, Milstein, Gallagher, and Leischow refer to systems thinking as a "general *conceptual* orientation concerned with the interrelationships between parts and their relationships to a functioning whole, often understood within the context of an even greater whole" (2006: 539). They developed a concept map of practical challenges that need to be addressed to encourage and support effective systems thinking in public health work. One of the concepts is to "Use Systems Measures and Models" and the practical challenge within the concept was "development of methods and tools that encourage systems approaches in research and evaluation" (Trochim et al., 2006: 543). In this chapter, we present analyses of health policies using *EquiFrame*, which is a framework that encourages a systems approach. The general conceptual orientation is that of health as a basic human right to be understood within the context of twenty-one core concepts related to equality, equity, and universal access (Table 26.1).

The Global Fund partnership mobilizes and invests approximately US $4 billion per year in support of AIDS, tuberculosis (TB), and malaria programs implemented by local experts and communities most in need (The Global Fund, 2016a). However, the prevalence of these three diseases remains significant, especially in low-income countries, and particularly in Africa. For example, in 2015, 1.1 million people globally died due to AIDS-related illnesses, and 470,000 of these people lived in eastern and southern Africa (UNAIDS, 2016). Importantly, these pandemics disproportionately affect the world's poorest and most marginalized people (Mathanga & Bowie, 2007; Harling, Ehrlich, & Myer, 2008; United Nations, 2011, 2012; Allotey, Verghis, Alvarez-Castillo, & Reidpath, 2012; Dybul, 2013; International HIV/AIDS Alliance, 2015; UNICEF, 2016; World Health Organization, 2012a, 2012b, 2013a, 2013b, 2014, 2016a, 2016b). It has been recognized that "vulnerable groups are key to addressing the ongoing HIV/AIDS pandemic" and "tackling the problem in these people is hampered by their exclusion from access to prevention and treatment" (Anonymous, 2010: 67). As vulnerable groups, such as people living in poverty, are also overrepresented and more at risk

Mutamad Amin, Malcolm MacLachlan, Hasheem Mannan, Durria M. Elhussein, Leslie Swartz, Alister Munthali, Gert Van Rooy, and Joanne McVeigh, *Human Rights and Social Inclusion in Health Policies* In: *Systems Thinking for Global Health.* Edited by: Fiona Larkan, Frédérique Vallières, Hasheem Mannan, and Naonori Kodate, Oxford University Press. © Oxford University Press 2023. DOI: 10.1093/oso/9780198799498.003.0026

Table 26.1 EquiFrame's core concepts of human rights

	Core Concept	Key Question	Key Language
1.	**Non-discrimination**	Does the policy support the rights of vulnerable groups with equal opportunity in receiving health care?	Vulnerable groups are not discriminated against on the basis of their distinguishing characteristics (i.e., Living away from services; Persons with disabilities; Ethnic minority or Aged).
2.	**Individualized Services**	Does the policy support the rights of vulnerable groups with individually tailored services to meet their needs and choices?	Vulnerable groups receive appropriate, effective, and understandable services.
3.	**Entitlement**	Does the policy indicate how vulnerable groups may qualify for specific benefits relevant to them?	People with limited resources are entitled to some services free of charge or persons with disabilities may be entitled to respite grant.
4.	**Capability-based Services**	Does the policy recognize the capabilities existing within vulnerable groups?	For instance, peer to peer support among women headed households or shared cultural values among ethnic minorities.
5.	**Participation**	Does the policy support the right of vulnerable groups to participate in the decisions that affect their lives and enhance their empowerment?	Vulnerable groups can exercise choices and influence decisions affecting their life. Such consultation may include planning, development, implementation, and evaluation.
6.	**Coordination of Services**	Does the policy support assistance of vulnerable groups in accessing services from within a single provider system (inter-agency) or more than one provider system (intra-agency) or more than one sector (inter-sectoral)?	Vulnerable groups know how services should interact where inter-agency, intra-agency, and inter-sectoral collaboration is required.
7.	**Protection from Harm**	Are vulnerable groups protected from harm during their interaction with health and related systems?	Vulnerable groups are protected from harm during their interaction with health and related systems.
8.	**Liberty**	Does the policy support the right of vulnerable groups to be free from unwarranted physical or other confinement?	Vulnerable groups are protected from unwarranted physical or other confinement while in the custody of the service system/provider.

(*continued*)

Table 26.1 Continued

	Core Concept	Key Question	Key Language
9.	**Autonomy**	Does the policy support the right of vulnerable groups to consent, refuse to consent, withdraw consent, or otherwise control or exercise choice or control over what happens to him or her?	Vulnerable groups can express "independence" or "self-determination". For instance, a person with an intellectual disability will have recourse to an independent third party regarding issues of consent and choice.
10.	**Privacy**	Does the policy address the need for information regarding vulnerable groups to be kept private and confidential?	Information regarding vulnerable groups need not be shared among others.
11.	**Integration**	Does the policy promote the use of mainstream services by vulnerable groups?	Vulnerable groups are not barred from participation in services that are provided for the general population.
12.	**Contribution**	Does the policy recognize that vulnerable groups can be productive contributors to society?	Vulnerable groups make a meaningful contribution to society.
13.	**Family Resource**	Does the policy recognize the value of the family members of vulnerable groups in addressing health needs?	The policy recognizes the value of family members of vulnerable groups as a resource for addressing health needs.
14.	**Family Support**	Does the policy recognize individual members of vulnerable groups may have an impact on the family members requiring additional support from health services?	Persons with chronic illness may have mental health effects on other family members, such that these family members themselves require support.
15.	**Cultural Responsiveness**	Does the policy ensure that services respond to the beliefs, values, gender, interpersonal styles, attitudes, cultural, ethnic, or linguistic aspects of the person?	(i) Vulnerable groups are consulted on the acceptability of the service provided. (ii) Health facilities, goods and services must be respectful of ethical principles and culturally appropriate, i.e., respectful of the culture of vulnerable groups.
16.	**Accountability**	Does the policy specify to whom, and for what, services providers are accountable?	Vulnerable groups have access to internal and independent professional evaluation or procedural safeguard.
17.	**Prevention**	Does the policy support vulnerable groups in seeking primary, secondary, and tertiary prevention of health conditions?	

Table 26.1 Continued

	Core Concept	Key Question	Key Language
18.	**Capacity Building**	Does the policy support the capacity building of health workers and of the system that they work in addressing health needs of vulnerable groups?	
19.	**Access**	Does the policy support vulnerable groups—physical, economic, and information access to health services?	Vulnerable groups have accessible health facilities (i.e., transportation; physical structure of the facilities; affordability and understandable information in appropriate format).
20.	**Quality**	Does the policy support quality services to vulnerable groups through highlighting the need for evidence-based and professionally skilled practice?	Vulnerable groups are assured of the quality of the clinically appropriate services.
21.	**Efficiency**	Does the policy support efficiency by providing a structured way of matching health system resources with service demands in addressing health needs of vulnerable groups?	

with regards to tuberculosis (Thomas & Rajagopalan, 2001; Barter, Agboola, Murray, & Bärnighausen, 2012; World Health Organization, 2012a, 2013a, 2013b, 2016a) and malaria (Mubyazi et al., 2010; World Health Organization, 2012b; Tusting et al., 2013), this argument concerning inclusion of vulnerable groups similarly applies.

Access to health for these vulnerable groups is increasingly recognized as a human rights issue. For example, it has been emphasized that "people who are marginalised in many societies and health systems are now central to the fight against HIV/AIDS. Only by improving the rights of these people can they have better access to prevention, treatment, and management" (Anonymous, 2010: 67). HIV-related human rights violations including stigma and discrimination increase the risk of HIV infection by preventing people from accessing prevention, treatment, care, and support services (World Health Organization, 2010). A principal component of a rights-based approach to HIV programming includes examining the policy environment in which programmes take place (Gruskin & Tarantola, 2008). The burden and social determinants of HIV/AIDS, TB and malaria are unequally distributed across regions and population groups (Dybul, 2013); this has important implications for program planning (The Global Fund, 2011b).

This chapter reports on the application of a new systematic and peer-reviewed policy analyses framework to HIV/AIDS, TB and malaria policies and policy-related documents across Namibia, Malawi, South Africa, and Sudan. *EquiFrame* evaluates the degree of explicit commitment of a policy to twenty-one core concepts of human rights and inclusion of twelve vulnerable groups, guided by the ethos of universal, equitable, and accessible health service provision. It is important to assess if human rights are promoted in health policies and, if so, if they are promoted in a manner that is socially inclusive (Mannan, Amin, MacLachlan, & the EquitAble Consortium, 2011). There is a dearth of research concerning communicable diseases among vulnerable groups, and particularly among persons with disabilities (Rohleder, Swartz, & Philander, 2009), and this was one focus of this research. For the Global Fund to enhance its effectiveness in addressing these diseases, health services must pay greater attention to promoting the human right of access to health, especially among vulnerable groups. Our goal was to identify the extent to which HIV/AIDS, TB, and malaria policies addressed the health-related human rights of vulnerable groups, and by so doing, distinguish best-practice policies and identify policies that may require urgent revision.

Methods

(i) *EquiFrame*

Although research is evident on the process of health policy development (Gilson, Buse, Murray, & Dickinson, 2008), there is paucity of frameworks that provide for an analysis of policy content, or policy "on the books" (Stowe & Turnbull, 2001). *EquiFrame* was developed as a framework for analyzing the actual content of health policies, with a particular relevance in low-income countries and in Africa particularly, and is guided by the ethos of universal, equitable, and accessible health services. Without assessing policy content, we risk privileging some groups over others, conceivably addressing the needs of dominant groups, particularly regarding services provided through international aid support (MacLachlan, Carr, & McAuliffe, 2010; Mannan et al., 2013).

EquiFrame evaluates policies' commitment to twenty-one core concepts of human rights and inclusion of twelve vulnerable groups. "Core concept" in this policy context may be defined as a "central, often foundational policy component generalized from particular instances (namely, literature reviews, analyses of statutes and judicial opinions, and data from focus groups and interviews)" (Umbarger, Stowe, & Turnbull, 2005: 201). *EquiFrame* outlines twenty-one core concepts of human rights, which are presented alongside key questions and key language tailored to clarify the particular core concept (Table 26.1). These core concepts represent an extensive range of prominent issues in realizing universal, equitable, and accessible healthcare.

Vulnerable groups may be defined as "social groups who experience limited resources and consequent high relative risk for morbidity and premature mortality" (Flaskerud & Winslow, 1998: 69). This definition of vulnerable groups chimes with the idea that vulnerability should be related to claims for special protection, including in health policies (Hurst, 2008). Eichler and Burke (2006) outline that social discrimination that arises based on such categories results from social hierarchies: similar exclusionary practices disempower different groups, undermining their human rights and their capacity to participate fully in society.

The World Report on Disability (World Health Organization & World Bank, 2011) estimates that over 1 billion people, approximately 15% of the global population, are living with disability. However, many people with disabilities do not have equal access to healthcare, education, and employment opportunities, do not receive needed disability-related services, and experience social exclusion (United Nations, 2006; World Health Organization & World Bank, 2011; Van Rooy, Amadhila, Mufune, Swartz, Mannan, H., & MacLachlan, 2012; Mannan & MacLachlan, 2013). Therefore, a particular interest of the research team was to assess the inclusion of persons with disabilities (identified by *EquiFrame* as a vulnerable group) in policies. Definitions for vulnerable groups are outlined in Table 26.2.

EquiFrame is directed toward health policy-oriented researchers and policymakers. The framework has been presented for the Ministry of Health in Malawi (Munthali, Mannan, & MacLachlan, 2010) and Ministry of Health in Sudan.

Table 26.2 EquiFrame's vulnerable groups definitions

	Vulnerable Group	Attributes or Definitions
1.	**Limited Resources**	Referring to poor people or people living in poverty.
2.	**Increased Relative Risk for Morbidity**	Referring to people with one of the top ten illnesses, identified by WHO, as occurring within the relevant country.
3.	**Mother Child Mortality**	Referring to factors affecting maternal and child health (0–5 years).
4.	**Women Headed Household**	Referring to households headed by a woman.
5.	**Children (with special needs)**	Referring to children marginalized by special contexts, such as orphans or street children.
6.	**Aged**	Referring to older age.
7.	**Youth**	Referring to younger age without identifying gender.
8.	**Ethnic Minorities**	Referring to non-majority groups in terms of culture, race, or ethnic identity.
9.	**Displaced Populations**	Referring to people who, because of civil unrest or unsustainable livelihoods, have been displaced from their previous residence.
10.	**Living Away from Services**	Referring to people living far from health services, either in time or distance.
11.	**Suffering from Chronic Illness**	Referring to people who have an illness, which requires continuing need for care.
12.	**Disabled**	Referring to persons with disabilities, including physical, sensory, intellectual, or mental health conditions, and including synonyms of disability.

Indeed, *EquiFrame* has been or is currently being used to develop or revise policies in South Africa (disability and rehabilitation policies), Malawi (National Health Policy and National Health Research Policy), Sudan (to guide future development of all health policies), Malaysia (Science and Technology Funding Policy), and policies in Cambodia and Timor-Leste, and has been adopted by several United Nations organizations (MacLachlan, Mannan, Huss, Munthali, & Amin, 2016). For further information on *EquiFrame* including its development, please see the *EquiFrame* manual (Mannan et al., 2011) and relevant publications (Amin et al., 2011; Andersen & Mannan, 2012; Eide, Amin, MacLachlan, Mannan, & Schneider, 2012, 2013; MacLachlan et al., 2012, 2016; Mannan, Amin, MacLachlan, & the EquitAble Consortium, 2012; Mannan, McVeigh, et al., 2012; Van Rooy, Amadhila, Mannan, et al., 2012; ; Van Rooy, Amadhila, Mufune, et al., 2012; Amadhila et al., 2013; Bedri et al., 2013; Mannan et al., 2013; O'Dowd, Mannan, & McVeigh, 2013; Schneider, Eide, Amin, MacLachlan, & Mannan, 2013; Ivanova, Draebel, & Tellier, 2015; Chinyama, MacLachlan, McVeigh, Huss, & Gawamadzi, 2018; O'Donovan et al., 2018).

Scoring. Each core concept received a score from 1 to 4. This was a rating of the quality of commitment to the core concept within the policy:

1 = Concept only mentioned.
2 = Concept mentioned and explained.
3 = Specific policy actions identified to address the concept.
4 = Intention to monitor concept expressed.

A core concept that was not relevant to the document context was recorded as not applicable. Two independent raters assessed each policy. For each policy, the presence of core concepts was assessed for each vulnerable group that was identified. If a vulnerable group was not mentioned but a core concept addressed the total population (such as "all people"), the core concept was recorded as "Universal." Total scores for core concepts and vulnerable groups were calculated for each document.

(ii) Summary indices

The four summary indices of *EquiFrame* are presented below:

1. **Core Concept Coverage**: A policy was assessed regarding the number of core concepts mentioned out of the twenty-one core concepts; and this ratio was expressed as a rounded-up percentage. Furthermore, the actual terminologies used to clarify the core concepts within each document were extracted for qualitative analyses and crosschecking between raters.
2. **Vulnerable Group Coverage**: A policy was assessed regarding the number of vulnerable groups mentioned out of the twelve vulnerable groups; and this ratio was expressed as a rounded-up percentage. Similarly, the actual terminologies used to clarify the vulnerable groups were extracted for qualitative analyses and crosschecking between raters.

3. **Core Concept Quality**: A policy was assessed regarding the number of core concepts within it that were rated as 3 or 4 (as either stating a specific policy action to address a core concept or an intention to monitor a core concept) out of the twenty-one core concepts; and this ratio was expressed as a rounded-up percentage. When there were numerous references to a core concept, the top-quality score received was recorded as the final quality scoring for the particular core concept.
4. An **Overall Summary Ranking** was assigned to each policy with regards to it being of *High*, *Moderate*, or *Low* standing with respect to the criteria below:
   (i) *High* = if the policy achieved ≥ 50% on all of the three summary indices above (Core Concept Coverage, Vulnerable Group Coverage, and Core Concept Quality).
   (ii) *Moderate* = if the policy achieved ≥ 50% on two of the three summary indices above.
   (iii) *Low* = if the policy achieved < 50% on two or three of the three summary indices above.

Selection of Policies

According to the World Health Report "Working Together for Health" (World Health Organization, 2006), Africa has the highest disease burden of any continent but has the weakest health services. The current analyses focus on four African countries that each experience distinctive challenges regarding equitable access to healthcare. These four countries allow us to address how access to healthcare systems for vulnerable groups can best be promoted in contexts where the population is greatly dispersed (Namibia); where chronic poverty and high disease burden compete for little resources (Malawi); where, notwithstanding relative wealth, universal and equitable access to healthcare is still to be realized (South Africa); and where a significant amount of the population is displaced (Sudan).

EquiFrame has been applied to analyze fifty-one health policies across Namibia, Malawi, South Africa, and Sudan. Health policies were included that met the following criteria: (i) health policies created by the Ministry of Health; (ii) policies that focused on health issues outside of the Ministry of Health; (iii) strategies that addressed health policies; and (iv) policies focusing on the top ten health conditions identified by the WHO within the particular country. Appropriate ministries, agencies, and libraries were contacted and asked to identify relevant policy documents. The total number of policy documents that met the inclusion criteria in the four countries were: Namibia: ten; Malawi: fourteen; South Africa: eleven; and Sudan: sixteen. These fifty-one policy documents comprised a range of health policies, including sexual and reproductive health policy, medicine policy, disability policy, rehabilitation policy, and mental health policy. Of these fifty-one policies, our analyses of nine policies relevant to HIV/AIDS, TB, and malaria are presented here.

Table 26.3 Core concept coverage and overall summary rankings for HIV/AIDS, TB, and malaria policies

Policy Type		Country Policy	Core Concept Coverage	Overall Summary Ranking
HIV/AIDS policies:	1.	Namibia National Policy on HIV/AIDS	100%	Moderate
	2.	South Africa HIV and AIDS and STI Strategic Plan for SA 2007–2011	81%	High
	3.	Sudan AIDS Policy	71%	Low
TB policies:	1.	Namibia National Guidelines for the Management of Tuberculosis	80%	Moderate
	2.	South Africa Tuberculosis Strategic Plan for SA 2007–2011	62%	Moderate
	3.	Sudan TB Policy	57%	Low
Malaria policies:	1.	Namibia National Malaria Policy	43%	Low
	2.	Malawi Malaria Policy	52%	Low
	3.	Sudan Malaria Policy	38%	Low

Findings

For the HIV/AIDS, TB, and malaria policies across Namibia, Malawi, South Africa, and Sudan, one document received an Overall Summary Ranking of *High* (see Table 26.3). This was the South Africa HIV and AIDS and STI Strategic Plan for SA 2007–2011. Three policies were evaluated as *Moderate*, while five policies were assessed as *Low*. Notably, all three Sudanese policies analyzed received an Overall Summary Ranking of *Low*, as did all three malaria policies analyzed.

With regards to Core Concept Coverage, the Namibian HIV/AIDS policy notably scored 100%, thereby explicitly mentioning all twenty-one core concepts (see Table 26.3). Conversely, the Sudanese malaria policy scored 38% and the Namibian malaria policy scored 43% for Core Concept Coverage. Further details of findings for the HIV/AIDS, TB, and malaria policies of Namibia, Malawi, South Africa and Sudan, including Vulnerable Group Coverage, are presented elsewhere (see MacLachlan et al., 2012).

Discussion

Considerable variability was identified in the extent to which core concepts of human rights and vulnerable groups feature in these health policies. Our analyses have highlighted country-specific patterns including critical weaknesses in Sudanese AIDS, TB, and malaria policies; serious shortcomings in others, in particular malaria policies; as well as highlighting a strong health policy, namely the South African HIV/AIDS policy. The Overall Summary Ranking of malaria policy documents across Namibia, Malawi, and Sudan was *Low*. This constitutes a striking finding when taking into consideration that malaria is one of the top ten diseases across all three countries (MacLachlan et al., 2012).

Our analyses highlight that less than 50% of core concepts of human rights were mentioned in the Namibian National Malaria Policy and the Sudanese Malaria Policy. Conversely, the Namibian National Policy on HIV/AIDS notably scored 100% for Core Concept Coverage, explicitly naming all twenty-one core concepts. While inclusive coverage of core concepts of human rights in health policies is valuable, Namibia's score for this policy implies that such coverage is also *viable*.

With the exception of the Namibian National Policy on HIV/AIDS, South African HIV and AIDS and STI Strategic Plan, and the South African Tuberculosis Strategic Plan, Vulnerable Group Coverage was less than 50% across the remaining health policies analyzed (see MacLachlan et al., 2012). This constitutes an alarming finding in light of literature asserting that vulnerable groups are critical to addressing the HIV/AIDS pandemic (Anonymous, 2010; WHO, UNAIDS, & UNICEF, 2011). As vulnerable groups are also overrepresented among those with TB and malaria (Thomas & Rajagopalan, 2001; Mubyazi et al., 2010; Barter et al., 2012; World Health Organization, 2012a, 2012b; Tusting et al., 2013), this argument relating to inclusion of all vulnerable groups similarly applies. If the aim of the Global Fund is to address these diseases, it is more likely to be successful if HIV/AIDS, TB, and malaria policies address all vulnerable groups, especially as the most vulnerable may be among the most at risk for these diseases and experience the greatest number of barriers to treatment.

The majority of health policies analyzed named only some, and usually only a small number, of vulnerable groups. For example, the vulnerable group of *Mother Child Mortality* was not explicitly mentioned in any of the Namibian policies analyzed. Failing to acknowledge maternal and child health in these health policies overlooks the critical intersection between this area of health and that of communicable diseases. HIV/AIDS is the leading direct and indirect cause of maternal mortality in health facilities in Namibia (World Health Organization, 2009). The 2014 National HIV Sentinel Survey reported the prevalence of HIV among pregnant women attending antenatal clinics in Namibia as approximately 16.9% (Ministry of Health and Social Services, Namibia, 2015). Further, among the most vulnerable groups to malaria in Namibia are pregnant women and children under five years of age (World Health Organization, 2009).

The United Nations Convention on the Rights of Persons with Disabilities (United Nations, 2006) has passed into international law, obliging all signatory countries to incorporate these human rights in all policies. Is there evidence of these rights being addressed in the health policies that we examined? All TB and malaria documents analyzed, alongside the Sudanese AIDS Policy, did not mention the vulnerable group of *Disabled* persons at all. According to the Global Burden of Disease Study 2010 (Horton, 2012; Murray et al., 2012), tuberculosis accounts for 2.0% of all DALYs (disability-adjusted life years), HIV/AIDS accounts for 3.3% of all DALYs, and malaria accounts for 3.3% of all DALYs.

Each of the countries examined in this study was included because it presented a specific challenge to health service provision. Accordingly, a number of important questions follow from this selection. Did Namibia, with a highly dispersed population, have policies that addressed the inclusion of those living away from services? No, persons *Living away from services* did not strongly feature in the Namibian HIV/AIDS, malaria, and TB documents, and in fact did not feature at all in the latter document. Did Malawi, with one of the highest burdens of disease in the world, have policies that addressed the inclusion of those *Suffering from chronic illness*? Persons *Suffering from chronic illness* were mentioned to a limited extent in the malaria policy. Did South Africa, with its history of apartheid and variation in income, have policies that addressed the inclusion of *Ethnic minorities?* Not for the HIV/AIDS policy. Further, did Sudan, with a high population of displaced people, have policies that addressed the inclusion of *Displaced populations*? Similarly, none of the Sudanese policies explicitly addressed this vulnerable group. Of course, we appreciate that each of these countries could be characterized in a different way, and that the issues identified above may not be considered by all to be priorities. Nonetheless, these issues are at least salient to the countries concerned. For example, culture and ethnicity are clearly significant issues for the transmission of HIV/AIDS (MacLachlan, 2006), and therefore we might expect them to be incorporated in policy in South Africa, and elsewhere.

Through conducting these policy analyses and through providing feedback of results to stakeholder workshops in all four project countries, a number of factors were specified that may be important to consider when interpreting findings. While the inclusion criteria outlined appropriate policy documents, several documents included for analyses were not official "policies" but were instead described as "guidelines," "programs," or "strategic plans." Accordingly, as these documents may not have been formulated with an equivalent purpose, it may be misleading to analyze and compare them as policies. To the extent that such documents are not policy-related, one could simply highlight the lack of a policy.

The indices used by *EquiFrame*—scores above 50% for all summary indices—could be revised to reflect alternate weighting regarding human rights, vulnerable groups, or specific actions to address core concepts or an explicit intention to monitor core concepts. As proposed by MacLachlan et al. (2012: 8), "ultimately, *EquiFrame* is a methodology for descriptive analysis that can provide quantitative indices that can be fine-tuned for the required purpose."

An important question is if all vulnerable groups are equally relevant across all policy types. However, it is important to be able to compare the inclusion of vulnerable groups across different spheres of policy, and to subsequently consider the contextual relevance of such analyses for the particular policies—without such data, such comparisons simply cannot be made. Furthermore, certain assumptions may give rise to conceptual foreclosure when analyzing some policies. For example, it might be contended that HIV/AIDS policies necessarily address the vulnerable group of *Increased relative risk for morbidity*, and therefore it may be deemed unnecessary to determine if such policies address this group. Nonetheless, the high comorbidity of HIV/AIDS and TB, particularly in sub-Saharan Africa (World Health Organization et al., 2011; World

Health Organization, 2012a, 2013b; African Union Commission, NEPAD Agency, & UNAIDS, 2013), indicates the value of conducting such analyses. Accordingly, policies that do not include groups with other serious comorbid conditions would be less effective than those that include these groups (MacLachlan et al., 2012).

Many of the social groups defined by The Global Fund (2011a) as underserved and most-at-risk populations are also included in *EquiFrame—Women headed household, Displaced populations*, those *Suffering from chronic illness*, those with *Increased relative risk for morbidity, Youth, Children (with special needs), Disabled* persons, *Ethnic minorities*, those with *Limited Resources*, and those *Living away from services*. However, the Global Fund also recognizes vulnerable groups further to those above-mentioned, potentially constituting a limitation of *EquiFrame*. However, this further highlights the objective and capability of *EquiFrame* as a methodology for guiding health policy content analyses to promote equitable and rights-based healthcare, presenting a range of indices that can be modified for the required purpose.

Supplementary analyses of the use of the word "all" and its synonyms in policies reveals that those documents that explicitly cite such "all-encompassing" terms also explicitly mention certain vulnerable groups to the exclusion of others (MacLachlan et al., 2012). It is therefore important to ascertain those vulnerable groups that are explicitly included, and those not explicitly included, as the use of all-embracing terminology does not necessarily address the specific health concerns and needs of different vulnerable groups (Mannan, Amin, et al., 2012). Even when "all" is frequently used in a document, the question remains of why only some vulnerable groups continue to be mentioned alongside it.

Alongside policies, *EquiFrame* can also be effectively applied to other types of planning documents, where human rights and inclusion of vulnerable groups are relevant (MacLachlan et al., 2012). Furthermore, *EquiFrame* may very effectively be used as a framework for evaluation, but also as a tool for ensuring human rights and social inclusion in the revision or development of policy documents. *EquiFrame* may highlight high-quality documents, and therefore guide policy-makers in the direction of best-practice documents. Further, it can provide a check-list of factors that may be considered for a relevant document, and provide specific terms related to equity and human rights (Van Rooy, Amadhila, Mannan, et al., 2012).

The Global Fund (2011b) emphasizes equity assessments of existing data to improve programmes supported through the Global Fund. Suggested data sources include demographic data, including censuses; data related to disease morbidity and mortality, such as vital registration; data on social determinants of health and risk factors, including population-based surveys; data on health service use, including health facility records; qualitative data, such as operational research; and grey sources, including information from civil society (The Global Fund, 2011b). Equity assessments of the above data sources are important, and as such represent prospects for future research. Notwithstanding the relevance of these data sources for assessments of equity, health policy as a data source for equity assessments—examining the extent to which health policy content is equitable—is an imperative enterprise.

The Global Fund has promoted a rights-based approach to health since its foundation (The Global Fund, 2016b). However, more recently, the Global Fund's Board has strengthened the Global Fund's mandate to promote human rights (Dybul, 2013).

EquiFrame provides an appropriate policy analyses framework to uphold this mandate by supporting policy development and revision for the promotion of health-related human rights. It is proposed that "the fight against HIV/AIDS is no longer a battle against the virus, it is, and will increasingly be, a battle for human rights" (Anonymous, 2010: 67). This is critically dependent upon the realization of health-related human rights for the most vulnerable and marginalized population groups, including access to healthcare.

Indeed, *EquiFrame* can provide vulnerable groups and their representative organizations with an analogous guiding list of core concepts of health-related human rights for which to advocate in policy development. While it is important to recognize that vulnerable groups are by no means homogenous in their health-related needs or aspirations, joint advocacy can serve to strengthen the participation of more vulnerable and marginalized groups in policy planning and development. Accordingly, such population groups can be effectively informed and guided regarding their health-related human rights but can also advocate for the same health-related human rights, strengthening advocacy through concerted effort and a unified voice, captured by the Ojibwa Native American saying "No tree has branches so foolish as to fight among themselves." If the Global Fund is to extend its reach to address the most vulnerable and marginalized, it should support a program of policy development and revision that incorporates the promotion of health-related human rights of vulnerable groups, including access to healthcare. In so doing, the Global Fund can contribute a vital step toward achieving the Sustainable Development Goals.

Acknowledgment

This research was funded by the European Commission Framework Programme 7; Project Title: Enabling Universal and Equitable Access to Healthcare for Vulnerable People in Resource Poor Settings in Africa; Grant Agreement No. 223501.

References

African Union Commission, NEPAD Agency, & UNAIDS. (2013). *Delivering results toward ending AIDS, tuberculosis and malaria in Africa: African Union accountability report on Africa-G8 Partnership commitments 2013.* Addis Ababa, Ethiopia. Retrieved from www.unaids.org/en/media/unaids/contentassets/documents/document/2013/05/20130525_AccountabilityReport_EN.pdf.

Allotey, P., Verghis, S., Alvarez-Castillo, F., & Reidpath, D. D. (2012). Vulnerability, equity and universal coverage—A concept note. *BMC Public Health, 12*(1), 1–3. doi:10.1186/1471-2458-12-S1-S2

Amadhila, E., Van Rooy, G., McVeigh, J., Mannan, H., MacLachlan, M., & Amin, M. (2013). Equity and core concepts of human rights in Namibian health policies. *Africa Policy Journal, 8*, 34–45. Retrieved from https://apj.hkspublications.org/equity-and-core-concepts-of-human-rights-in-namibian-health-policies/

Amin, M., MacLachlan, M., Mannan, H., El Tayeb, S., El Khatim, A., Swartz, L., ... Schneider, M. (2011). EquiFrame: A framework for analysis of the inclusion of human rights and vulnerable groups in health policies. *Health and Human Rights, 13*(2), 1–20.

Andersen, A., & Mannan, H. (2012). Assessing the quality of European policies on disability and development cooperation: A discussion of core concepts of human rights and coherence. *Disability and International Development, 1*, 16–24.

Anonymous. (2010). Rights of vulnerable people and the future of HIV/AIDS. *Lancet Infectious Diseases, 10*(2), 67–138. doi:10.1016/S1473-3099(10)70013-X

Barter, D. M., Agboola, S. O., Murray, M. B., & Bärnighausen, T. (2012). Tuberculosis and poverty: The contribution of patient costs in sub-Saharan Africa—a systematic review. *BMC Public Health, 12*(980), 1–21. doi10.1186/1471-2458-12-980

Bedri, N., Amin, M., El Khatim, A., Gamal Eldin, A., MacLachlan, M., & Mannan, H. (2013). Core concepts of human rights and vulnerable groups in Nutrition Policy of Sudan. *International Journal of Nutrition and Food Sciences, 2*(6), 352–359. doi:10.11648/j.ijnfs.20130206.24

Chinyama, M. J., MacLachlan, M., McVeigh, J., Huss, T., & Gawamadzi, S. (2018). An analysis of the extent of social inclusion and equity consideration in Malawi's national HIV and AIDS policy review process. *International Journal of Health Policy and Management, 7*(4), 297–307. doi:10.15171/IJHPM.2017.87

Dybul, M. (2013). *Better health, better human rights*. Geneva: The Global Fund to Fight AIDS, Tuberculosis and Malaria.

Eichler, M., & Burke, M. A. (2006). The BIAS FREE Framework: A new analytical tool for global health research. *Canadian Journal of Public Health, 97*(1), 63–68.

Eide, A. H., Amin, M., MacLachlan, M., Mannan, H., & Schneider, M. (2012). Human rights, social inclusion and health equity in international donors' policies. *Disability, CBR and Inclusive Development, 23*(4), 24–40. doi:10.5463/DCID.v23i4.144

Eide, A. H., Amin, M., MacLachlan, M., Mannan, H., & Schneider, M. (2013). Addressing equitable health of vulnerable groups in international health documents. *ALTER—European Journal of Disability Research, 7*(3), 153–162.

Flaskerud, J. H., & Winslow, B. J. (1998). Conceptualizing vulnerable populations health-related research. *Nursing Research, 47*(2), 69–78. doi:10.1097/00006199-199803000-00005

Gilson, L., Buse, K., Murray, S. F., & Dickinson, C. (2008). Future directions for health policy analysis: A tribute to the work of Professor Gill Walt. *Health Policy and Planning, 23*(5), 291–293. doi:10.1093/heapol/czn025

The Global Fund. (2011a). *Policy on eligibility criteria, counterpart financing requirements, and prioritization of proposals for funding from the Global Fund (Twenty-third Board Meeting, Geneva, Switzerland, May 11–12, 2011)*. Geneva: The Global Fund to Fight AIDS, Tuberculosis and Malaria.

The Global Fund. (2011b). *Matching resources to need: Opportunities to promote equity; information note*. Geneva: The Global Fund to Fight AIDS, Tuberculosis and Malaria.

The Global Fund. (2016a). *The Global Fund*. Geneva: The Global Fund to Fight AIDS, Tuberculosis and Malaria. Retrieved from http://www.theglobalfund.org/en/.

The Global Fund. (2016b). *35th board meeting. The Global Fund strategy 2017–2022: investing to end epidemics*. Geneva: The Global Fund to Fight AIDS, Tuberculosis and Malaria. Retrieved from https://www.theglobalfund.org/media/1176/bm35_02-theglobalfundstrategy2017-2022investingtoendepidemics_report_en.pdf.

Gruskin, S., & Tarantola, D. (2008). Universal access to HIV prevention, treatment and care: Assessing the inclusion of human rights in international and national strategic plans. *AIDS, 22*(2), S123–S132. doi:10.1097/01.aids.0000327444.51408.21

Harling, G., Ehrlich, R., & Myer, L. (2008). The social epidemiology of tuberculosis in South Africa: A multilevel analysis. *Social Science & Medicine, 66*(2), 492–505. DOI: 10.1016/j.socscimed.2007.08.026

Horton, R. (2012). GBD 2010: Understanding disease, injury, and risk. *The Lancet, 380*(9859), 2053–2054. doi:10.1016/S0140-6736(12)62133-3

Hurst, S. A. (2008). Vulnerability in research and health care: Describing the elephant in the room? *Bioethics, 22*(4), 191–202. doi:10.1111/j.1467-8519.2008.00631.x

International HIV/AIDS Alliance. (2015). *Alliance charter and linking agreement 2015–2017.* Hove: International HIV/AIDS Alliance.

Ivanova, O., Draebel, T., & Tellier, S. (2015). Are sexual and reproductive health policies designed for all? Vulnerable groups in policy documents of four European countries and their involvement in policy development. *International Journal of Health Policy and Management, 4*(10), 663–671. doi:10.15171/ijhpm.2015.148

MacLachlan, M. (2006). *Culture and health: A critical perspective towards global health* (2nd ed.). West Sussex: John Wiley & Sons Ltd.

MacLachlan, M., Carr, S. C., & McAuliffe, E. (2010). *The aid triangle: Recognizing the human dynamics of dominance, justice and identity.* London: Zed Books.

MacLachlan, M., Mannan, H., Huss, T., Munthali, A., & Amin, M. (2016). Policies and processes for social inclusion: Using EquiFrame and EquIPP for policy dialogue; Comment on "Are sexual and reproductive health policies designed for all?" Vulnerable groups in policy documents of four European countries and their involvement in policy development. *International Journal of Health Policy and Management, 5*(3), 193–196. doi:10.15171/ijhpm.2015.200

MacLachlan, M., Amin, M., Mannan, H., El Tayeb, S., Bedri, N., Swartz, L., … McVeigh, J. (2012). Inclusion and human rights in health policies: Comparative and benchmarking analysis of 51 policies from Malawi, Sudan, South Africa and Namibia. *PLoS One, 7*(5), e35864. doi:10.1371/journal.pone.0035864

Mannan, H., & MacLachlan, M. (2013). Disability and health: A research agenda. *Social Inclusion, 1*(1), 37–45. doi:10.12924/si2013.01010037

Mannan, H., Amin, M., MacLachlan, M., & the EquitAble Consortium. (2011). *The EquiFrame manual: A tool for evaluating and promoting the inclusion of vulnerable groups and core concepts of human rights in health policy documents.* Dublin: Global Health Press.

Mannan, H., Amin, M., MacLachlan, M., & the EquitAble Consortium. (2012). Non-communicable disease priority actions and social inclusion. *The Lancet, 379*(9812), e17–e18. doi:10.1016/S0140-6736(12)60106-8

Mannan, H., MacLachlan, M., McVeigh, J., & the EquitAble Consortium. (2012). Core concepts of human rights and inclusion of vulnerable groups in the United Nations Convention on the Rights of Persons with Disabilities. *ALTER—European Journal of Disability Research, 6*(3), 159–177. doi:10.1016/j.alter.2012.05.005

Mannan, H., El Tayeb, S., MacLachlan, M., Amin, M., McVeigh, J., Munthali, A., & Van Rooy, G. (2013). Core concepts of human rights and inclusion of vulnerable groups in the mental health policies of Malawi, Namibia, and Sudan. *International Journal of Mental Health Systems, 7*(1), 1–13. doi:10.1186/1752-4458-7-7

Mannan, H., McVeigh, J., Amin, M., MacLachlan, M., Swartz, L., Munthali, A., & Van Rooy, G. (2012). Core concepts of human rights and inclusion of vulnerable groups in the disability and rehabilitation policies of Malawi, Namibia, Sudan, and South Africa. *Journal of Disability Policy Studies, 23*(2), 67–81. doi:10.1177/1044207312439103

Mathanga, D. P., & Bowie, C. (2007). Malaria control in Malawi: Are the poor being served? *International Journal for Equity in Health, 6*(22), 1–6. doi:10.1186/1475-9276-6-22

Ministry of Health and Social Services, Namibia. (2015). *The Namibia AIDS response progress report 2015. Reporting period 2013–2014.* Windhoek, Namibia: Namibia Ministry of Health and Social Services. Retrieved from https://www.unaids.org/sites/default/files/country/documents/NAM_narrative_report_2015.pdf.

Mubyazi, G. M., Bloch, P., Magnussen, P., Olsen, Ø. E., Byskov, J., Hansen, K. S., & Bygbjerg, I. C. (2010). Women's experiences and views about costs of seeking malaria chemoprevention and other antenatal services: a qualitative study from two districts in rural Tanzania. *Malaria Journal, 9*(54), 1–13. doi:10.1186/1475-2875-9-54

Munthali, A., Mannan, H., & MacLachlan, M. (2010). Social inclusion and health policies: National workshop for health policy makers and policy analysts, Lilongwe, Malawi, November 8–9, 2010.

Murray, C. J. L., Vos, T., Lozano, R., Naghavi, M., Flaxman, A. D., Michaud, C., ... Lopez, A. D. (2012). Disability-adjusted life years (DALYs) for 291 diseases and injuries in 21 regions, 1990–2010: a systematic analysis for the Global Burden of Disease Study 2010. *The Lancet, 380*(9859), 2197–2223. doi:10.1016/S0140-6736(12)61689-4

O'Donovan, M-A., Mannan, H., McVeigh, J., McCarron, M., McCallion, P., & Byrne, E. (2018). Core human rights concepts in Irish health and housing policy documents: In search of equity for people with ID. *Journal of Policy and Practice in Intellectual Disabilities, 15*(4), 307–313. doi:10.1111/jppi.12274

O'Dowd, J., Mannan, H., & McVeigh, J. (2013). India's disability policy—Analysis of core concepts of human rights. *Disability, CBR, and Inclusive Development, 24*(4), 69–90. doi:105463/DCID.v24i4.277

Rohleder, P., Swartz, L., & Philander, J. (2009). Disability and HIV/AIDS: A key development issue. In M. MacLachlan & L. Swartz (Eds.), *Disability & international development: Towards inclusive global health* (pp. 137–148). New York, NY: Springer.

Schneider, M., Eide, A. H., Amin, M., MacLachlan, M., & Mannan, H. (2013). Inclusion of vulnerable groups in health policies: regional policies on health priorities in Africa. *African Journal of Disability, 2*(1), 1–9. doi:10.4102/ajod.v2i1.40

Stowe, M. J., & Turnbull, H. R. (2001). Tools for analyzing policy "on the books" and policy "on the streets". *Journal of Disability Policy Studies, 12*(3), 206–214. doi:10.1177/104420730101200306

Thomas, T. Y., & Rajagopalan, S. (2001). Tuberculosis and aging: A global health problem. *Clinical Infectious Diseases, 33*(7), 1034–1039. doi:10.1086/322671

Trochim, W. M., Cabrera, D. A., Milstein, B., Gallagher, R. S., & Leischow, S. J. (2006). Practical challenges of systems thinking and modeling in public health. *American Journal of Public Health, 96*(3), 538–546. doi:10.2105/AJPH.2005.066001

Tusting, L. S., Willey, B., Lucas, H., Thompson, J., Kafy, H. T., Smith, R., & Lindsay, S. W. (2013). Socieconomic development as an intervention against malaria: a systematic review and meta analysis. *The Lancet, 382*(9896), 963–972. doi:10.1016/S0140-6736(13)60851-X

Umbarger, G. T., Stowe, M. J., & Turnbull, H. R. (2005). The core concepts of health policy affecting families who have children with disabilities. *Journal of Disability Policy Studies, 15*(4), 201–208. doi:10.1177/10442073050150040201

UNAIDS (Joint United Nations Programme on HIV/AIDS). (2010). *Getting to zero: UNAIDS 2011–2015 strategy.* Geneva: UNAIDS. Retrieved from https://www.unaids.org/

en/resources/documents/2010/20101221_JC2034_UNAIDS_Strategy#:~:text=This%20Strategy%20has%20been%20developed,and%20the%20Millennium%20Development%20Goals.

UNAIDS. (2016). *UNAIDS fact sheet 2016*. Geneva: UNAIDS.

United Nations Children's Fund. (2016). *Malaria*. New York, NY: UNICEF.

United Nations. (2006). *Convention on the Rights of Persons with Disabilities*. New York, NY: United Nations. Retrieved from https://www.un.org/development/desa/disabilities/convention-on-the-rights-of-persons-with-disabilities/convention-on-the-rights-of-persons-with-disabilities-2.html

United Nations. (2011). *Political Declaration on HIV and AIDS: Intensifying our efforts to eliminate HIV and AIDS (Resolution adopted by the General Assembly][A/Res/65/277)*. New York, NY: United Nations. Retrieved from http://www.unaids.org/en/media/unaids/contentassets/documents/document/2011/06/20110610_UN_A-RES-65-277_en.pdf.

United Nations. (2012). *The Millennium Development Goals report 2012*. New York, NY: United Nations. Retrieved from https://mdgs.un.org/unsd/mdg/Resources/Static/Products/Progress2012/English2012.pdf.

Van Rooy, G., Amadhila, E., Mannan, H., McVeigh, J., MacLachlan, M., & Amin, M. (2012). Core concepts of human rights and inclusion of vulnerable groups in the Namibian policy on orthopaedic technical services. *Disability, CBR and Inclusive Development, 23*(3), 24–47. doi:10.5463/DCID.v23i3.132

Van Rooy, G., Amadhila, E. M., Mufune, P., Swartz, L., Mannan, H., & MacLachlan, M. (2012). Perceived barriers to accessing health services among people with disabilities in rural northern Namibia. *Disability & Society, 27*(6), 761–75. doi:10.1080/09687599.2012.686877

World Health Organization. (2006). *Working together for health: The world health report 2006*. Geneva: World Health Organization. Retrieved from https://www.who.int/whr/2006/whr06_en.pdf

World Health Organization. (2009). *Bringing it all together: Annual report 2008 (Namibia)*. Windhoek, Namibia: World Health Organization. Retrieved from https://www.afro.who.int/publications/bringing-it-all-together-annual-report-2008-who-namibia

World Health Organization. (2010). *UNAIDS report on the global AIDS epidemic 2010*. Geneva, Switzerland: UNAIDS.

World Health Organization. (2012a). *Global tuberculosis report 2012*. Geneva,: World Health Organization. Retrieved from https://www.who.int/tb/publications/global_report/gtbr12_main.pdf.

World Health Organization. (2012b). *World malaria report 2012*. Geneva: World Health Organization. Retrieved from https://www.who.int/malaria/publications/world_malaria_report_2012/wmr2012_full_report.pdf.

World Health Organization. (2013a). *Global TB programme*. Geneva: World Health Organization.

World Health Organization. (2013b). *HIV-associated TB facts 2013*. Geneva: World Health Organization. Retrieved from https://www.who.int/tb/challenges/hiv/tbhiv_factsheet_2013_web.pdf.

World Health Organization. (2014). *MDG 6: Combat HIV/AIDS, malaria and other diseases*. Geneva: World Health Organization.

World Health Organization. (2016a). *Tuberculosis*. Geneva: World Health Organization.

World Health Organization. (2016b). *Malaria*. Geneva: World Health Organization.

World Health Organization, UNAIDS, & UNICEF. (2011). *Global HIV/AIDS response: Epidemic update and health sector progress towards universal access. Progress report 2011.* Geneva: World Health Organization. Retrieved from https://apps.who.int/iris/handle/10665/44787.

World Health Organization, & World Bank. (2011). *World report on disability.* Geneva: World Health Organization. Retrieved from http://www.who.int/disabilities/world_report/2011/en/index.html.

27
Stillbirth
The Hidden Global Mortality Burden

Margaret M. Murphy, Rakhi Dandona, Hannah Blencowe, Paula Quigley, Susannah Hopkins Leisher, Claire Storey, Dimitrios Siassakos, Alexander Heazell, and Vicki Flenady, on behalf of the International Stillbirth Alliance

Introduction

Stillbirth is defined as the birth of a baby showing no signs of life. Each year, 2 million babies greater than twenty-eight weeks' gestation are stillborn around the world (Hug et al., 2021). Low-income countries have the greatest burden of stillbirth with 42% of the global total occurring in Sub-Saharan Africa and 34% in Southern Asia. Six countries in the world account for half of all stillbirths: India, Pakistan, Nigeria, Democratic Republic of the Congo, China, and Ethiopia (United Nations, 2020). These numbers may be an underestimate, as stillbirths are often unreported (United Nations, 2020). The World Health Organization (WHO) ICD (International Classification of Diseases) defines stillbirth as twenty-two or more completed weeks (but it uses twenty-eight weeks for international comparisons).

Although global stillbirth numbers are commensurate with numbers of newborn deaths (deaths of babies up to twenty-seven days following live birth), stillbirth has remained largely invisible at the global policy level. It is estimated that numbers of stillbirths are rising in Sub-Saharan Africa, up from 0.77 million in 2000 to 0.82 million in 2019 (Hug et al., 2021). Despite the acknowledged global mortality burden and impact, stillbirth was absent from the Millennium Development Goals and the Sustainable Development Goals (SDGs) (United Nations Inter-agency Group for Child Mortality Estimation, 2020). Stillbirth remains hidden because these births are not counted in the vital registration system, particularly in countries where the burden is the highest. They are not counted because they are not considered as important as those infants who are born live. The world needs a paradigm shift from fatalism to considering a stillborn baby as the loss of a future productive member of society and the enormity of the loss to women and families. Importantly, the past few years have seen small but important changes in global policies. For example, the United Nations' Global Strategy for Women's, Children's, and Adolescents' Health (United Nations, 2015) and WHO/United Nations Children's Fund's (2014) Every Newborn Action Plan (ENAP) have brought attention to stillbirths and some countries now have stillbirth reduction targets (Blencowe et al., 2021).

Margaret M. Murphy, Rakhi Dandona, Hannah Blencowe, Paula Quigley, Susannah Hopkins Leisher, Claire Storey, Dimitrios Siassakos, Alexander Heazell, and Vicki Flenady, *Stillbirth* In: *Systems Thinking for Global Health.* Edited by: Fiona Larkan, Frédérique Vallières, Hasheem Mannan, and Naonori Kodate, Oxford University Press.
DOI: 10.1093/oso/9780198799498.003.0027

The global stillbirth situation is disappointing because a great number of stillbirths are preventable with the provision of safe, high-quality maternity care. In fact, many of the interventions that reduce neonatal mortality could also reduce the mortality from stillbirth. However, the apathy within the health system and of health providers continues to drive ignorance of stillbirths. There is also perpetuation of stigma, isolation, and neglect of women, babies, and their families, even some reported cases in South America resulting in imprisonment of women following stillbirth (Viterna & Bautista, 2017). These babies' deaths have a profound and long-lasting impact on women, their partners, families, communities, and wider society (Heazell et al., 2016).

Bereaved parents are key to bringing about change. The International Stillbirth Alliance (ISA) as an example is an organization uniting bereaved parents and other family members, health professionals, and researchers to drive global change for the prevention of stillbirth and newborn death and provision of bereavement support for all those affected. ISA is an alliance of member organizations and individual supporters with over fifty member organizations and individual supporters on every continent. ISA's mission is to raise awareness and promote global collaboration for the prevention of stillbirth and newborn death and provision of appropriate respectful care for all those affected. ISA does this through various channels, including stillbirth advocacy, prevention, and bereavement working groups, and hosting global conferences annually. ISA contributes to global policy such as ENAP and UNICEF publications, participates in relevant global events, such as Align MNH: Collective action for maternal newborn health, and publishes commentaries on issues of significance (Leisher et al., 2020; Homer et al., 2021).

Using the WHO Health Systems Framework (World Health Organization, 2010), this chapter will outline the challenges facing global communities in reducing stillbirth. It will discuss challenges common to all settings: high-, middle-, and low-income countries. It will seek to unpack the potential shared solutions, using a systems-thinking approach necessary to confront the global stillbirth mortality statistics.

Background

Stillbirth is inequitably distributed, and prevention is rarely integrated into social welfare policy. Sub-Saharan Africa, South East Asia, and South America carry the greatest stillbirth burden with 98% of cases (Figure 27.1). Stillbirth remains a concern for high-income countries too with about one in 200 pregnancies ending in stillbirth There are well-recognized healthcare inequalities evident in high-income settings with women of color (in largely white societies), marginalized populations, and women from ethnic minorities, and low-income households over-represented in the mortality statistics. Women with comorbidities and social disadvantages are also overrepresented in the stillbirth statistics (Draper et al., 2020).

Stillbirth follows the death of a baby *in utero*, yet prevention is rarely explicitly integrated in antenatal care services. Antenatal care is designed to identify women at increased risk and prevent, where possible, adverse pregnancy outcomes. Though

Substantial disparities between regions

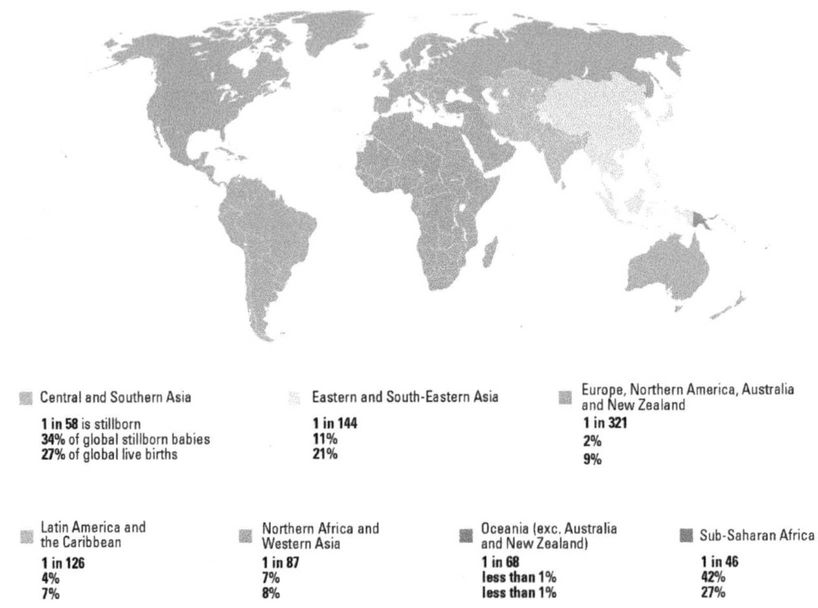

Figure 27.1 Global stillbirth burden (UN IGME, 2020)

antenatal care is known to reduce neonatal mortality and the coverage of at least one antenatal care visit has improved in recent years to 87% of pregnant women globally, fewer than three in five (59%) pregnant women receive at least four antenatal care visits (United Nations Children's Fund, 2021). Furthermore, it is estimated that 40% of women give birth without midwifery care or at a minimum a trained birth attendant globally (United Nations Children's Fund, 2021). Babies may die *in utero* before labor begins or may be alive at the commencement of labor but die during the process. Access to midwife or healthcare-delivered interventions have been estimated to potentially reduce stillbirths by 26% globally (Nove et al., 2021). With good quality maternity care, in particular access to emergency obstetric care the recognition and treatment of prolonged or obstructed labor, the death of a baby during labor is often a preventable event.

The effects of stillbirth impact more than mothers but this is rarely reflected in family care and community engagement. Stillbirths affect the woman, her partner, their families, society, and wider communities (Burden et al., 2021) with health, social, and economic impacts (Heazell et al., 2016). However, policies to support and engage families are virtually non-existent in most low-resource countries and at best cursory even in high-resource settings. Respectful bereavement care after stillbirth is a human rights issue with its foundations in respectful maternity care (White Ribbon Alliance, 2019), yet stillbirth is absent from human rights policy. Women, their partners, and families deserve respectful bereavement care allied to the respectful maternity care movement as outlined by the World Health Organization (2014). The manner in which women and families are cared for at and after stillbirth has a profound and long-lasting effect on parents (Ellis et al., 2016).

Stillbirth Challenges

Interventions and programs that can be implemented to prevent the global burden of newborn death are also pertinent for the reduction of deaths from stillbirth. These would not require much additional input, rather a reframing of mindset to consider these preventable deaths. Utilizing the WHO Health Systems Framework's (World Health Organization, 2010) six building blocks, leadership and governance, health-care information, financing, human resources, access to medicines and technology, and service delivery, provides a very useful method of framing the discussion of ending preventable stillbirths. This section will look at each of these building blocks in turn and discuss the challenges and potential solutions to address them. The section contents are outlined in Table 27.1. Governance and health information systems provide the basis for the overall policy and regulation of all the other health system blocks so they are a good place to begin.

(i) Leadership and governance

Leadership and governance are needed at every level and facet to tackle the stillbirth crisis from the global (United Nations/WHO), national (Ministry-level leadership), community, and health service facility levels, to individual practitioners. There needs to be a whole-of-society approach taken to address the issues that need to be examined to address prevention of stillbirths and supporting families after stillbirth. The global community can learn from the success achieved by Australia in engaging the leadership to address stillbirths.

Engaging with parents and civic society is another key component of governance. It is important to recognize parent voices when discussing such a devastating personal event as the death of a baby. This principle is a key cornerstone of the ISA which collaborates with and involves bereaved parents at all levels of the organization. The ISA has harnessed their unique position in the development of the Parents Voices Initiative, which aims to establish a registry of global parent support organizations and the development of stillbirth advocacy toolkits for providers and parents in India and Kenya. Another vital role for parents is in the annual ISA international conferences held across the globe with parents' committee and contribution as key features in all the conferences. ISA conferences have been held in Spain, Uruguay, Vietnam, Netherlands, Scotland, Ireland, and in 2021 was held in Australia.

Another component of governance is increasing global advocacy to raise awareness about stillbirth. Through the establishment of the Stillbirth Advocacy Working Group (SAWG), ISA in partnership with London School for Hygiene & Tropical Medicine seeks to develop and support a network that advocates for stillbirth prevention and care within the existing global architecture, ensuring key evidence and data are made

Table 27.1 Ending preventable stillbirths (adapted from WHO 2010 Health Systems Framework; Storey 2020, adapted from Barton & Grant 2006)

GOVERNANCE	INFORMATION	FINANCING	HUMAN RESOURCES	MEDICINES & TECHNOLOGY	SERVICE DELIVERY
Leadership needed at global (UN/WHO), national (Ministry-level leadership), community and health service facility levels. Identify champions Learn from successes e.g., Australian Stillbirth CRE story	**Counting/Stillbirth** Registration Agreed definitions.	**Stillbirth: low priority** little funding is available for stillbirth research.	**Skills, Availability, and Accountability** Education programs for health and social care professionals.	**Identification and Prevention of Stillbirth** Clinical factors e.g., Previous stillbirth, Parity, Maternal age, comorbidities. Packages of Care to prevent stillbirth e.g., Safe Baby Bundles.	**Accessibility, Availability, & Quality** Affordable and accessible healthcare. Availability of healthcare in rural setting. Increase healthcare facility capabilities.
Engaging with parents and civic society Recognize parent voices Increased global advocacy	**Classification** Agreed classification systems. **Develop and prioritize mortality review** Perinatal death reviews and audits. **Risk Factors** Identification of risk factors for occurrence and recurrence of stillbirth. **Bereavement Care** Recognized and accepted standards of care. **Information Sharing and Research Collaboration** **Reciprocal Learning.**	**Investment needed:** Maternity Services Social determinants of health Health and nutritional care Preventative programs e.g., Malaria, HIV, STIs Healthcare training Data collection	**Population education programs:** Stigma Fatalism Religious/cultural beliefs about birth and stillbirth Family support Domestic abuse		

visible for key audiences. It is hoped to link to accountability at country level and globally, seize key moments to advocate for stillbirth prevention and care, and empower "bottom-up" advocacy from parents and parent groups.

(ii) Healthcare information systems

One of the biggest challenges facing the global community in addressing stillbirth is the lack of reliable data. Therefore, obtaining core indicators on health information is a key priority in ending preventable stillbirths (de Bernis et al., 2016). There are several facets that need to be considered here in turn which all contribute to the overall structure. These include agreeing on a definition for stillbirth and associated terms, counting stillbirths, registering the number of stillbirths, and agreeing on the classification of the causes of stillbirths. The need to develop and conduct perinatal mortality audits and reviews is also important as is the identification of risk factors for occurrence and recurrence of stillbirth. Finally, the development of recognized bereavement care standards and the necessity for reciprocal learning throughout the global community through research collaboration and information sharing.

Poor-quality data availability has hampered initiatives to reduce the global stillbirth burden. The United Nations (UN) established an Inter-agency Group for Child Mortality Estimation (UNIGME). Along with its Technical Advisory Group and Core Stillbirth Estimation Group, UNIGME has developed robust methods to estimate stillbirths and in 2020 produced its first report (United Nations Inter-agency Group for Child Mortality Estimation, 2020). This report recommends gestational age as the single criterion to define stillbirth and use the International Classification of Diseases definition of stillbirth as "late gestation fetal deaths" as deaths occurring at or after twenty-eight weeks of gestation. This definition allowed for an international comparison of 171 countries with data around the world (United Nations, 2020).

Having an agreed stillbirth definition is one thing, ensuring that countries accurately record all instances of stillbirth is another challenge. Stillbirth needs to be included in each country's health metrics alongside live birth data and the data need to be captured accurately to improve data quality relating to the actual information itself and the statistical systems employed (World Health Organization, 2010). Capturing accurate stillbirth rates is problematic due to misclassification or omission and relies on accurate assessment of vital status at birth and birthweight or gestational age. There may be a reluctance on the part of health services to record stillbirths if doing so reflects poorly on the "quality" of the maternity service provided. For example, as intrapartum stillbirth rate is a key performance indicator for quality maternity care (Lawn et al., 2009), some professionals may misclassify intrapartum stillbirth (death during labor) as antepartum stillbirth (death during pregnancy) to give the impression of optimal performance. Furthermore, it is estimated that more than 40 million women give birth unattended at home each year, which places them at increased risk of intrapartum stillbirth *and* prevents these loses from being counted. Blencowe et al., (2021), in their cross-sectional population-based survey of women of reproductive age in five health and demographic surveillance system sites in Bangladesh, Ethiopia,

Ghana, Guinea-Bissau, and Uganda, suggest further investment is needed to improve the measurement and reporting of vital status at birth, birthweight, and gestational age by health providers to improve health systems stillbirth data. In addition, as many low- and middle-income settings rely on maternal recalled pregnancy outcomes, this information must be communicated clearly to women and barriers to women reporting adverse events addressed.

Determining the cause of stillbirth is important both in terms of providing answers to parents as to why their baby died but also in identifying conditions that may be preventable in future pregnancies and may prevent other perinatal deaths. Classification of the causes of stillbirth is currently problematic due to the lack of accurate data collection, as outlined earlier, the lack of access to trained perinatal pathology services resulting in many stillbirth causes being based upon clinical presentation and history only, and finally the multitude of classification systems that exist. A systematic review by Leisher et al. (2016) identified eighty-one systems for classification of causes of stillbirth and newborn deaths between 2009 and 2014. Having various classification systems with lack of agreement on key characteristics contributes further confusion to the data metrics. The review concluded that there is an urgent need to standardize a globally acceptable classification system (Leisher et al., 2016). The ISA Prevention Working Group is addressing this gap. Reinebrant et al. (2018) further found the majority of stillbirths globally are classified as unexplained using the current systems, which continues to remain a major barrier for prevention of stillbirths.

Another key component of effective care and to improve services is to conduct audits and reviews of stillbirths. These, in conjunction with robust stillbirth classifications can assist in reducing preventable stillbirths. Thus far, collated and published, anonymized audits are a feature of perinatal death reporting in countries with well-established data collection systems. A recently published review outlined the varying approaches for service improvement including national audits, local reviews, confidential enquiries, and other in-depth reviews (Helps, Leitao, Greene, & O'Donoghue, 2020). A recent development has been parental involvement in perinatal review processes. A study on parental involvement in perinatal review processes from the UK PARENTS 2 study. Eighty-one parents took part in the study which found that parental contributions to perinatal reviews were perceived to improve safety and future care for mothers and babies, as well as being useful for the bereaved parents themselves (Burden et al., 2021).

The development of evidence-based bereavement care standards is important in providing appropriate care to parents. Several high-income countries have developed evidence-based standards for bereavement care including Ireland, United Kingdom, Australia (Health Service Executive, 2016; NBCP UK, 2020; Flenady et al., 2020). The RESPECT study, an international Delphi study by Shakespeare et al. (2020) developed global consensus on a set of evidence-based core principles for bereavement care after stillbirth: stigma reduction, respectful maternity care for the bereaved, supporting women and families to make informed decisions, to investigate and identify cause of death, acknowledge normal grief responses, offer appropriate postnatal support, provide information on future pregnancy planning and follow-up, and enable high-quality bereavement care by training and supporting healthcare professionals (Shakespeare et al., 2020).

However, there are often disparities in parents' experiences of care offered after stillbirth as was found in a large international online survey of high- and middle-income countries (Horey et al., 2021). There is considerable variation between high- and low-resource countries and even between different settings in high-resource countries. Only one country, the Netherlands, offered all bereavement care practices that were explored in this study. There is much work still remaining in this area in high- and middle-income countries and even greater work to establish these standards for low-income countries.

There is a growing need for reciprocal learning throughout the global community through research collaboration and information sharing due to the fact that stillbirth remains an under-resourced area of health and social care, and little research funding is allocated globally compared to newborn research, for instance. This is where multidisciplinary organizations such as the ISA can contribute greatly to the global work in this area by facilitating collaboration of parents, researchers, clinicians, advocates, epidemiologists, and supporters across all continents with one aim, the reduction of the global stillbirth burden.

(iii) Financing

Stillbirth has had a low priority for research investment compared to newborn research therefore little funding was traditionally available for stillbirth research. Funding typically came from the charitable sector in high-income settings such as SANDS UK, Tommy's UK, Red Nose Australia, Star Legacy Foundation USA, or Féileacáin Ireland, among many others. The contributions of these charitable funders helped researchers explore the lived experiences of bereaved parents and the development and piloting of small intervention studies. However, funders in recent years have been looking at the stillbirth area and providing larger research grant awards.

Regardless of location, financial investment is consistently required in maternity services. investment is necessary in low-income settings to ensure all women have access to safe and high-quality maternity care throughout the antenatal period to recognize risk factors and in the intrapartum period to prevent stillbirth in labor (United Nations Children's Fund, 2021). Investment is also needed to address health inequalities in high-income settings where women from marginalized groups are over-represented in the perinatal mortality statistics (Draper et al., 2020). Financial investment would also be beneficial to address the social determinants of health including safe working conditions, urban/rural divide, transportation to facilities, nutrition, sanitation, clean water, smoking, alcohol, and substance misuse. Preventative programs require investment and financing and can have an impact upon stillbirth outcomes, for example in malaria, HIV, sexually transmitted infections (STIs) which are all major contributors to antenatal stillbirth deaths globally (World Health Organization, 2014).

Beyond the frontline investment in direct healthcare costs financial investment is required in adequate healthcare training (Ellis et al., 2016) to ensure an educated and prepared workforce and to invest in the collation of accurate vital statistics across all health systems (World Health Organization, 2010).

(iv) Human resources

In order to deliver high-quality maternity care to women, trained health providers are needed with the necessary skills to provide high-quality care, and an accountability mechanism to ensure compliance to appropriate standards. It is important to ensure an adequate number of health workers per head of population to deliver such maternity service (World Health Organization00, 2010). Human resources include clinical staff, such as midwives, nurses, and doctors, as well as management and support staff. Although access to essential health services is improving, with greatest increases seen in low- and lower-middle-income countries, still less than one-half of the world's population was able to access essential health services in 2017 (World Health Organization, 2020). Indeed, great inequity remains between those living in the wealthiest and the poorest nations. The relative shortage of doctors, nurses, and midwives is still most acute in Sub-Saharan Africa with eighty-three countries facing a health worker crisis. This is currently one of the major obstacles to achieving the SDGs and other international health goals, including universal health coverage. The Global Health Workforce Alliance works with a group of "champions," prominent people from the health and development community who agreed to contribute their knowledge, wisdom, and leadership toward highlighting the essential role of health workers.

Education of health workers is vital to ensure that women are in receipt of respectful maternity care as disrespectful care during childbirth is very prevalent across the globe. Based on human rights principles, *Respectful Maternity Care: The Universal Rights of Women and Newborns* was drafted by the White Ribbon Alliance (2019). The adoption of this rights-based approach to maternity care is valuable for all women but especially for women experiencing stillbirth. Once ingrained in health worker education it can be disseminated across wider societal populations.

(v) Access to medicines and technology

Equitable access to essential medicines and technologies are vital in ensuring a well-functioning health system which is capable of delivering on goals such as the reduction of stillbirth (World Health Organization, 2010). *The Lancet* has published two series on stillbirth in 2011 and 2016. The 2016 series was titled "ending preventable stillbirths." A key component of the global strategy in stillbirth reduction is first, the identification of risk factors and clinical conditions likely to predispose women to stillbirth and to treat those conditions. Secondly, the prevention of stillbirth necessitates the introduction of packages of care designed to prevent stillbirth in the first instance (de Bernis et al., 2016).

Identification of risk factors and clinical conditions likely to predispose a woman to stillbirth include history of previous stillbirth, parity, maternal age, comorbidities, particularly obesity and diabetes. Prevention of stillbirth may be achieved by the introduction of packages of care; for example, the Saving Babies Lives (UK) and Safer Baby Bundle (Australia) are evidence-based packages of care consists of elements designed to reduce stillbirth rates after twenty-eight weeks' gestation. The Safer Baby Bundle, for example, includes:

Element 1: Supporting women to stop smoking during pregnancy.
Element 2: Improving detection and management of fetal growth restriction.
Element 3: Raising awareness and improving care for women with decreased fetal movements.
Element 4: Improving awareness of maternal safe going-to-sleep position in late pregnancy.
Element 5: Improving decision-making about the timing of birth for women with risk factors for stillbirth.

The primary targets for these Safer Baby Bundles are midwives, doctors, health service managers, nurses, and other healthcare providers providing maternity care and for women accessing maternity care (Centre of Research Excellence, 2019). Adoption of these bundles have been associated with significant (~20%) reduction in stillbirth rate in high-income settings (Widdows, Roberts, Camacho, & Heazell, 2021).

(vi) Service delivery

Strengthening service delivery for maternity care is crucial to all SDGs and reducing the global stillbirth incidence. Ensuring a high-quality, affordable, and accessible maternity care which is available across a variety of urban and rural settings is challenging for many nations (World Health Organization, 2010). The service delivery principles include comprehensiveness, accessibility, coverage, continuity, high-quality person-centeredness coordination, accountability, and efficiency (World Health Organization, 2010: 3). The women of reproductive age group should be provided with a comprehensive range of services, appropriate to their needs at that time, including preventative and curative services and health promotion activities. Pregnant women should be provided continuum of care from the antenatal care period to the postnatal care period, and the activities of care bundles in the United Kingdom and Australia address this principle. How these bundles may be rolled out to pregnant women in more countries or the appropriateness of the bundles for specific populations needs exploration as the work thus far has been in high-income settings with relatively homogenous populations.

"Stillbirth is associated with substantial direct, indirect, psychological, and social costs to women, and to their families, society, and government" (Heazell et al., 2016: 611). Population education programs may be useful to address the wider cultural issues surrounding stillbirth. They include but are not limited to social isolation, stigma and fatalism, religious or cultural beliefs about birth and stillbirth, the role that women and mothers play in society, family support structures and who provides them, and the role of gender-based violence and violence against children, for example feticide of female infants or induced termination of pregnancy due to sex preference (Kochar et al., 2014). These are very complex, intricate systems to navigate and go beyond the mere provision of clinical care. It requires therefore an integrated, systems-thinking approach to work in partnership with all stakeholders at all levels to address the common goal of stillbirth reduction, possibly the area that is least developed in terms of research and investment to date. However, there are excellent examples of work taking place globally including the ISA Parents Voices Initiative.

Examples to improve service delivery for stillbirth include appointing a stillbirth/perinatal death champion in each health facility, having dedicated stillbirth prevention and follow-up clinics, employing dedicated bereavement and loss midwives, and undertaking local perinatal mortality reviews. Local successes in high resource countries in tackling stillbirth and bereavement have relied on having individuals who tend to drive service improvement and coordinate action (Ellis et al., 2016). Local area health service networks are actively coordinated, across types of provider, types of care, levels of service delivery, and for both routine and emergency preparedness. A means of quantifying these principles when it comes to stillbirth prevention is the development of a core dataset such as the Ending Preventable Stillbirths Scorecard (Stillbirth Advocacy Working Group 2018) which was developed from *The Lancet's* "Ending preventable stillbirth series call to action" (De Bernis et al., 2016). The scorecard developed by this initiative is a means of tracking progress at a global level toward this call to action which covers three distinct areas: (i) 2030 mortality targets, (ii) universal health care coverage targets, and (iii) global and national milestones for improving care and outcomes for all mothers and their babies (as specified by ENAP) and specifically for women and families affected by stillbirth.

Conclusion

Ending the global burden of 2 million annual stillbirths is a challenge that requires multisystems thinking. It requires a whole-system approach, sharing and collaboration of learning and resources to tackle the health and systemic inequities that contribute to the enduring deaths. Twenty million babies are projected to be stillborn in the next decade, if trends observed between 2000 and 2019 in reducing the stillbirth rate continue (United Nations Inter-agency Group for Child Mortality Estimation, 2020: 6). Yet humanity can achieve wonderous things when it is willing to do so; dealing with the COVID-19 pandemic is an example of such collaborative endeavors. Women, infants, and their families require similar energy to be directed toward preventing stillbirth.

References

Blencowe, H., Bottecchia, M., Kwesiga, D., Akuze, J., Haider, M. M., Galiwango, E., Dzabeng, F., Fisker, A. B., Enuameh, Y. A., Geremew, B. M., & Nareeba, T. (2021). Stillbirth outcome capture and classification in population-based surveys: EN-INDEPTH study. *Population Health Metrics, 19*, 1–9. Retrieved from https://doi.org/10.1186/s12963-020-00239-8

Burden, C., Bakhbakhi, D., Heazell, A. E., Lynch, M., Timlin, L., Bevan, C., Storey, C., Kurinczuk, J. J., & Siassakos, D. (2021). Parents' Active Role and ENgagement in the review of their stillbirth/perinatal death 2 (PARENTS 2) study: A mixed-methods study of implementation. *BMJ Open 2021*, 11(3), e044563. doi:10.1136/bmjopen-2020-044563

Centre of Research Excellence Stillbirth. (2019). *Safer baby bundle handbook and resource guide: Working together to reduce stillbirth.* Mater Research Institute, Brisbane, Australia: Centre of Research Excellence Stillbirth.

Barton, H., & Grant, M. (2006). A health map for the local human habitat. *The Journal for the Royal Society for the Promotion of Health, 126*(6), 252–253.

De Bernis, L., Kinney, M. V., Stones, W., ten Hoope-Bender, P., Vivio, D., Leisher, S. H., . . . Franco, L. (2016). Stillbirths: Ending preventable deaths by 2030. *The Lancet, 387*(10019), 703–716.

Draper, E. S., Gallimore, I. D., Smith, L. K., Fenton, A. C., Kurinczuk, J. J., Smith, P. W., . . . on behalf of the MBRRACE-UK Collaboration. (2020). *MBRRACE-UK perinatal mortality surveillance report, UK perinatal deaths for births from January to December 2018.* Leicester: The Infant Mortality and Morbidity Studies, Department of Health Sciences, University of Leicester.

Ellis, A., Chebsey, C., Storey, C., Bradley, S., Jackson, S., Flenady, V., . . . Siassakos, D. (2016). Systematic review to understand and improve care after stillbirth: A review of parents' and healthcare professionals' experiences. *BMC Pregnancy Childbirth, Jan 25;16*(16), 1–11. doi:10.1186/s12884-016-0806-2. PMID: 26810220; PMCID: PMC4727309.

Flenady, V., Oats, J., Gardener, G., Masson, V., McCowan, L., & Kent, A. (2020). *Clinical practice guideline for care around stillbirth and neonatal death.* Brisbane, Brisbane, Australia: NHMRC Centre of Research Excellence in Stillbirth. Retrieved from https://sanda.psanz.com.au/clinical-practice/clinical-guidelines/.

Health Service Executive. (2016). *National standards for bereavement care following pregnancy loss and perinatal death.* Dublin: Health Service Executive. Retrieved from https://www.hse.ie/eng/services/list/3/maternity/bereavementcare/national-standards-for-bereavement-care-following-pregnancy-loss-and-perinataldeath.pdf.

Heazell, A. E., Siassakos, D., Blencowe, H., Burden, C., Bhutta, Z. A., Cacciatore, J., . . . Gold, K. J. (2016). Stillbirths: Economic and psychosocial consequences. *The Lancet, 387*, 604–616.

Helps, A., Leitao, S., Greene, R., & O'Donoghue, K., (2020). Perinatal mortality audits and reviews: Past, present and the way forward. *European Journal of Obstetrics & Gynecology and Reproductive Biology, 250*, 24–30.

Homer, C. S., Leisher, S. H., Aggarwal, N., Akuze, J., Babona, D., Blencowe, H., . . . Dandona, R. (2021). Counting stillbirths and COVID 19—There has never been a more urgent time. *The Lancet Global Health, 9*(1), e10–e11.

Horey, D., Boyle, F. M., Cassidy, J., Cassidy, P. R., Erwich, J. J., Gold, K. J., Gross, M. M., Heazell, A. E., Leisher, S. H., Murphy, M., & Ravaldi, C. (2021). Parents' experiences of care offered after stillbirth: An international online survey of high and middle-income countries. *Birth.*

Hug, L., You, D., Blencowe, H., Mishra, A., Wang, Z., Fix, M., Wakefield, J., Moran, A. C., Gaigbe-Togbe, V., Suzuki, E., & Blau, D. M. (2021). *Global, regional, and national levels and trends in stillbirths from 2000 to 2019: A systematic assessment.* Retrieved from http://dx.doi.org/10.2139/ssrn.3796098.

Kochar, P. S., Dandona, R., Kumar, G. A., & Dandona, L. (2014). Population-based estimates of still birth, induced abortion and miscarriage in the Indian state of Bihar. *BMC Pregnancy Childbirth, 14*, 1–9. Retrieved from https://doi.org/10.1186/s12884-014-0413-z.

Lawn, J. E., Kinney, M., Lee, A. C., Chopra, M., Donnay, F., Paul, V. K., . . . Darmstadt, G.L. (2009). Reducing intrapartum-related deaths and disability: Can the health system deliver? *International Journal of Gynecology & Obstetrics, 107*, S123–S142. Retrieved from https://doi.org/10.1016/j.ijgo.2009.07.021.

Leisher, S. H., Kinney, M., Blencowe, H., Sexton, J., Cassidy, P., Christiansen-Lindquist, L., . . . Jayaratne, K. (2020). Leaving no one behind: Where are 2.6 million stillbirths? *British Medical Journal, 368*(16986).

Leisher, S. H., Teoh, Z., Reinebrant, H., Allanson, E., Blencowe, H., Erwich, J. J., Frøen, J. F., Gardosi, J., Gordijn, S., Gülmezoglu, A. M., & Heazell, A. E. (2016). Seeking order amidst chaos: A systematic review of classification systems for causes of stillbirth and neonatal death, 2009–2014. *BMC Pregnancy and Childbirth, 16*(1), 1–7.

National Bereavement Care Pathway, UK. (2017). https://nbcpathway.org.uk/about-nbcp/national-bereavement-care-pathway-background-project.

National Bereavement Care Pathway, UK. (2020). https://nbcpathway.org.uk/professionals/nbcp-pathways-material

Nove, A., Friberg, I. K., de Bernis, L., McConville, F., Moran, A. C., Najjemba, M., ten Hoope-Bender, P., Tracy, S., & Homer, C. S. (2021). Potential impact of midwives in preventing and reducing maternal and neonatal mortality and stillbirths: A Lives Saved Tool modelling study. *The Lancet Global Health, 9*(1), e24–32.

Reinebrant, H. E., Leisher, S. H., Coory, M., Henry, S., Wojcieszek, A. M., Gardener, G., . . . Blencowe, H. (2018). Making stillbirths visible: A systematic review of globally reported causes of stillbirth. *British Journal of Obstetrics & Gynaecology, 125*(2), 212–224.

Shakespeare, C., Merriel, A., Bakhbakhi, D., Blencowe, H., Boyle, F. M., Flenady, V., . . . Murphy, M. M. (2020). The RESPECT Study for consensus on global bereavement care after stillbirth. *International Journal of Gynecology & Obstetrics, 149*(2), 137–147.

Stillbirth Advocacy Working Group. (2018). *The ending preventable stillbirths scorecard, International Stillbirth Alliance and the London School of Hygiene & Tropical Medicine, founded by the Partnership for Maternal, Newborn and Child Health.* Retrieved from https://www.healthynewbornnetwork.org/hnn-content/uploads/Stillbirth-Global-scorecard_overview.pdf.

United Nations. (2015). *The global strategy for women's, children's, and adolescents' health (2016–2030)*. New York, NY: United Nations.

United Nations Children's Fund. (2021). *Antenatal care dataset.* Retrieved from https://data.unicef.org/topic/maternal-health/antenatal-care/#:~:text=Globally%2C%20while%2087%20per%20cent,least%20four%20antenatal%20care%20visits.

United Nations Inter-agency Group for Child Mortality Estimation. (2020). *A neglected tragedy: The global burden of stillbirths.* New York, NY: United Nations Children's Fund

Viterna, J., & Bautista, J.S.G. (2017). Pregnancy and the 40-year prison sentence: How "abortion is murder" became institutionalized in the Salvadoran judicial system. *Health and Human Rights, 19*(1), 81.

White Ribbon Alliance. (2019). *Respectful maternity care: The universal rights of women and newborns.* Washington, DC: White Ribbon Alliance.

Widdows, K., Roberts, S. A., Camacho, E. M., & Heazell, A. E. P. (2021). Stillbirth rates, service outcomes and costs of implementing NHS England's Saving Babies' Lives care bundle in maternity units in England: A cohort study. *PLoS One, 16*(4), e0250150.

World Health Organization. (2010). *Monitoring the building blocks of health systems: A handbook of indicators and their measurement strategies.* Geneva: World Health Organization.

World Health Organization/United Nations Children's Fund. (2014). *Every newborn: An action plan to end preventable deaths.* Geneva: World Health Organization/United Nations Children's Fund.

World Health Organization. (2016). *Global strategy on human resources for health: Workforce 2030.* Geneva: World Health Organization.

World Health Organization. (2020). *The world health report 2020—Monitoring health for the SDGs*. Geneva: World Health Organization. Retrieved from https://www.who.int/data/gho/publications/world-health-statistics.

Web Resources

International Stillbirth Alliance
https://www.stillbirthalliance.org/
UK NHS Saving Babies Lives
https://www.england.nhs.uk/mat-transformation/saving-babies/
Australian Centre of Stillbirth Excellence in Stillbirth
https://www.stillbirthcre.org.au/safer-baby-bundle/

Index

Tables, figures and boxes are indicated by *t*, *f* and *b* following the page number.

ABM (Agent-Based Modelling) 12*t*
Abstinence, Be faithful, and Condom (ABC) (Ethiopia) 250
Academy of Health Sciences (AHS), Sudan 46
Access to Infant and Maternal Health (AIM-Health Programme), Community Health Committee 92*b*
accountability, EquiFrame 344*t*
ACT (artemisinin combined therapy) 312
Action on Smoking and Health (ASH)
  Thailand 260
  USA 261
active case finding (ACF) 335
active surveillance 325–6
active workforce stage, Sudan 47–8
actors
  community health 88
  war health needs 124–5, 125*f*, 127–8
acute multi-organ toxicity, radioactivity 267
ADA (American with Disabilities Act) 203
Afghanistan, Comprehensive National Disability Policy (2003) 112
AFPTC (ASEAN Focal Points on Tobacco Control) 257, 260
Africa
  Charter on the Rights and Welfare of the Child (1990) 299
  Commission for Human and Peoples' Rights 298
  Eliminating Meningitis Across Africa's Meningitis Belt 289
African Network for Evidence to Action and Disability (AfriNEAD) 220, 227
"After Now Project" 206
aging in place 189
Agency for Medical Research and Development (Japan) 191
Agent-Based Modelling (ABM) 12*t*
agents of change, reproductive health 139
Alliance for Health Policy and Systems (WHO) 179–80
Alma-Ata declaration 86
  reproductive health 134
alternative service delivery models 113
American Speech Language Hearing Association (ASHS) 205
American with Disabilities Act (ADA) 203
Amref Health Africa 79
*Analytical Framework for Inclusive Policy Design (*United Nations Educational, Scientific and Cultural Organization) 175–6
antenatal care 361–2
Anti-Ballistic Missile Treaty 270
antimicrobial resistance 336
anti-retroviral treatment (ART) 236
  scaling up of 243–4
  South Africa 98
AP (assistive products) 107
APPLICABLE (Malawi) 113*b*
Argentina, Plan Nacer 289
armed conflict *see* war health needs
ART *see* anti-retroviral treatment (ART)
artemisinin combined therapy (ACT) 312
ASEAN *see* Association of Southeast Asian Nations (ASEAN)
ASEAN Focal Points on Tobacco Control (AFPTC) 257, 260
ASH (Action on Smoking and Health)
  Thailand 260
  USA 261
ASHS (American Speech Language Hearing Association) 205
Assistive Product List (APL) 116
assistive products (AP) 107
assistive technology 107–19, 110*t*, 194–5
  alternative service delivery models 113
  challenges 115–16
  definition 107–8
  diverse stakeholders 111
  element inter-connectedness 114–15, 115*f*
  global leadership/needs 111

assistive technology (*cont.*)
  human resources 114
  implementation 196
  policy guidance 112–13
  socio-economic contexts 110–11
  see also robotics-aided care
Assistive Technology Embedded Systems Thinking (ATEST) Model 108, 109*f*
Assistive Technology Systems (ATS) 107–8
Association of Southeast Asian Nations (ASEAN) 253
  ASEAN Focal Points on Tobacco Control 253
  Socio-Cultural Community Blueprints (2016-2030) 258
  Tobacco Control Atlas 260
  tobacco use control 254
AT2030 112*b*
ATEST (Assistive Technology Embedded Systems Thinking) Model 108, 109*f*
ATS (Assistive Technology Systems) 107–8
Australia
  Cancer Control Australia 261
  Safer Baby Bundle 368–9
  stillbirth leadership & governance 363
autonomy, EquiFrame 344*t*

balancing loop 122*f*
balancing processes 14
Bangladesh, mental health in emergencies 147
behaviour-over-time graph 14
behaviour, supportive supervision 58
BERA (British Educational Research Association) 79
bereavement care, stillbirth 362–3
bias, case studies 285
Bill and Melinda Gates foundation 258, 259
birth registration 294, 299
blast waves, nuclear weapons 267
blended learning courses 162
Bloomberg Foundation 258
Bloomberg Initiative to Reduce Tobacco use 259
Botswana, Mass Antiretroviral Therapy Program 289
boundaries
  communities 89
  social inclusion 178–9
  systems of 2
British Educational Research Association (BERA) 79
budgets *see* finances

CAFS (conflict-affected fragile states) 134–5
Cambodia, Population Movement Framework 313–14
Campaign for Tobacco Control (Thailand) 289
Campaign for Tobacco-Free Kids (CTFK) 261
Cancer Control Australia 261
capability-based services
  disability 209–12
  EquiFrame 343*t*
capacity-building program
  EquiFrame 345*t*
  Health Workforce Transformation Initiative (Sudan) 45
  refugee education pathways 160
Care and Treatment Centres (CTC) 100
Care Dependency grants, South Africa 224
care homes *see* robotics-aided care
CARE (Concepts for Applying Resilience Engineering) model 193, 193*f*
Care Quality Commission (CQC) 197
care settings, assistive technology 194–5
case management, mental health in emergencies 154–5
case studies 285–92
  bias 285
  collection 290–1
  collection of 290–1
  definition 285–6
  evidential strength 285
  examples in global health 288–91
  global health 286–91
  global health applications 286–8
  HIV/AIDS epidemic 291
  International Campaign to Abolish Nuclear Weapons 279
  low- and middle-income countries 290
  malaria 291
  malnutrition 291
  mental health in emergencies 150, 152–3
  narratives 285
  positive synergy 290
  program design 287–8
  reproductive health 135–6
  Sustainable Development Goals 289–90

teaching 288
teaching cases 288
tropical diseases 291
tuberculosis 291
CASP (Critical Appraisal Skills Program) criteria 19
CASs *see* Complex Adaptive Systems (CASs)
catastrophe theory 11*t*
causal loop diagrams (CLDs) 12*t*
Indian disease surveillance 332, 333*f*
causal modelling, social inclusion 179–80
CBR (Community Based rehabilitation) 221
CCM (Country Coordinating Mechanism), Sub-Saharan Africa 237, 238
Center for Global Development, *Millions Saved* 288–9
Centers for Victims of Torture (CVTs) 148
centralization–decentralization dilemma 5
change management history 13*t*
chaos theory 11*t*
charitable response, disability 202
Checklist for TB Surveillance (WHO) 329–30
chemical weapons 272
Chemical Weapons Convention 272
CHEWs (community health extension workers) 78
children
mobile community health workers 81
statelessness 297, 298–9
Child Support Grant (South Africa) 289
China, stillbirth rates 360
CHIs *see* complex health interventions (CHIs)
chronic homelessness 180–1
chronic illness, Namibian HIV/AIDS policy 352
CHWs *see* community health workers (CHWs)
Citizen Rights Initiative in Africa (CRAI) 297
Citizenship and Immigration Act (Kenya) 160
civil rights movements, disability 203
civil society
stillbirth 363
tobacco use control 254–5
Treaty on the Prohibition of Nuclear Weapons 275
class, South African disabled 226–7
CLDs *see* causal loop diagrams (CLDs)
climate change
disability 208
malaria control 315–16
post-nuclear war 268–70
clinic attendance, Health Information Systems 100
closed systems
Complex Adaptive Systems 175
open systems *vs.* 175
collaborative decision-making, reproductive health 137
collection, case studies 290–1
colonialism, statelessness 298
comfort, robotics-aided care 190*t*
CommCare 58
COMMs (Community Committees), AIM-Health Programme 92*b*
communication
disabilities 223–4
disability 209
reproductive health 138
robotics-aided care 190*t*
communication robots 194*t*
alerting system 192*f*
communities 86–95
assistive technology 110*t*, 113
community health workers 57
complexity 88–9
definitions of 87–8
disease surveillance 334
engagement 91
Ethiopian healthcare 251
health interventions 88
importance of 86–7
South African disabled 227
war health needs 126
Community Based rehabilitation (CBR) 221
Community Committees (COMMs), AIM-Health Programme 92*b*
community health 90–3
definition 88
Ethiopian pastoral care 249
community health extension workers (CHEWs) 78
Community Health Framework 91
community health workers (CHWs) 54–66, 90
deficit of 56
human resources 56–7
Kenya 77–85 *see also* mobile community health workers (mCHW)

community health workers (CHWs) (*cont.*)
mobile application design & implementation 79–81
product resupply procedures 59–60
supportive supervision 55, 56 *see also* supportive supervision
tuberculosis surveillance 329
Community Systems Strengthening (CSS) Framework 92, 92*b*
Complex Adaptive Systems (CASs) 174–5
social inclusion 175–7
complex health interventions (CHIs) 88
self-organizing system as 88–9
complex systems 5
Comprehensive Helmet Law (Vietnam) 289
Comprehensive National Disability Policy (2003) (Afghanistan) 112
Concepts for Applying Resilience Engineering (CARE) model 193, 193*f*
concerns, communities 87
conflict-affected fragile states (CAFS) 134–5
conflicting goals 5
conflicts
disability 208–9
preparedness 126–7
constraints, refugee education 160–2
contextualization, social inclusion 176–7
continuing professional development (CPD), Sudan health services 47
contribution, EquiFrame 344*t*
conventional (default) approaches, assistive technology 114
Convention of Parties (COP) 255
Convention on the Rights of the Child (1989) 298
disabilities 221
Convention Relating to the Status of Stateless Persons (1954) 296
Conversational Framework 79
COP (Convention of Parties) 255
Core Concept Coverage 350, 350*t*
Equiframe 348
core concepts, Equiframe 346, 349
countries
assistive technology 110*t*
cooperation in assistive technology 109–10
Country Coordinating Mechanism (CCM), Sub-Saharan Africa 237, 238
COVID-19 pandemic 188, 322
care homes 197
disability 208, 209
ID testing and 335–6
mental health and psychological support 152–3
supportive supervision 61–2
CPD (continuing professional development), Sudan health services 47
CRAI (Citizen Rights Initiative in Africa) 297
Critical Appraisal Skills Program (CASP) criteria 19
CRPD *see* United Nations Convention on the Rights of Persons with Disabilities (UNCRPD)
CSS (Community Systems Strengthening) Framework 92, 92*b*
CTC (Care and Treatment Centres) 100
CTFK (Campaign for Tobacco-Free Kids) 261
culture
communication in reproductive health 138
EquiFrame 344*t*
Curbing the epidemic–governments and the economics of tobacco control (1999) (World Bank) 259
CVTs (Centers for Victims of Torture) 148
cybernetics 11*t*

Dadaab (Kenya) 159
DAH (development assistance for health) 258
data
Health Information Systems 101–3
Indian ID surveillance system 325–6
refugee education pathways 162–3
war health needs 129
decentralization, health services *see* health service decentralization
definition of systems thinking 1, 120, 342
delay 122*f*
Democratic Republic of the Congo, stillbirth rates 360
Democratic Republic of Timor-Leste (RDTL)
National Action Plan for People with Disabilities 2014-2018 182
National Disability Policy 181–3
Strategic Development Plan 182
Department for International Development (DFID) 78

development assistance for health (DAH) 258
development education 299–302
  definition 300
  statelessness 294
DFID (Department for International Development) 78
digitization, malaria control 316
dignity
  disability care 211
  robotics-aided care 197
Directly Observed Short Course (DOTS) 331
disability
  capability approach 209–12
  definition 202
  Democratic Republic of Timor-Leste 181
  epidemiology 218
  global challenges 207–9
  health care provision 218–19
  health problems and 221
  health *vs.* 202–4
  human rights 209–12
  impairment *vs.* 221
  normative view 206
  prevalence estimates 206–7
  South Africa *see* South African disabled
  theoretical models of 220–1
  see also United Nations Convention on the Rights of Persons with Disabilities (UNCRPD)
disability-adjusted life years (DALYs) 253
disability aid systems 202–17
  regional construct as 205–7
Disability and development report (UN) 210
disability rights 221–2
  South Africa 223
Disabled Persons Organization, South Africa 226
Disasters Emergency Committee 127–8
discrimination prohibition 219
disease outbreaks, global health 286–7
displaced populations 149
  Namibian HIV/AIDS policy 352
  see also refugees
district councils, Malawi health services 70–1
District Health Management Teams (Malawi) 70
district-level designated microscopy center (DMCs) 331
diverse stakeholders, assistive technology 111
documentation, Ethiopian healthcare 250
Doomsday Clock 271
DOTS (Directly Observed Short Course) 331
double burden of disease 243–4
double loop learning 10
drug-resistance tuberculosis 335
dynamic approach, Health Information Systems 99
dynamic thinking 6
  Health Information Systems 97–8
dynamism, social inclusion 176

earthquakes, Nepal 151
Ebola outbreak (2014-2015) 58
Economic and Social Research Council (ESRC) 78
Economic Co-operation and Development 133
economics
  Sudan health services 49
  Treaty on the Prohibition of Nuclear Weapons 276
  see also finances
education
  development education *see* development education
  Ethiopian pastoral care 249
  feminist pedagogy 294
  refugee education pathways 165–7
  refugees *see* refugee education pathways
  Sudan health services 42, 46
efficiency, EquiFrame 345*t*
EHRP (Emergency Human Resources Programme) 69
electromagnetic pulse (EMP), nuclear weapons 267
electronic ART patient tracking 241
electronic medical record (EMR) systems 99
element inter-connectedness, assistive technology 114–15, 115*f*
Eliminating Meningitis Across Africa's Meningitis Belt 289
Eliminating Polio (Haiti) 289
emergencies
  mental health *see* mental health in emergencies
  obstetric care 249
  supportive supervision 58

Emergency Human Resources Programme (EHRP) 69
EMP (electromagnetic pulse), nuclear weapons 267
empowerment, reproductive health 138–9
EMR (electronic medical record) systems 99
ENAP (Every Newborn Action Plan) 360
Ending Preventable Stillbirths Scorecard 370
End TB Surveillance (WHO) 329–30, 335
entitlement, EquiFrame 343*t*
entry stage, Sudan health services 46–7
environment
  disability 208
  disruption 265
epidemics 286–7
EquiFrame 346–8
  core concepts 346
  health policy analysis 349
  human rights 343–5*t*
  planning documents 353
  summary indices 348–9
  vulnerable group definition 347*t*
ESRC (Economic and Social Research Council) 78
Ethiopia 246–52
  Federal Ministry of Health 248
  Health Extension Program 246
  Health Sector Development Program 248
  Health Sector Transformation Plan 248
  health services 248–9
  Health Systems Directorate 248–49
  Pastoral Community Development Program 250
  stillbirth rates 360
ethnic minorities
  Namibian HIV/AIDS policy 352
  statelessness 298
evaluation, reproductive health 139
Every Newborn Action Plan (ENAP) 360
evidence
  Health Workforce Transformation Initiative (Sudan) 45
  Sudan health services 50
evidence-based bereavement care 366
evidential strength, case studies 285
exit stage, Sudan health services 48

face-to-face interviews, reproductive health 139–40
factor thinking
  Health Information Systems 98
  operational thinking *vs.* 101–3
families
  changes in 189
  EquiFrame 344*t*
  stillbirth effects 362
FAO (Food and Agriculture Organization) 250
FCA (Framework Convention Alliance) 260–1
Federal Ministry of Health (Ethiopia) 248
feedback
  distortion 5
  social inclusion 176
Féileacain, Ireland 367
feminism 301
  development education 294–5
  pedagogy 294
feminization of poverty 301
finances
  Framework Convention on Tobacco Control 257–8, 257*f*, 258
  Global Health Initiatives 238–9, 242*t*
  health system strengthening 323
  Indian ID surveillance system 324–5
  malaria control 316
  Malawi health services 70–1
  mental health in emergencies 149
  social inclusion 182–3
  South African disabled 226
  stillbirth prevention 367
  WHO building block of health 306, 313
  see also economics
fires, post-nuclear war 268
fissile materials 266–7
focus
  community health 88
  health systems design 35
Food and Agriculture Organization (FAO) 250
food production, post-nuclear war 269
Food Security Information Network (FSIN) 123
forest thinking 6
  Health Information Systems 98
  tree-by-tree thinking *vs.* 99–101
formal health systems, community health workers 58

Forrester, Jay 3
  world model 10
4 Ws (Who, Where, When, What) 148
Framework Convention Alliance (FCA) 260–1
Framework Convention on Tobacco Control (FCTC) 253–64
  Convention of Parties (COP) 255
  financing 258
  governance 254–5
  information & financing 257–8, 257*f*, 259–61
  interference by tobacco industry 255–7, 256*f*
  philanthropic foundations 258–9
  South East Asia 253
"Framework for Action" 323
frameworks, health system design 34
FSIN (Food Security Information Network) 123
functional impairments
  assistive technology 114
  disability 188
Future Health Systems 91

GATE (Global Cooperation on Assistive Technology) 111, 112*b*
GDP (gross domestic product), Sudan 41
gender discrimination, statelessness 298
general systems theory 11*t*
Geneva Convention (1949) 122
Geographic Information Systems (GIS) 336
geography
  communities 87
  health workers in Malawi 73
  South African disabled 226–7
  Sudan health services 47
Georgia 59
Gestalt school 3
GFTAM (Global Fund to Fight AIDS, Tuberculosis and Malaria) 234, 313
Ghana, community health workers 57
GINI coefficient, South Africa 226
GIS (Geographic Information Systems) 336
Global Alliance for Vaccines and Immunization 234
Global Burden of Diseases Survey 351–2
  disability 204
Global Code of Practice for International Recruitment of Health Personnel 48
Global Cooperation on Assistive Technology (GATE) 111, 112*b*
Global Disability Action Plan 2014-2021 (WHO) 204
Global Fund 342
  Community Systems Strengthening 91
  data equity assessment 353–4
  social group definitions 353
Global Fund to Fight AIDS, Tuberculosis and Malaria (GFTAM) 234, 313
global health
  case studies 286–91
  disease outbreaks 286–7
  policy formation 286
Global Health Initiatives (GHIs) 241–2*t*
  country leadership 243
  double burden of disease 243–4
  effects of 235–41
  financing 238–9, 242*t*
  governance 237–8, 242*t*
  health system interdependence 243
  health workforce 235–7, 241*t*
  HIV/AIDS 243–4
  impact in Sub-Saharan African countries 235
  information systems 241, 242*t*
  leadership 237–8, 242*t*
  mechanisms 235
  medical supply chains 240
  medicine & technology supply 240, 242*t*
  service delivery 239–40, 242*t*
  short-term *vs.* long-term effects 242–3
  see also Sub-Saharan Africa (SSA)
Global Health Partnership, Treaty on the Prohibition of Nuclear Weapons 276–8
Global Health Systems Symposium on Health Systems Research 134
Global Leprosy Programme 234
global level, assistive technology 111, 113
Global Polio Eradication Initiative 128
global population aging 207
global stockpiles, highly-enriched uranium 266–7
governance
  Framework Convention on Tobacco Control 254–5
  Global Health Initiatives 237–8, 242*t*
  health system strengthening 323

governance (*cont.*)
Indian ID surveillance system 324–5
Malawi healthcare 70
mental health in emergencies 146–7
refugee education pathways 160
refugees 167–8
robotics-aided care 197
stillbirth 363, 365
supportive supervision 60–1
WHO building block of health 306
governments, WHO building block of health 313–14
gross domestic product (GDP), Sudan 41
group risks, social inclusion 177

Haiti, Eliminating Polio 289
Hard System Approach (HAS) 4
hard systems 4
quantitative research 5
health
disability *vs.* 202–4
problems and disability 221
social determinants 206
HealthBridge Canada 261
healthcare
access 219, 345*t*
digitized information systems 241
information systems in stillbirth 365–7
personnel lack in malaria control 316
statelessness exclusion 293–6
Healthcare in Danger Project (International Committee of the Red Cross) 128
health centers, Ethiopian pastoral care 250
Health Extension Program (HEP) 246
Health in All Policies 258
Health Information Management Systems (HMIS) 147–8
Health Information Systems (HIS) 96–107
data quality 101–3
low- and middle-income countries 103
standardization 97
static to dynamic thinking 98–9
tree-by-tree thinking *vs.* forest thinking 99–101
Health Policy and Systems Research (HPSR) (WHO) 90
health professionals
nuclear weapon eradication 278, 280, 281–3*t*
South African disabled 226
health promotion
communities 89–90
disability 208
tobacco use 260
health risk behaviour counselling 208
Health Sector Development Program (HSDP) (Ethiopia) 248
Health Sector Strategic Plan II (HSSP) (2017-2022) (Malawi) 69
Health Sector Transformation Plan (HSTP) (Ethiopia) 248
health service decentralization 67–76
definition 67
future work 72–3
health financing 70–1
health worker shortages 69
human resources 68–9
information systems 71
leadership & governance 70
service delivery 71–2
Sudan health services 46, 49
health surveillance assistants (HSAs) 70
health systems
assistive technology 113
interdependence in sub-Saharan Africa 243
supportive supervision in financing 60
Health Systems Directorate (Ethiopia) 250
health systems strengthening
assistive technology 110*t*
definition 18
systematic review 18–38, 20–32*t*
health workforce
development 39–53 *see also* Sudan health services
Global Health Initiatives 235–7, 241*t*
health system strengthening 323
Indian ID surveillance system 325–7
non-governmental organizations, migrations to 237
refugee education pathways 163–9
shortages in Malawi 69
WHO building block of health 306, 311
Health Workforce Transformation Initiative (Sudan) 43, 44–5
HEP (Health Extension Program) 246
HEU (highly-enriched uranium) 266–7
hierarchical levels, systems thinking 7–8, 7*f*

high-income countries (HIC) 110
highly-enriched uranium (HEU) 266–7
HIS *see* Health Information Systems (HIS)
historical dependency, social inclusion 176
history of systems thinking 2–3
HIV/AIDS Clinics 100
HIV/AIDS epidemic
  birth registration issues 302
  case studies 291
  Core Concept Coverage 350*t*
  Ethiopian pastoral care 250
  financing 238–9
  Global Fund to Fight AIDS, Tuberculosis and Malaria 234, 313
  Global Health Initiatives 243–4
  global response to 238
  human rights violations 345
  Malawi 69
  mother-to-child transmission prevention *see* prevention of mother-to-child transmission of HIV (PMTCT)
  Namibia 351
  service sustainability 240
  South Africa 98, 223, 225
  Sub-Saharan Africa 234, 235, 236, 237
HMIS (Health Information Management Systems) 147–8
holarchy 108
holistic response, social inclusion 177–8
hospital design 249
Housing First 180–1
HPSR (Health Policy and Systems Research) 90
HRH (Human Resources for Health) 68–9
HRMIS (Human Resources Management Information System) 71
HSAs (health surveillance assistants) 70
HSDP (Health Sector Development Program) 248
HSSP (Health Sector Strategic Plan II) 69
humanitarian emergencies, mental health *see* mental health in emergencies
human resources
  assistive technology 114
  community healthcare workers 80
  community health workers 56–7
  Malawi health service decentralization 68–9
  mental health in emergencies 150
  refugee education pathways 160–2
  social inclusion 182–3
  stillbirth 368
Human Resources for Health (HRH) (Malawi) 68–9
Human Resources Management Information System (HRMIS) (Malawi) 71
human rights 342–59
  disability 209–12
  EquiFrame 343–5*t*
  linear thinking monitoring 227
  policy selection 349
Human Rights Watch 295

IASC (Inter-Agency Standing Committee) 124
ICAN *see* International Campaign to Abolish Nuclear Weapons (ICAN)
iceberg hierarchy 7–8, 7*f*
ICF (International Classification of Functioning, Disability and Health) 191, 205, 221
ICN (International Council of Nurses) 278
ICRC *see* International Committee of the Red Cross (ICRC)
ICT *see* information and communications technology (ICT)
IDEA (Irish development Education Association) 300
ID surveillance system (India) 324–7
IFMIS (integrated financial management information systems) 71
IHL (international humanitarian law) 122
IHR (International Health Regulations) (WHO) 322
IMC (International Medical Corps) 146, 149
impairment, disability *vs.* 221
incentive staff, refugees 160
independence support, robotics 190*t*
India
  ID surveillance system 324–7
  infectious disease surveillance 322–41
  Initiative for Promoting Affordable and Quality Tuberculosis Tests 331, 332
  measles surveillance 328, 329*f*
  Ministry of Health and Family Welfare 322
  National AIDS Control Programme 306
  National Apical Advisory Committee for National Disease Surveillance and Response System 324

India (*cont.*)
National Surveillance Programme for Communicable Diseases 324–5
National Tuberculosis Elimination Program 329
National Vector Borne Disease Control Programme 306
Revised National Tuberculosis Control 306
stillbirth rates 360
surveillance interrelationships 332
tuberculosis surveillance 329–31, 330*f*
indiscriminate weapons 271–2
individual risks, social inclusion 177
individual systems
assistive technology 110*t*
EquiFrame 343*t*
Indonesia
Total Sanitation and Sanitation Marketing Program 289
see also Association of Southeast Asian Nations (ASEAN)
infant mortality rate, Sudan 41
infectious disease surveillance, India 322–41
information
Framework Convention on Tobacco Control 257–8, 257*f*, 259–61
Global Health Initiatives 241, 242*t*
Health Workforce Transformation Initiative (Sudan) 45
Indian ID surveillance system 325–7
Kenyan community healthcare workers 80
Malawi health service decentralization 71
mental health in emergencies 147–8
systems thinking 8–9
war health needs 121, 129
WHO building block as 96, 306, 311–12
information and communications technology (ICT) 166
disability 209
disease surveillance 336
infrastructure, refugee education 161
Initiative for Promoting Affordable and Quality Tuberculosis Tests (India) 331, 332
innovation history 13*t*
Innovative Participatory Health Education (IPHE) 136
insecticide-treated nets (ITNs) 312
Integrated Disease Surveillance and Response (ISDR) (WHO) 322
integrated financial management information systems (IFMIS) 71
Integrated Refugee Health Information System (iRHIS) 148–9
Integrated Refugee Health Information System (UNHCR) 148–9
integration
community health 88
EquiFrame 344*t*
Inter-agency Emergency Health Kit 152
Inter-Agency Standing Committee (IASC) 124
Intermediate Nuclear Forces Treaty 270
International Campaign to Abolish Nuclear Weapons (ICAN)
case study 279
Treaty on the Prohibition of Nuclear Weapons 276
International Classification of Functioning, Disability and Health (ICF) 191, 205, 221
International Committee of the Red Cross (ICRC) 122
Healthcare in Danger Project 128
Treaty on the Prohibition of Nuclear Weapons 275
International Council of Nurses (ICN) 278
International Court of Justice 272
International Covenant on Economic, Social and Cultural Rights 221
International Health Regulations (IHR) (WHO) 322
international humanitarian law (IHL) 122
International Medical Corps (IMC) 146, 149
International Physicians for the Prevention of Nuclear War (IPPNW) 278, 279
International Stillbirth Alliance (ISA) 361
inter-sectorial nature, assistive technology 112
interviews, assistive technology 194–5
investor–state dispute settlement (ISDS) 256–7
IPHE (Innovative Participatory Health Education) 136
IPPNW (International Physicians for the Prevention of Nuclear War) 278, 279
iRHS (Integrated Refugee Health Information System) 148–9
Irish development Education Association (IDEA) 300

ISA (International Stillbirth Alliance) 361
ISDR (Integrated Disease Surveillance and Response) (WHO) 322
ISDS (investor–state dispute settlement) 256–7
ITNs (insecticide-treated nets) 312

Japan
Agency for Medical Research and Development 191
care homes *see* robotics-aided care
Ministry of Health, Labour and Welfare 189
Office for Nursing Care Robot Development 189
Social Welfare Corporation 190–1
job creation, Sudan health services 46
job satisfaction, community health workers 55, 57
joined-up policies, social inclusion 178

Kenya
Citizenship and Immigration Act 160
community health workers 77–85 *see also* mobile community health workers (mCHW)
HIV/AIDS 236
Human Rights Commission 159
refugee movement 168
School-Based Deworming Program 289
Social Cash Transfer Program 289
Kiduichatta sheet 196–7, 197*t*
knowledge brokerage, reproductive health 140–1, 141*f*
Kyrgyzstan, supportive supervision case study 59

laboratory surveillance 326
quality differences 334–5
lack of predictability 5
landmines 271–2
language 5–6
leadership
Global Health Initiatives 237–8, 242*t*
health systems in sub-Saharan Africa 243
health system strengthening 323
Indian ID surveillance system 324–5
Malawi healthcare 70
mental health in emergencies 146–7
stillbirth 363, 365
supportive supervision 60–1
WHO building block of health 306, 313–14
learning analysis, refugee education pathways 162
learning organizations theory 11*t*
Lebanon
mental health 146, 150, 154–5
Ministry of Public Health 146
National Mental Health Programme 146
leprosy
eradication in India 323
Global Leprosy Programme 234
leverage points 8
liberty
disability care 211
EquiFrame 343*t*
Liechtenstein v. Guatemala [1955] ICJ 296
literature reviews 309–10*t*
malaria control 307, 308*f*
LMICs *see* low- and middle-income countries (LMICs)
Local Government Act, Malawi 68
Local Government Services Commission (Malawi) 71
locations, community health 88
loop analysis, malaria control 315
loop diagrams 14
loop thinking 6
low- and middle-income countries (LMICs)
assistive technology 110
case studies 290
community health 90–1
community healthcare workers 77
Health Information Systems 96, 103
mental health in emergencies 148
tobacco use control 255
vertical disease surveillance 323

malaria 99, 306–21
case studies 291
climate change 315–16
Core Concept Coverage 350*t*
loop analysis 315
Namibia 350
Roll-Back Malaria framework 314–15
Sub-Saharan Africa 237
Malawi
assistive technology 113*b*
District Health Management Teams 70

Malawi (*cont.*)
Health Sector Strategic Plan II 69
health service decentralization *see* health service decentralization
HIV/AIDS 236
Human Resources Management Information System 71
National Community Health Workers Strategy 73
National Decentralization Program 68
policy selection 349
Malawi Developmental Assessment Tool (MDAT) 79
malnutrition 291
managers, refugee education 164
MAPW (Medical Association for Prevention of War) 279
marginalization
social inclusion 179
statelessness 294
Mass Antiretroviral Therapy Program (Botswana) 289
mass screening programs 312
Maternal and Child Programme (USAID) 91
maternal, newborn, and child health (MNCH) 133
maternity services, financing 367
Maximizing Positive Synergies Collaborative Group 290
mCHW *see* mobile community health workers (mCHW)
MDAT (Malawi Developmental Assessment Tool) 79
MDGs *see* Millennium Development Goals (MDGs)
MDR (multidrug-resistant) tuberculosis 98–9
measles 328, 335
Medical Association for Prevention of War (MAPW) 279
medical products
access in emergencies 152–3
access in stillbirth 368–9
assistive technology 108
Global Health Initiatives 242*t*
resupply procedures 59–60
supply chains 240
supportive supervision 59–60
medical technology
health system strengthening 323
Kenyan community healthcare workers 80
WHO building block of health 306, 312
mental health and psychological support (MHPSS) 145–6
funding in Lebanon 150
Nepal, task-sharing 151
mental health Gap Action Programme (mhGAP) 148, 154
mental health in emergencies 145–57
case example 147, 148–9, 151, 154–5
case management 154–5
case study 150, 152–3
financing 149
human resources 150
information systems 147–8
leadership & governance 146–7
medical product access 152–3
service delivery 153–4, 153*f*
mental health information systems (MHIS) 147–8
mental, neurological and substance abuse (MNS) 148
mentorship, Global Health Initiatives 236
methods of systems thinking 11, 11–13*t*, 14
mHealth (mobile health) technology 58
mhGAP (mental health Gap Action Programme) 148, 154
MHIS (mental health information systems) 147–8
MHPSS *see* mental health and psychological support (MHPSS)
micro-environments, communities 89
midwives 362
migrants/migration
healthcare access 295
statelessness 298
Millennium Development Goals (MDGs)
community health workers 54
disability care 210
Ethiopian health system 247
malaria control 314
Sudan 41
Millions Saved (Center for Global Development) 288–9
Millions Saved, Center for Global Development 288–9
Ministry of Health and Family Welfare (MoHFW) (India) 322
Ministry of Health, Labour and Welfare (Japan) 189

Ministry of Public Health (Lebanon) 146
MNCH (maternal, newborn, and child health) 133
  see also reproductive health
MNS (mental, neurological and substance abuse) 148
mobile community health workers (mCHW) 78–9
  integration of 81–2
  quality 81
  service delivery 82–3
  systems-thinking approach 80–1, 80*f*
mobile health (mHealth) technology 58
mobility, refugees 167–8
Model List of Essential Medicines (WHO) 152
models, systems thinking 9–10
MoHFW (Ministry of Health and Family Welfare) (India) 322
monitoring sensors, robotics 195*t*
morbidity, Namibian HIV/AIDS policy 352–3
Mother Child Mortality 351
motivation, community health workers 55, 57
movement barriers, statelessness 298
Mozambique, war health needs 123
Multi-country AIDS Programme, World Bank 234
multidrug-resistant (MDR) tuberculosis 98–9
multi-level thinking, robotics 192–3
multimorbidity, disability 207
multiple levels
  communities 89
  social inclusion 177
multi-stakeholders, Sudan 50

Namibia
  HIV/AIDS policy 351, 352
  malaria policy 350
  National Malaria Policy 351
  policy selection 349
narratives, case studies 285
National Action Plan for People with Disabilities 2014-2018 (NAP) 182
National AIDS Control Programme (India) 306
National Animal Disease Reporting System 336
National Apical Advisory Committee for national Disease Surveillance and Response System (India) 324
National Community Health Workers Strategy (Malawi) 73
National Council for Health Care Coordination (Sudan) 45
National Decentralization Program (Malawi) 68
National Disability Policy (Timor-Leste) 181–3
National Disability Policy for inclusion and Promotion of the Rights of People wit Disabilities (Democratic Republic of Timor-Leste) 182
national governments, war health needs 126
national guidelines, war health needs 125
nationality 297–8
National Malaria Policy (Namibia) 351
National Malaria Policy (Sudan) 351
National Mental Health Programme (NMHP) (Lebanon) 146
national policies, assistive technology 112
National Polio Surveillance Program (WHO-NPSP) 328
National Surveillance Programme for Communicable Diseases (NSPC) (India) 324–5
National Tuberculosis Elimination Program (NTEP) (India) 329, 335
National Vector Borne Disease Control Programme (India) 306
NATO (North Atlantic Treaty Organization), Treaty on the Prohibition of Nuclear Weapons 274
needs, communities 87
neonatal care 249
Nepal, mental health in emergencies 151
net primary production (NPP) 269
Network Analysis 12*t*
NGOs *see* non-governmental organizations (NGOs)
Nigeria
  health system leadership 243
  HIV/AIDS financing 239
  stillbirth rates 360
NMHP (National Mental Health Programme) (Lebanon) 146
non-communicable diseases, Malawi 68
non-discrimination, EquiFrame 343*t*

non-governmental organizations (NGOs)
community health workers 54
health worker migration 237
mental health in emergencies 146
refugee education pathways 159
reproductive health 139
Rwanda 236
war health needs 124, 126, 127
non-health professionals 236
non-linearity
social inclusion 176
systems of causality 2
non-skilled workers, refugees 165
non-state actors 121
Norwegian Cancer Society 261
NPP (net primary production) 269
NPT (nuclear non-proliferation treaty) 272–3
nuclear famine 268–70
nuclear non-proliferation treaty (NPT) 272–3
nuclear war 270–1
nuclear weapon eradication 265–84
current status 272–3
health professionals 278, 280, 281–3*t*
public health 281*b*
nuclear weapons 266–7
acute effects 267–8
climate impact 268–70

Office for Nursing Care Robot Development (Japan) 189
OI (patient identification) 102
"One Health" principle 248, 250
online forums, refugee education 162
online surveys, refugee education 162
Open Skies Treaty 270
Open Society Justice Initiative (2016) 299
open systems
closed systems *vs.* 175
Complex Adaptive Systems 175
operational thinking 6
factor thinking *vs.* 101–3
Health Information Systems 98

Pakistan
Global Polio Eradication Initiative 128
stillbirth rates 360
parents, stillbirth 363
participation, EquiFrame 343*t*
Participatory Ethnographic Evaluation Research (PEER) 136, 139
Participatory Impact Pathway Analysis (PIPA) 13*t*
participatory research, reproductive health 137–9
partnership, assistive technology 108
passive surveillance 326
Pastoral Community Development Program (Ethiopia) 250
pastoral health 246–52
definition 246
health service provision 247
holistic features 250–1
improvement opportunities 250
service provision 248–9
pastoral livelihoods, Ethiopian healthcare 250–251
path dependency theory 11*t*
Pathways to Housing (PtH) 181
patient identification (PI) 102
patients, reproductive health 134
PEER (Participatory Ethnographic Evaluation Research) 136, 139
people, assistive technology 108
People-centred Health model (WHO) 91
PEPFAR (President's Emergency Plan for AIDS Relief) 234, 238, 290
performance
community health workers 55, 57
Sudan health services 49
persecution, statelessness 293–4
personnel, assistive technology 108
PFA (psychological first aid) training 151
PHCCs *see* primary healthcare centers (PHCCs)
PHC (Primary Health Care) for All 86
philanthropic foundations, Framework Convention on Tobacco Control 258–9
Philippines *see* Association of Southeast Asian Nations (ASEAN)
photo elicitation exercise 78
physical barriers, South African disabled 224–5
physical delay, systems thinking 8
physical support, robotics 190*t*
PIPA (Participatory Impact Pathway Analysis) 13*t*
place, assistive technology 108
planetary collisions 265
Plan Nacer (Argentina) 289

planning documents, EquiFrame 353
plutonium 266
PMTCT *see* prevention of mother-to-child transmission of HIV (PMTCT)
PNC (postnatal care) services 249
policies
  assistive technology 108, 112–13
  global health 286
  human rights 349
polio, eradication of 128
politics
  leadership in Sub-Saharan Africa 238
  Sudan health services 50
  Treaty on the Prohibition of Nuclear Weapons 276
poly pharmacy, disability 207
population education programs 369–70
Population Movement Framework (Cambodia) 313–14
positive synergy, case studies 290
postgraduate training, Sudan health services 47–8
postnatal care (PNC) services 249
poverty
  birth registration issues 302
  feminization of 301
  malaria and 306
  United Nations Convention on the Rights of Persons with Disabilities 224
power, assistive technology 108
predictability lack 5
prenatal care training 161
President's Emergency Plan for AIDS Relief (PEPFAR) (USA) 234, 238, 290
President's Malaria Initiative (USA) 234
presumptive surveillance 326
prevention, EquiFrame 344*t*
prevention of mother-to-child transmission of HIV (PMTCT) 98, 100
  clinics 101
  Tanzania 102
primary healthcare centers (PHCCs)
  Indian ID surveillance system 326
  mental health in emergencies 154
Primary Health Care (PHC) for All 86
primary preventative healthcare 208
privacy, EquiFrame 344*t*
private health services
  Indian tuberculosis surveillance 331
  Sudan 49
private sector, disease surveillance 336
proactive attitudes, assistive technology 196–7
process mapping 13*t*
procurement, assistive technology 108
productivity
  disability 202
  Sudan health services 49
program design, case studies 287–8
promotion, assistive technology 108
protection from harm, EquiFrame 343*t*
psychological first aid (PFA) training 151
psychotropic medications 152
PtH (Pathways to Housing) 181
public attitudes to disability 207
public health
  disease surveillance 334
  nuclear weapon eradication 281*b*
  officers of 81
public policies, disability care 210
public–private partnerships 313
punctuated equilibrium 12*t*
purpose, systems of 1–2

quality, EquiFrame 345*t*
quality of care
  disabilities 219
  South African disabled 225
quantitative research, hard systems 5
quantitative simulation models 35–6

race
  South African disabled 226–7
  statelessness 298
radioactive materials 266–7
radioactivity 267
rapid diagnostic testing (RDT) 311, 312
rapid response teams (RRTs) 327, 329
RDTL *see* Democratic Republic of Timor-Leste (RDTL)
recruitment, Sudan health services 46
Red Crescent 276
Red Cross 276
  see also International Committee of the Red Cross (ICRC)
Red Nose Australia 367
reductionism 3
REFER app. 3, 79, 80
refugee education pathways 158–72
  blended learning courses 162

refugee education pathways (*cont.*)
constraints 160–2
data collection & analysis 162–3
educational needs 165–7
governance 160
health workers entrance 163–9
human resources 160–2
limitations 169
technology 165–7
training 165–7
see also Dadaab (Kenya)
refugees 149
repatriation 167
see also displaced populations
regional guidelines, war health needs 125
regulation, Sudan health services 46–7, 49
reinforcing loop 122*f*
reinforcing processes 14
relationality, social inclusion 176
repatriation, refugees 167
Report on the Global Tobacco Epidemic (WHO) 259
reproductive health 133–44
access barriers 133
case study 135–6 *see also* South Sudan
collaborative decision-making 137–41
exclusion from healthcare systems 134–5
knowledge brokering platforms 140–1, 141*f*
stakeholder capacity development 139–40
Reproductive Health Project Management (RHPM) 136–7
research, Ethiopian healthcare 250
resistance to change 2
resources
community health workers 55
Health Information Systems 102–3
Respectful Maternity Care: The Universal Rights of Women and Newborns (White Ribbon Alliance) 368
respect, robotics-aided care 197
RESPECT study 366
retention strategy, Sudan health services 47
retirement age 48
Revised National Tuberculosis Control (India) 306
RHPM (Reproductive Health Project Management) 136–7
Rights of Persons with Disabilities (South Africa) 228
risks, social inclusion 177
robotics-aided care 188–201, 190*t*
communication robots 192*f*, 194*t*
monitoring sensors 195*t*
pilot testing 191–3
socially assisted robots 191
systems approach 193–4
see also assistive technology
Rockefeller Foundation 258–9
Roll-Back Malaria
framework 314–15
Monitoring and Evaluation Reference Group 314
partnership 234
RRTs (rapid response teams) 327, 329
rural populations, statelessness 297
Rwanda
HIV/AIDS 236
non-governmental organizations 236

Safeguarding Health in Conflict Coalition 128
Safer Baby Bundle (Australia) 368–9
safety monitoring, robotics 190*t*
SAHRC (South African Human Rights Commission) 223
SANDS UK 367
SARs (socially assisted robots) 191
Saving Babies Lives (UK) 368–9
SAWG (Stillbirth Advocacy Working Group) 363, 365
scenario planning 12*t*
School-Based Deworming Program (Kenya) 289
SDGs *see* Sustainable Development Goals (SDGs)
SEAR *see* South East Asia Region (SEAR)
SEATCA (Southeast Asia Tobacco Control Alliance) 257, 260
self-organization
social inclusion 175–6, 177
systems of 2
sentinel surveillance 325–6
service access
EquiFrame 343*t*
Namibian HIV/AIDS policy 352
war health needs 122–3
service delivery
Global Health Initiatives 239–40, 242*t*
health system strengthening 323

Indian ID surveillance system 325–7
Kenyan community healthcare workers 80
Malawi health service decentralization 71–2
mental health in emergencies 153–4, 153*f*
mobile community health workers 82–3
stillbirth 369–70
supportive supervision 59
WHO building block of health 306, 310–11
sexually transmitted diseases (STDs) 161
simple systems 5
skill mix imbalance, Sudan health workers 42–3
smallpox 323
smartphones, mobile community health workers 81–2
smoke coverage, post-nuclear war 268–9
social care system, assistive technology 113
Social Cash Transfer Program (Kenya) 289
social determinants of health 206
social grants, South African disabled 224
social groups 353
social inclusion 173–87, 342–59
boundaries 178–9
causal modelling 179–80
chronic homelessness 180–1
Complex Adaptive System as 175–7
definition 173
disability 212
holistic response 177–8
interventions for 177–80
self-organization 175–6
social interactions, communities 87
socially assisted robots (SARs) 191
social mobility 164
social models, disability 204, 220–1
Social Network Analysis 12*t*
social systems, assistive technology 110*t*
Social Welfare Corporation (SWC) 190–1
socio-economic contexts, assistive technology 110–11
soft systems 4
Soft Systems Approach 4–5
Soft Systems Methodology (SSM) 4–5
Somalia 167–8
health education barriers 168
refugee movement 168
South Africa
Bill of Rights 223
Care Dependency grants 224
Child Support Grant 289
Equiframe 348
Health Information Systems 101
HIV/AIDS epidemic 98, 223, 236
HIV/AIDS policies 351
migrant healthcare access 295
Rights of Persons with Disabilities 228
tuberculosis 98–9
Tuberculosis Strategic Plan 351
South African disabled 222–5
Care Dependency grants 224
epidemiology 222–3
rights movement 223
Rights of Persons with Disabilities 228
systems thinking 225–8
South African Human Rights Commission (SAHRC) 223
South America, stillbirth rates 361
South East Asia Region (SEAR)
IDSP 323
stillbirth rates 361
Southeast Asia Tobacco Control Alliance (SEATCA) 257, 260
Southern Asia, stillbirth rates 360
South Sudan
health systems 135–6
reproductive health case study 135–6, 136*f*, 137*t*, 138*f*
SSM (Soft Systems Methodology) 4–5
stability, systems of 2
stakeholders
capacity development in reproductive health 139–40
communities 90
Health Workforce Transformation Initiative (Sudan) 45
Indian disease surveillance 332
Sudan health services 49
Star Legacy Foundation USA 367
state borders, statelessness 298
statelessness 293–305
causes 297–8
children 297, 298–9
definition 293, 296–9
epidemiology 296–7
healthcare exclusion 293–6
impact 296–9
persecution 293–4
prevalence 296–9

static thinking, Health Information Systems 97–8
STDs (sexually transmitted diseases) 161
stillbirth 360–73
  audits and reviews 366
  causes 366
  challenges about 363, 365–70
  classification systems 366
  definition 360, 365
  global burden 362*f*
  preventative programs 367
  prevention 361
  WHO prevention strategies 364*t*
Stillbirth Advocacy Working Group (SAWG) 363, 365
stock and flow diagrams 13*t*, 14
Stop TB Partnership 234
Strategic Development Plan, Democratic Republic of Timor-Leste 182
strategic thinking, war health needs 126
structure duplication, Sub-Saharan Africa 238
Sub-Saharan Africa (SSA)
  Country Coordinating Mechanism 237
  double burden of disease 243–4
  healthcare worker shortages 368
  stillbirth rates 360, 361
  see also Global Health Initiatives (GHIs)
subsystems, health systems 35
Sudan
  Health Workforce Transformation Initiative 43, 44–5
  National Malaria Policy 351
Sudan health services 39–53
  active workforce stage 47–8
  challenges 49–50
  entry stage 46–7
  exit stage 48
  health worker mobility 48
  Health Workforce Development 45–6
  Health Workforce Transformation Initiative 43, 44–5
  National Malaria Policy 351
  reform & transformation 43
  workforce 41–3, 44*b*
Sudan Medical Council (SMC) 42
summary indices, Equiframe 348–9
supply shortages, Ethiopian pastoral health 247–8
supportive supervision
  community health workers 55, 56
  COVID-19 61–2
  Global Health Initiatives 236
  health information 57–9
  health system financing 60
  leadership & governance 60–1
  medical products 59–60
  service delivery 59
surveillance 325–6
  ID surveillance system 324–7
  infectious disease surveillance 322–41
  laboratory surveillance *see* laboratory surveillance
  National Polio Surveillance Program 328
Sustainable Development Goals (SDGs)
  assistive technology 109–10
  case studies 289–90
  community health workers 54
  disability care 210
  Malawi 69, 72–3
  social inclusion 173
  Sudan health services 39
  tobacco use *see* Framework Convention on Tobacco Control (FCTC)
SWC (Social Welfare Corporation) 190–1
syndromic (symptom-based) surveillance 326
systems
  archetypes 13*t*
  classification 4–5
  definition of 1–2
  dynamic modelling 12*t*
systems-as-cause thinking 6
Systems Engineering Initiative for Patient Safety (SEIPS) 9*f*, 10
Systems Thinking for Health Systems Strengthening (WHO) 3–4, 8, 90

TACTS (Technology-Assisted Cascaded Training and Supervision system) 58
Tanzania
  community health programs 91–2
  HIV/AIDS 100, 102, 236
  prevention of mother-to-child transmission of HIV 102
TAPS (tobacco advertising, promotion and sponsorship) 255
TBT (Technical Barriers to Trade) Committee 256–7
teaching case studies 288
teamwork, robotics-aided care 197

Technical Advisory Group and Core Stillbirth Group 365
Technical Barriers to Trade (TBT) Committee 256–7
technology
  Global Health Initiatives 242*t*
  Indian ID surveillance system 325–7
  refugee education pathways 165–7
  stillbirth 368–9
  supply chains 240
Technology-Assisted Cascaded Training and Supervision system (TACTS) 58
10,000-meter thinking 6–7
terminology 6
Thailand
  Campaign for Tobacco Control 289
  Health Promotion Foundation 260
  Universal Coverage Scheme 289
  see also Association of Southeast Asian Nations (ASEAN)
theories of systems thinking 11, 11–13*t*, 14
thinking skills 6–7
tobacco advertising, promotion and sponsorship (TAPS) 255
tobacco industry 255–7, 256*f*
tobacco use 260
Tommy's UK 367
tools in systems thinking 11, 11–13*t*, 13–14
Total Sanitation and Sanitation Marketing Program (Indonesia) 289
toxicity, fissile materials 266
TPNM *see* Treaty on the Prohibition of Nuclear Weapons (TPNW)
Trade-Related Aspects of Intellectual Property (TRIPS) 256–7
Trading Tobacco for Health Initiative (2000-2004) 259
traditional health systems 58
training
  Global Health Initiatives 236, 237
  refugee education pathways 160, 165–7
transactional delay, systems thinking 8
Transcultural Psychosocial Organization Nepal (TPO) 151
transformational leadership 61
transportation, South African disabled 225
Treaty on the Prohibition of Nuclear Weapons (TPNW) 273–6, 278
  Global Health Partnership 276–8
  process of acheiving 274–6, 277*b*
tree-by-tree thinking
  forest thinking *vs.* 99–101
  Health Information Systems 98
tropical diseases 291
tuberculosis (TB)
  case studies 291
  Core Concept Coverage 350*t*
  drug-resistance tuberculosis 335
  End TB Surveillance 329–30, 335
  South Africa 98–9, 351
  Sub-Saharan Africa 237
  surveillance of 329–31, 335
Tuberculosis Strategic Plan (South Africa) 351

'ubuntu' 224, 227–8
UDHR (Universal Declaration on Human Rights) 203, 221
Uganda
  HIV/AIDS 236
  HIV community care 91
UHC *see* Universal Health Coverage (UHC)
UK PARENTS 2 study 366
UN *see* United Nations (UN)
UNCRPD *see* United Nations Convention on the Rights of Persons with Disabilities (UNCRPD)
UNHCR *see* United Nations High Commission for Refugees (UNHCR)
Union of Physically Impaired Against Segregation (UPIAS) 203
United Kingdom (UK)
  SANDS UK 367
  Saving Babies Lives 368–9
  Tommy's UK 367
  UK PARENTS 2 study 366
United Nations (UN)
  Convention on the Rights of the Child (1989) 299, 302
  Disability and development report 210
  Educational, Scientific and Cultural Organization 175–6
  Global Strategy for Women's Children's and Adolescents; Health 360
  mental health in emergencies 146
United Nations Children's Fund (UNICEF) 240, 360
  birth registration 299
  mental health in emergencies 146

United Nations Convention on the Rights of Persons with Disabilities (UNCRPD) 182, 203–4, 218, 221–2, 228, 351–2
barriers to 219, 223–4
implementation 222, 225–6
social models 222
United Nations General Assembly (UNGA)
nuclear weapon eradication 272–3
Treaty on the Prohibition of Nuclear Weapons 275–6
United Nations High Commission for Refugees (UNHCR) 159, 298
Integrated Refugee Health Information System 148–9
refugee education 165
United Nations Inter-agency Group for Child Mortality Estimation (UNIGME) 365
United Nations Partnership for the Rights of People with Disability (UNPRPD) 220
United States Agency for International Development (USAID) 91
United States of America (USA)
President's Emergency Plan for AIDS Relief 234, 238, 290
President's Malaria Initiative 234
universal birth registration 301–2
Universal Coverage Scheme (Thailand) 289
Universal Declaration on Human Rights (UDHR) 203, 221
Universal Health Coverage (UHC) 175, 291
Malawi 69
Sudan 39
"Unlocking Communities Capabilities" (Future Health Systems) 91
unsustainability 97
UPIAS (Union of Physically Impaired Against Segregation) 203
uranium 266–7

vaccines, supportive supervision 59–60
vertical disease control programs 306, 317
Vietnam
Comprehensive Helmet Law 289
Steering Committee on Smoking and Health 260
see also Association of Southeast Asian Nations (ASEAN)
violence, disability 208–9
visual languages 6
voluntary return, refugees 159
vulnerable groups
access to health services 345
definition of 346–7, 347*t*
Equiframe 348
policies 352
vulnerable populations, statelessness 297

WAD (work as done) 193, 195
WAI (work as imagined) 193, 195
war health needs 120–32
actor potential 127–8
conflict preparedness 126–7
data & health information 129
history 122–4
improvements in 124–6
risks to health workers 128
WFPHA (World Federation of Public Health Associations), Treaty on the Prohibition of Nuclear Weapons 276, 278
WHA (World Health Assembly), Global Code of Practice for International Recruitment of Health Personnel 48
White Ribbon Alliance, *Respectful Maternity Care: The Universal Rights of Women and Newborns* 368
WHO *see* World Health Organization (WHO)
WMA (World Medical Association), Treaty on the Prohibition of Nuclear Weapons 276, 278
work as done (WAD) 193, 195
work as imagined (WAI) 193, 195
work engagement, community health workers 55, 57
working lifespan approach (WHO) 40
Working Lifespan framework (WHO) 45–6
World Bank
Curbing the epidemic–governments and the economics of tobacco control 259
Multi-country AIDS Programme 234
World Report on Disability 347
World Federation of Public Health Associations (WFPHA), Treaty on the Prohibition of Nuclear Weapons 276, 278
World Health Assembly (WHA), Global Code of Practice for International Recruitment of Health Personnel 48
World Health Organization (WHO)
Alliance for Health Policy and Systems 179–80

Checklist for TB Surveillance 329–30
Children's Fund 360
community health workers
supervision 55
decentralization 67
disability definition 188
End TB strategy 335
End TB Surveillance 329–30
Global Cooperation on Assistive
Technology 111, 112*b*
Global Disability Action Plan 2014-2021 204
Health Policy and Systems Research 90
health system building blocks 4, 4*f*
health systems strengthening 18
information as building block 96
Integrated Disease Surveillance and
Response 322
International Health Regulations 322
Maximizing Positive Synergies
Collaborative Group 290
measles elimination 328–9
mental health in emergencies 146
mhGAP Intervention Guide 154
Model List of Essential Medicines 152
National Polio Surveillance Program 328
People-centred Health model 91
Report on the Global Tobacco Epidemic 259
six building blocks of health
strengthening 33, 306, 308, 308*f*, 310–14, 316, 323
stillbirth prevention 364*t*
Systems Thinking for Health Systems Strengthening 3–4, 8, 90
systems thinking framework 34
tobacco use control 254
working lifespan approach 40
Working Lifespan framework 45–6
World Report on Disability 206, 207, 304, 347
World Medical Association (WMA),
Treaty on the Prohibition of Nuclear
Weapons 276, 278
World Report on Disability (WHO) 204, 206, 207, 347
World Report on Health Policy and Systems
Research 175
World systems, assistive technology 110*t*

YPO (Transcultural Psychosocial
Organization Nepal) 151

Zambia
health system leadership 243
HIV/AIDS 236
zoonotic diseases, Ethiopia 247